INSTRUCTOR'S RESOURCE MANUAL

Principles and Practice of Psychiatric Nursing

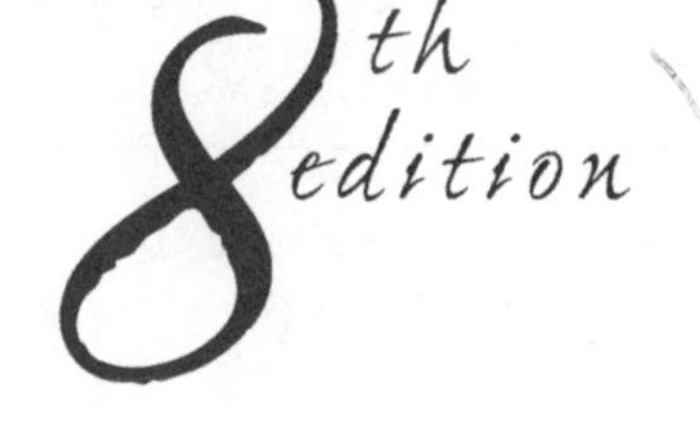

GAIL WISCARZ STUART, PHD, APRN, BC, FAAN
Dean and Professor, College of Nursing
Professor, College of Medicine
Department of Psychiatry and Behavioral Sciences
Medical University of South Carolina
Charleston, South Carolina

MICHELE T. LARAIA, PHD, RN
Associate Professor
Director, Advanced Practice Nursing Programs
School of Nursing
Oregon Health and Science University
Portland, Oregon

Test Bank written by

MARY ANN HOGAN, RN, CS, MSN
Clinical Assistant Professor
School of Nursing
University of Massachusetts
Amherst, Massachusetts

LEE MURRAY, RN, MS, CS, CADAC
Associate Professor
Holyoke Community College
Holyoke, Massachusetts

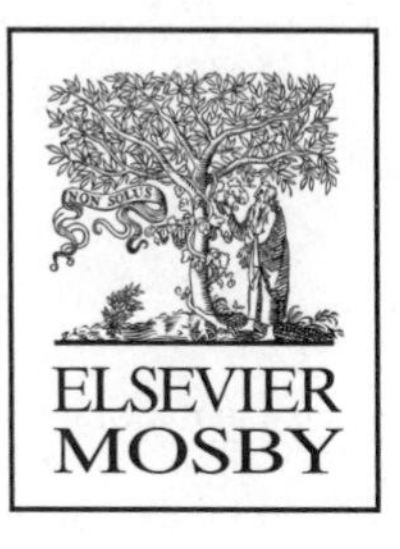

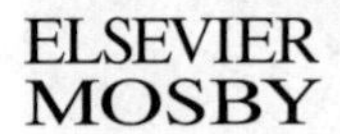

11830 Westline Industrial Drive
St. Louis, Missouri 63146

INSTRUCTORS RESOURCE MANUAL TO ACCOMPANY
PRINCIPLES AND PRACTICE OF PSYCHIATRIC NURSING

ISBN 0-323-03298-2

NOTICE

Nursing is an ever-changing field. Standard safety precautions must be followed, but as new research and clinical experience broaden our knowledge, changes in treatment and drug therapy may become necessary or appropriate. Readers are advised to check the most current product information provided by the manufacturer of each drug to be administered to verify the recommended dose, the method and duration of administration, and contraindications. It is the responsibility of the licensed prescriber, relying on experience and knowledge of the patient, to determine dosages and the best treatment for each individual patient. Neither the publisher nor the author assumes any liability for any injury and/or damage to persons or property arising from this publication.

Previous editions copyrighted 2001, 1998, 1995, 1991, 1987, 1983

International Standard Book Number 0-323-03298-2

Acquisitions Editor: Tom Wilhelm
Developmental Editor: Jill Ferguson
Publishing Services Manager: Gayle May
Project Manager: Joseph Selby
Senior Book Designer: Julia Dummitt

Printed in the United States of America

Last digit is the print number: 9 8 7 6 5 4 3 2 1

PREFACE

The Instructor's Resource Manual for *Principles and Practice of Psychiatric Nursing*, 8th Edition is designed to help you, the instructor, develop lectures, reinforce teaching through classroom and clinical activities, and evaluate student comprehension.

Adapted Course Outlines. Course outlines are provided as suggestions for adapting the book's chapters to courses of varying length. Suggestions are provided for a 6-week course, a 9-week course, a 15-week course, and a graduate course for advanced practice.

Chapter by Chapter Teaching Aids. There are 40 chapters in this manual, one for each respective text chapter. Each chapter contains the following sections: *Critical Thinking Questions*, *Critical Thinking Activities*, and *Research Agenda for Evidence-Based Practice*.

Test Bank. The *Test Bank* includes over 1,000 completely revised multiple-choice, NCLEX-style test questions. The *Answers to Test Bank* section includes the following categories of information for each test question: correct answer, rationale, cognitive level, nursing process step, NCLEX label, and text page reference.

An **Instructor's Resource (CD-ROM)** is also included in this manual. The *Instructor's Manual* section of the CD-ROM includes the sample course outlines as well as critical thinking questions and activities and research topics for each chapter of the text. The *PowerPoint/Image Collection* offers presentations with more than 200 slides, including four-color images from the text. The *Computerized Test Bank* provides the full bank of over 1,000 questions in ExamView, allowing you to generate and customize tests and perform online testing.

We hope you find this manual to be an outstanding resource to supplement your journey in the pursuit of psychiatric nursing teaching excellence.

Gail Wiscarz Stuart
Michele T. Laraia

Table of Contents

ADAPTED COURSE OUTLINES

The following course outlines are provided as suggestions for adapting the book's chapters to courses of varying length. Suggestions are provided for a 6-week course, a 9-week course, a 15-week course, and a graduate course for advanced practice.

6-WEEK COURSE

Week 1
- Chapter 1: Roles and Functions of Psychiatric Nurses: Competent Caring
- Chapter 2: Therapeutic Nurse-Patient Relationship
- Chapter 4: The Stuart Stress Adaptation Model of Psychiatric Nursing Care
- Chapter 5: Evidence-Based Psychiatric Nursing Practice

Week 2
- Chapter 6: Biological Context of Psychiatric Nursing Care
- Chapter 7: Psychological Context of Psychiatric Nursing Care
- Chapter 8: Social, Cultural, and Spiritual Context of Psychiatric Nursing Care

Week 3
- Chapter 10: Legal and Ethical Context of Psychiatric Nursing Care
- Chapter 11: Families as Resources, Caregivers, and Collaborators
- Chapter 12: Implementing the Nursing Process: Standards of Care and Professional Performance
- Chapter 14: Crisis Intervention

Week 4
- Chapter 16: Anxiety Responses and Anxiety Disorders plus pages 573-577 on Antianxiety and Sedative-Hypnotic Drugs from Chapter 27: Psychopharmacology
- Chapter 18: Self-Concept Responses and Dissociative Disorders
- Chapter 22: Social Responses and Personality Disorders
- Chapter 23: Cognitive Responses and Organic Mental Disorders

Week 5
- Chapter 19: Emotional Responses and Mood Disorders plus pages 577-587 on Antidepressant Drugs and Mood-Stabilizing Drugs from Chapter 27: Psychopharmacology
- Chapter 20: Self-Protective Responses and Suicidal Behavior
- Chapter 21: Neurobiological Responses and Schizophrenia and Psychotic Disorders plus pages 587-592 on Antipsychotic Drugs from Chapter 27: Psychopharmacology

Week 6
- Chapter 17: Psychophysiological Responses and Somatoform and Sleep Disorders
- Chapter 24: Chemically Mediated Responses and Substance-Related Disorders
- Chapter 25: Eating Regulation Responses and Eating Disorders
- Chapter 26: Sexual Responses and Sexual Disorders

9-WEEK COURSE

Week 1
Chapter 1: Roles and Functions of Psychiatric Nurses: Competent Caring
Chapter 2: Therapeutic Nurse-Patient Relationship
Chapter 4: The Stuart Stress Adaptation Model of Psychiatric Nursing Care
Chapter 5: Evidence-Based Psychiatric Nursing Practice

Week 2
Chapter 6: Biological Context of Psychiatric Nursing Care
Chapter 7: Psychological Context of Psychiatric Nursing Care
Chapter 8: Social, Cultural, and Spiritual Context of Psychiatric Nursing Care

Week 3
Chapter 10: Legal and Ethical Context of Psychiatric Nursing Care
Chapter 11: Families as Resources, Caregivers, and Collaborators
Chapter 12: Implementing the Nursing Process: Standards of Care and Professional Performance
Chapter 13: Mental Health Promotion and Illness Prevention

Week 4
Chapter 14: Crisis Intervention
Chapter 30: Preventing and Managing Aggressive Behavior
Chapter 31: Cognitive Behavioral Treatment Strategies

Week 5
Chapter 16: Anxiety Responses and Anxiety Disorders plus pages 573-577 on Antianxiety and Sedative-Hypnotic Drugs from Chapter 27: Psychopharmacology
Chapter 17: Psychophysiological Responses and Somatoform and Sleep Disorders
Chapter 18: Self-Concept Responses and Dissociative Disorders

Week 6
Chapter 19: Emotional Responses and Mood Disorders plus pages 577-587 on Antidepressant Drugs and Mood-Stabilizing Drugs from Chapter 27: Psychopharmacology
Chapter 20: Self-Protective Responses and Suicidal Behavior
Chapter 28: Somatic Therapies

Week 7
Chapter 21: Neurobiological Responses and Schizophrenia and Psychotic Disorders plus pages 587-592 on Antipsychotic Drugs from Chapter 27: Psychopharmacology
Chapter 15: Psychiatric Rehabilitation and Recovery

Week 8
Chapter 22: Social Responses and Personality Disorders
Chapter 25: Eating Regulation Responses and Eating Disorders
Chapter 26: Sexual Responses and Sexual Disorders

Week 9
Chapter 13: Mental Health Promotion and Illness Prevention
Chapter 24: Chemically Mediated Responses and Substance-Related Disorders
Chapter 39: Care of Survivors of Abuse and Violence

15-WEEK COURSE

Week 1
Chapter 1: Roles and Functions of Psychiatric Nurses: Competent Caring
Chapter 2: Therapeutic Nurse-Patient Relationship

Week 2
Chapter 4: The Stuart Stress Adaptation Model of Psychiatric Nursing Care
Chapter 5: Evidence-Based Psychiatric Nursing Practice
Chapter 11: Families as Resources, Caregivers, and Collaborators

Week 3
Chapter 6: Biological Context of Psychiatric Nursing Care
Chapter 7: Psychological Context of Psychiatric Nursing Care
Chapter 8: Social, Cultural, and Spiritual Context of Psychiatric Nursing Care

Week 4
Chapter 12: Implementing the Nursing Process: Standards of Care and Professional Performance
Chapter 13: Mental Health Promotion and Illness Prevention

Week 5
Chapter 14: Crisis Intervention
Chapter 15: Psychiatric Rehabilitation and Recovery

Week 6
Chapter 31: Cognitive Behavioral Treatment Strategies
Chapter 16: Anxiety Responses and Anxiety Disorders plus pages 573-577 on Antianxiety and Sedative-Hypnotic Drugs from Chapter 27: Psychopharmacology

Week 7
Chapter 17: Psychophysiological Responses and Somatoform and Sleep Disorders
Chapter 18: Self-Concept Responses and Dissociative Disorders

Week 8
Chapter 19: Emotional Responses and Mood Disorders plus pages 577-587 on Antidepressant Drugs and Mood-Stabilizing Drugs from Chapter 27: Psychopharmacology
Chapter 20: Self-Protective Responses and Suicidal Behavior
Chapter 28: Somatic Therapies

Week 9
Chapter 21: Neurobiological Responses and Schizophrenia and Psychotic Disorders plus pages 587-592 on Antipsychotic Drugs from Chapter 27: Psychopharmacology

Week 10
Chapter 23: Cognitive Responses and Organic Mental Disorders
Chapter 38: Geropsychiatric Nursing

Week 11
Chapter 22: Social Responses and Personality Disorders
Chapter 25: Eating Regulation Responses and Eating Disorders

Week 12
Chapter 24: Chemically Mediated Responses and Substance-Related Disorders
Chapter 26: Sexual Responses and Sexual Disorders

Week 13
Chapter 39: Care of Survivors of Abuse and Violence
Chapter 29: Complementary and Alternative Therapies

Week 14
Chapter 30: Preventing and Managing Aggressive Behavior
Chapter 32: Therapeutic Groups

Week 15
Chapter 9: Environmental Context of Psychiatric Nursing Care
Chapter 10: Legal and Ethical Context of Psychiatric Nursing Care

GRADUATE COURSE

Most graduate courses are 15 weeks in length and therefore the following course outline is recommended. In addition, readings for each of these weeks should be supplemented by selected research and clinical articles listed in the References at the end of each chapter of the textbook and the Annotated Suggested Readings provided on the Evolve website. Students should also be encouraged to access designated information from the many resources on the Evolve website and Student Study CD-ROM accompanying the text.

Week 1	Chapter 1: Roles and Functions of Psychiatric Nurses: Competent Caring Chapter 2: Therapeutic Nurse-Patient Relationship Chapter 4: The Stuart Stress Adaptation Model of Psychiatric Nursing Care Chapter 5: Evidence-Based Psychiatric Nursing Practice
Week 2	Chapter 3: Conceptual Models of Psychiatric Treatment Chapter 7: Psychological Context of Psychiatric Nursing Care Chapter 8: Social, Cultural, and Spiritual Context of Psychiatric Nursing Care
Week 3	Chapter 6: Biological Context of Psychiatric Nursing Care Chapter 27: Psychopharmacology Chapter 28: Somatic Therapies
Week 4	Chapter 9: Environmental Context of Psychiatric Nursing Care Chapter 10: Legal and Ethical Context of Psychiatric Nursing Care Chapter 11: Families as Resources, Caregivers, and Collaborators
Week 5	Chapter 12: Implementing the Nursing Process: Standards of Care and Professional Performance Chapter 40: Psychological Care of Patients with Life-Threatening Illness
Week 6	Chapter 13: Mental Health Promotion and Illness Prevention Chapter 14: Crisis Intervention Chapter 15: Psychiatric Rehabilitation and Recovery
Week 7	Chapter 30: Preventing and Managing Aggressive Behavior Chapter 31: Cognitive Behavioral Treatment Strategies Chapter 29: Complementary and Alternative Therapies
Week 8	Chapter 16: Anxiety Responses and Anxiety Disorders Chapter 17: Psychophysiological Responses and Somatoform and Sleep Disorders Chapter 18: Self-Concept Responses and Dissociative Disorders
Week 9	Chapter 19: Emotional Responses and Mood Disorders Chapter 20: Self-Protective Responses and Suicidal Behavior
Week 10	Chapter 21: Neurobiological Responses and Schizophrenia and Psychotic Disorders Chapter 23: Cognitive Responses and Organic Mental Disorders
Week 11	Chapter 22: Social Responses and Personality Disorders Chapter 25: Eating Regulation Responses and Eating Disorders
Week 12	Chapter 24: Chemically Mediated Responses and Substance-Related Disorders Chapter 26: Sexual Responses and Sexual Disorders
Week 13	Chapter 34: Hospital-Based Psychiatric Nursing Care Chapter 35: Community Psychiatric Nursing Care

Week 14	Chapter 32: Therapeutic Groups Chapter 33: Family Interventions Chapter 39: Care of Survivors of Abuse and Violence
Week 15	Chapter 36: Child Psychiatric Nursing Chapter 37: Adolescent Psychiatric Nursing Chapter 38: Geropsychiatric Nursing

ROLES AND FUNCTIONS OF PSYCHIATRIC NURSES: COMPETENT CARING

1

CRITICAL THINKING QUESTIONS

1. In 1951, Bennet and Eaton identified these three problems affecting psychiatric nurses: the scarcity of qualified psychiatric nurses, the partial use of their abilities, and the performance of little real psychiatric nursing in psychiatric hospitals and units. Do you believe these problems exist at present? Support your position.
2. Compare each of the philosophical beliefs described in Chapter 1 with your own philosophical beliefs. Describe any differences, problems, or dilemmas that arise for you.
3. Explain how a psychiatric nurse's level of performance is influenced by one's qualifications, including education, work experience, and certification.
4. Explain how personal competence and initiative affect a nurse's level of functioning.
5. While you are at home on vacation, a relative notices your textbook on psychiatric nursing. She says she's surprised at its size, because psychiatric nurses "merely carry out the orders of psychiatrists and don't really do anything unique or different." How would you respond to her and support your position?

CRITICAL THINKING ACTIVITIES

1. Write a newspaper article or letter to the editor that presents a positive image of psychiatric nursing.
2. Give examples of settings in which psychiatric nurses currently work in your community.
3. Obtain a copy of your state's nurse practice act. After reading it, describe the legal limits of nursing practice and ways in which the nurse practice act may be made more congruent with the evolving role of the psychiatric nurse.
4. Investigate whether home health agencies in your community provide mental health services. If not, discuss the reasons for this. If so, discuss the services that are provided by nurses in these agencies.
5. Identify an issue related to mental health care that is currently being addressed by your state legislature. Analyze the issue and develop a position paper. Write a letter or visit your own legislator explaining your position.
6. Design a television public service announcement that would present a positive image of the psychiatric nurse.
7. View the film "Psychiatric Nursing: Profiles in Compassion" (Fanlight Productions, Boston, MA) and critique the image, relevancy, and accuracy of the content.

RESEARCH AGENDA FOR EVIDENCE-BASED PRACTICE

The following are some of the nursing research problems raised in Chapter 1 that merit further study by psychiatric nurses:

1. Factors associated with the recruitment of nurses into the field of psychiatric nursing
2. The perceptions of other mental health professionals and the public of advanced practice psychiatric nursing
3. The amount of time nurses spend in each of the three domains of contemporary psychiatric nursing practice and whether these activities vary by education or setting
4. Clinical, functional, financial, and perceptual outcomes associated with psychiatric nursing care
5. Nontraditional settings and the parameters of practice of psychiatric nurses
6. The extent to which psychiatric nurses are practicing in primary care settings along with their activities and clinical outcomes
7. The leadership roles enacted by psychiatric nurses
8. Political action and advocacy efforts by psychiatric nurses in each state

2 THERAPEUTIC NURSE-PATIENT RELATIONSHIP

CRITICAL THINKING QUESTIONS

1. Evaluate how well you would display Rogers' characteristics of a helping relationship by asking yourself his 10 questions posed in the introduction of Chapter 2.
2. Do you think that during the socialization process into nursing, the nurse's spontaneity is destroyed and she or he becomes alienated from the true self? Support your position.
3. Explain the steps one would take in the process of increasing self-awareness.
4. Describe the cognitive, affective, and behavioral criteria used in the value clarification process.
5. Identify some of your own feelings, fantasies, and fears about working with psychiatric patients.
6. Explain what is meant by a "facade of professionalism."
7. Think back to the last time you needed to ask someone for help. How did you feel at the time? What things would have made you feel more or less comfortable?
8. Review significant losses you have experienced in your life. How have you handled them? What are your unresolved feelings about them? How might they affect the quality of your termination with patient relationships?
9. Analyze empathic understanding, including how it develops and how it differs from sympathy.
10. Describe the specific verbal and nonverbal behaviors that the nurse displays to convey to a patient the responsive dimensions of genuineness, respect, empathic understanding, and concreteness.
11. Discuss the way in which the responsive and action dimensions interrelate in maintaining a therapeutic relationship.
12. Evaluate your use of the responsive and action dimensions in the therapeutic relationship. Validate your analysis with your instructor or supervisor. Set goals for future growth.
13. Identify a countertransference reaction you experienced. Think about how it developed, and evaluate how you resolved it.
14. Review the common boundary violations described in this chapter. Have you seen nurses engaged in any of them? What would you say to a colleague who is involved in one of these violations?
15. Review the techniques of crisis intervention presented in Chapter 14. Compare these with the therapeutic communication techniques, responsive dimension, and action dimensions described in this chapter. Note areas of similarity, difference, and modification.
16. Use the process of value clarification to increase your self-understanding and discover your own values in the area of human sexuality (Chapter 26).
17. Explain why self-awareness and the personal qualities of the nurse as helper are crucial in working with abusive and violent families (Chapter 39) and patients with life-threatening illness (Chapter 40).

CRITICAL THINKING ACTIVITIES

1. Begin the process of self-analysis by answering the following questions and setting specific goals for your future growth:
   A. Who am I?
   B. What is important to me, and what do I value?
   C. Am I open to my feelings, and can I express them?
   D. What type of role model am I?
   E. Why do I want to help others?
   F. What are my personal beliefs about patient welfare and social responsibility, and do I act on these beliefs?
2. Review the literature on "therapeutic touch" in nursing. What evidence exists to support its mechanism of action and effectiveness? Identify questions for future research.
3. Arrange to have your next small-group seminar or supervision session videotaped. Play it back and analyze your own nonverbal behavior using the five categories of nonverbal communication described in the chapter.
4. Use the videotape recorded in Activity 3 or tape record your next small group or supervision session. Analyze your own process of communication using either the structural or transactional analysis models.
5. Review the advantages and disadvantages of, and your own comfort with, the various methods of recording nurse-patient interactions. After trying out each method, decide on the particular method you prefer.

6. Tape record one of your sessions with a patient. Evaluate your communication skills by identifying specific therapeutic and nontherapeutic techniques you used in the interaction. Validate your analysis with your instructor or supervisor. Set goals for future growth.
7. Engage in some role-playing in a small-group seminar. At the end of it, discuss how and when it can be useful in helping patients resolve conflicts and increase self-awareness.

RESEARCH AGENDA FOR EVIDENCE-BASED PRACTICE

The following are some of the nursing research problems raised in Chapter 2 that merit further study by psychiatric nurses:

1. The extent to which psychiatric nurses possess the personal qualities associated with being able to help others
2. The levels of openness, authenticity, and empathic understanding in student-teacher relationships in nursing
3. The validity of Burgess and Burns' description of reasons why patients seek psychiatric care and which nursing approaches would be effective with each
4. The affective and behavioral patient outcomes associated with the nurse's use of personal space and spatial parameters
5. Valid and reliable instruments to measure the responsive and action dimensions of a therapeutic nurse-patient relationship
6. The extent to which psychiatric nurses demonstrate the responsive dimensions of genuineness, respect, empathic understanding, concreteness, and resulting therapeutic outcomes
7. The extent to which psychiatric nurses demonstrate the action dimensions of confrontation, immediacy, nurse self-disclosure, catharsis, role-playing, and resulting therapeutic outcomes
8. The most common boundary violations that occur in psychiatric nursing practice and ways in which they can be anticipated and prevented

3 Conceptual Models of Psychiatric Treatment

CRITICAL THINKING QUESTIONS

1. Discuss the ways in which the interpretation of the following behaviors would differ depending on the sociocultural setting in which they occur. Include "normal" and "abnormal" interpretations for each behavior:
   A. Carrying a loaded shotgun
   B. Removing one's clothing in the presence of others
   C. Sitting motionless and staring into space
   D. Laughing
2. Compare and contrast the therapeutic process for any two of the following conceptual models: psychoanalytical, interpersonal, existential, or supportive.
3. One function of the medical model is to avoid placing blame for deviant behavior. Discuss the implications of this for the care of patients with mental disorders.
4. Identify the conceptual model of psychiatric care that is most congruent with your personal philosophy of nursing. Discuss the reasons for your choice.
5. Psychoanalytical theory is viewed with skepticism by many contemporary mental health care providers. Yet its influence on Western culture is pervasive. Identify three ways in which the influence of psychoanalytical theory is apparent in contemporary culture.
6. Some people believe that, in the future, the supportive therapy model will be the one used most often by clinicians. Why do you think this is so?
7. Which models best lend themselves to a multicausal view of psychiatric illness?
8. Which model do you think is most culture-bound? Which is most culture-free?

CRITICAL THINKING ACTIVITIES

1. Select and read the works of any two proponents of the existential model of psychiatric care (e.g., Perls, Glasser, Ellis). Discuss the similarities and differences between the therapeutic approaches. Identify the reason for their classification as existential.
2. Szasz believes that deviant behavior is defined by culture. Watch a popular television show and identify behaviors that could be considered deviant if they occurred in another context.
3. Review recent articles that have appeared about psychiatric care in *Time* magazine. Identify which model of treatment they endorse.
4. Describe to a colleague how managed care is influencing psychiatric treatment and the use of various conceptual models.

RESEARCH AGENDA FOR EVIDENCE-BASED PRACTICE

The following are some of the nursing research problems raised in Chapter 3 that merit further study by psychiatric nurses:

1. The costs and clinical outcomes associated with each of the various conceptual models of psychiatric treatment
2. A description of the treatment models used by psychiatric nurses, based upon their educational background and work setting
3. An assessment of the conceptual models of psychiatric treatment taught in psychiatric nursing graduate programs
4. The effectiveness of interdisciplinary teams in which members use similar or divergent models of psychiatric care
5. The level of consumer awareness of the various treatment models and the extent to which this influences choice of provider
6. The portrayal in the media of various models of psychiatric treatment and the impact the media have on the public perception of psychiatric care
7. The models of psychiatric treatment that are most frequently used in managed care settings
8. The ethical issues raised by the various conceptual models of psychiatric care

THE STUART STRESS ADAPTATION MODEL OF PSYCHIATRIC NURSING CARE

4

CRITICAL THINKING QUESTIONS

1. Some people believe that the idea of any single criterion of mental health should be abandoned. Do you agree? Support your position.
2. Evaluate yourself using Rogers' traits of the "fully functioning person."
3. Compare and contrast health-illness, conformity-deviance, and adaptation-maladaptation.
4. Cite specific examples of biological, psychological, and sociocultural predisposing or conditioning factors.
5. Explain why, in assessing a patient's stressors, it is necessary to consider their nature, origin, timing, and number.
6. From a theoretical and clinical point of view, compare the following types of precipitation stressors: major life changes, chronic unsatisfactory conditions of living, and daily hassles.
7. Describe how you would distinguish between constructive and destructive coping mechanisms.
8. You are attending a team planning conference about your psychiatric patient. After you describe your nursing care plan, a medical student comments, "All those nursing plans are a bit premature because no medical diagnosis has been made yet." How would you respond to him?
9. How does "neurosis" differ from "psychosis"? Which type of mental illness do you believe is more prevalent in contemporary American society?
10. Identify and briefly describe each of the five axes used for diagnostic classification according to the *DSM-IV-TR*.
11. Describe the four possible patient treatment stages and identify nursing activities related to each one.
12. Analyze how the stress-adaptation model would be adapted if one's focus were on a: (a) family, (b) group, and (c) community.

CRITICAL THINKING ACTIVITIES

1. Maslow identified the following people as being self-actualized: Abraham Lincoln, Thomas Jefferson, Walt Whitman, Ludwig von Beethoven, Franklin D. Roosevelt, Albert Einstein, and Eleanor Roosevelt. Read about the life of one of these individuals, and support or refute Maslow's conclusion.
2. It has been observed that the attributes of challenge, commitment, and control are qualities of stress-resistant people. Think of someone you know who tolerates stress well, and talk to him or her about these attributes.
3. Observe the coping resources used by your friends and family when they are under stress. Evaluate whether they are constructive or destructive and which ones might be helpful to you.
4. Make a list of the settings that your school uses to teach psychiatric nursing. Identify which psychiatric treatment stage is emphasized in each setting.
5. Research one "culture-bound syndrome" identified by the *DSM-IV-TR* and report on it to your class.

RESEARCH AGENDA FOR EVIDENCE-BASED PRACTICE

The following are some of the nursing research problems raised in Chapter 4 that merit further study by psychiatric nurses:

1. The theoretical basis for practice used by psychiatric nurses
2. Attitudes of psychiatric nurses regarding the health-illness and conformity-deviance conceptions of mental illness
3. The role of psychiatric nurses in the delivery of mental health care to cultural, sexual, and ethnic minorities
4. The validity and reliability of tools used to collect data about coping strategies used by healthy and ill individuals
5. Methods to evaluate the effectiveness of coping strategies
6. The direct and interactive efforts related to the nature, origin, timing, and number of stressors
7. Variables that intervene between stressful life events and maladaptive coping responses
8. Stressful life events, chronic strains, and daily hassles relevant to various high-risk groups
9. The role of social attribution in an individual's response to threat
10. The types of coping resources associated with adaptive responses and their mechanism of action
11. Correlation between NANDA nursing diagnoses and *DSM-IV-TR* diagnoses

12. The amount of time psychiatric nurses spend in activities related to each stage of treatment—crisis, acute, maintenance, and health promotion
13. The specific nursing interventions implemented by nurses in each stage of treatment—crisis, acute, maintenance, and health promotion
14. The specific outcomes achieved by nurses in each stage of treatment—crisis, acute, maintenance, and health promotion

5 Evidence-Based Psychiatric Nursing Practice

CRITICAL THINKING QUESTIONS

1. Discuss the public attention that the Surgeon General's report on mental health received, compared with his report on smoking. What differences do you observe?
2. How has the World Wide Web changed access to information for both the lay person and the professional?
3. Identify some of your own biases that influence the psychiatric care you provide.
4. Think of a situation you experienced recently in which scientific evidence was not available to help you in your clinical decision making. What other resources did you rely on?
5. Why are randomized controlled trials (RCTs) considered to be the "gold standard" of research methodologies?
6. How do clinical algorithms compare and contrast with practice guidelines?
7. What outcomes are routinely assessed in your clinical setting? How comfortable are you with participating in the outcome measurement process?
8. Why do you think psychiatric patients consistently report high levels of satisfaction with the care they receive?

CRITICAL THINKING ACTIVITIES

1. Select a psychiatric nursing journal and review the articles in it. Sort them by the hierarchy of research evidence presented in Box 5-1.
2. Obtain one of the many practice guidelines for psychiatric care. Look carefully at the references cited at the end of the guidelines that support the recommendations. Determine how many, if any, of the references are from the nursing literature. Discuss the implications of your findings with your classmates.
3. On an average clinical day in psychiatric nursing, record your various nursing interventions. At the end of the day categorize them into one of the four bases of nursing practice described in Chapter 5.
4. Go online to the Cochrane Library—http://www.cochrane.org. Find out what systematic reviews they have for the various psychiatric illnesses. What value might this library have for your practice as a nurse?

RESEARCH AGENDA FOR EVIDENCE-BASED PRACTICE

The following are some of the nursing research problems raised in Chapter 5 that merit further study by psychiatric nurses:

1. The impact of the Surgeon General's report in funding of both mental health services and mental health research
2. The extent to which psychiatric nurses access the World Wide Web for professional information, and the nature of such access
3. The relative degree to which psychiatric nursing interventions have a traditional, regulatory, philosophical, or evidence basis for practice
4. The extent to which psychiatric nurses use practice guidelines in any form in their practice
5. Outcomes associated with the use of practice guidelines
6. Effective ways of disseminating practice guidelines to psychiatric nurses
7. Clinical, functional, satisfaction, and financial outcomes associated with psychiatric nursing care
8. The patient satisfaction indicators that are directly related to nursing care
9. Evidence supporting the efficacy of the basic elements of the nurse-patient relationship
10. Evidence supporting the efficacy of the Nursing Intervention Classification (NIC) codes

6 BIOLOGICAL CONTEXT OF PSYCHIATRIC NURSING CARE

CRITICAL THINKING QUESTIONS

1. It has been said that psychiatric nurses need an understanding of the brain in the same way that cardiac care nurses need an understanding of the heart. Support or refute this statement.
2. Compare and contrast adoption, twin, and family studies as they are used to understand the genetics of psychiatric illnesses.
3. You overhear your minister telling an older woman that her depression will be relieved if she prays to God for strength and forgiveness. As a nurse, how can you intervene in this situation?
4. A friend tells you that she thinks mental illness is just a social explanation for unacceptable behavior. Based on your knowledge of contemporary psychiatric theory, how would you respond?
5. Some people believe that biology determines behavior and that people are therefore not responsible for what they do. Interpret this belief in light of the Decade of the Brain.
6. Your co-worker refuses to do shift work any longer because she says it takes too long to recover. How would you respond to this?
7. Your patient asks you whether her children are more at risk for mental illness because their parent is mentally ill, or because they were raised by a symptomatic parent. How would you respond?
8. Your patient asks you why she has to take medications instead of getting gene therapy for her mental illness. How would you respond?

CRITICAL THINKING ACTIVITIES

1. Describe the structures and processes underlying neurotransmission, using drawings of brain structures and functions as appropriate.
2. Make a chart tracking your own body rhythms related to sleep, eating, and energy levels. Compare it with that of a friend.
3. It has been suggested that there is a link between one's psychological state and the development of cancer. Review the literature in this area and support or refute this observation.
4. Conduct a biological assessment of a psychiatric patient, using the essential elements presented in Box 6-3. Identify your areas of strength and weakness.
5. Compare the impact of the Decade of the Brain with that of the Human Genome Project on our understanding of and interventions for mental illness.
6. Hold a debate in class. One person defends retaining the driver's license and another supports suspending it for an individual who seems to suffer from time interval delays as the reason he has repeatedly received tickets for driving through red and yellow lights and nearly missing pedestrians in intersections.
7. Develop a brief primer on the impact of the Human Genome Project relevant for your psychiatric patients.

RESEARCH AGENDA FOR EVIDENCE-BASED PRACTICE

The following are some of the nursing research problems raised in Chapter 6 that merit further study by psychiatric nurses:

1. The amount of neuroscience and psychobiology content included in nursing programs at the associate, baccalaureate, and master's level
2. The proficiency of psychiatric nurses in the biological assessment of patients
3. Biological predictors of treatment strategies for the various psychiatric illnesses
4. The degree to which the findings from genetic research are included in patient and family education with regard to psychiatric illnesses
5. Psychiatric nurses' familiarity with brain imaging techniques, how they work, and what they show
6. The degree to which psychiatric nurses understand neurotransmission and the role of brain chemicals, such as neurotransmitters, in the normal and abnormal function of the brain
7. The effects of interval time disabilities on safety related to using sharp instruments such as knives, machinery, and even child-care activities
8. How the Human Genome Project findings affect patient teaching by psychiatric nurses related to the potential for inheritance of mental illnesses
9. The relationship of environmental factors with genetically vulnerable individuals and the effect on risk of or protection against mental illnesses
10. How genetic vulnerability to mental illness will affect treatment selection

Psychological Context of Psychiatric Nursing Care 7

CRITICAL THINKING QUESTIONS

1. Identify the theoretical knowledge and specific skills required of the nurse to perform a mental status exam.
2. Identify three clinical settings in which the nurse could use the psychiatric history and mental status examination in the formulation of nursing diagnoses.
3. Describe the essential characteristics of the interviewer that enhance effective data collection.
4. Select a patient for whom you have performed a nursing assessment. Describe how you would integrate the components of mental status examination into that assessment.
5. Discuss how one determines priorities in the psychiatric interview that require further exploration.
6. Discuss the importance of the medical history and its correlation to the presenting problem and the subsequent formulation of the nursing care plan. Give examples.
7. In the overall assessment process, discuss the significance of the family and personal history in the formulation of a nursing care plan.
8. Define the components of the mental status examination that relate to alterations in cognitive function.
9. Discuss the importance of assessing the patient's judgment in the overall analysis of a mental status examination.
10. Identify several ancillary data resources in the analysis of patient behavior. Give clinical examples of how these are used in the nursing assessment.
11. Correlate three nursing diagnoses with *DSM-IV-TR* diagnoses. Discuss how these were derived from the psychiatric evaluation.
12. Discuss the significance of the patient's perception and degree of reality testing in response to nursing intervention. Give examples.
13. Explore the possible medicolegal implications of an undiagnosed psychiatric problem.
14. What advantages and disadvantages do computerized assessments bring to the field?

CRITICAL THINKING ACTIVITIES

1. Conduct a mental status examination on a fellow student, a friend or family member, and a person with a diagnosed psychiatric illness. Identify how these examinations differ in both process and content.
2. Talk with a patient who has a psychotic disorder and note the types of thought content and thought process problems expressed.
3. From among the people you know, identify separate individuals each of whom displays one of the seven types of intelligence listed in the Critical Thinking About Contemporary Issues box on page 115. Do any of them display more than one type of intelligence? How does their type of intelligence relate to their personal happiness, career success, and perceived social status?
4. Review the behavioral rating scales listed in Appendix C. Select two that interest you and obtain copies of them. Learn how to use them in your practice.
5. If one of your psychiatric settings uses computerized assessments or rating scales, ask to take one of them on the computer. Describe your reaction to it.

RESEARCH AGENDA FOR EVIDENCE-BASED PRACTICE

The following are some of the nursing research problems raised in Chapter 7 that merit further study by psychiatric nurses:

1. Effectiveness of the psychiatric nurse in patient evaluation and triage
2. Effects of cultural diversity on patient presentation of symptoms and interviewer interpretation
3. Qualities of the interview process that affect the accurate collection of data
4. Responsive and active dimensions of the nurse that influence the self-disclosure of the patient
5. Effects of the availability of technology on the quality, costs, and outcomes of the mental status exam
6. Early identification of suicidal ideation in patients at risk for self-destructive behavior
7. The impact of the nurse-patient rapport on the quality of data collected during the mental status exam

8. Comparison of patient and interviewer perceptions of the presenting problem and its effect on patient compliance with the treatment plan
9. The extent of the use of behavioral rating scales by psychiatric nurses
10. The degree to which nurses in nonpsychiatric settings include elements of the mental status exam in their evaluation of patients

SOCIAL, CULTURAL, AND SPIRITUAL CONTEXT OF PSYCHIATRIC NURSING CARE

8

CRITICAL THINKING QUESTIONS

1. Do you think there is a difference between the terms "culturally sensitive" and "culturally competent?" Discuss how these differences might apply to nursing.
2. It has been observed that more people who suffer from schizophrenia are in the low-income portion of the population. Why do you think this is so? What does it reflect about the mental health care delivery system in this country?
3. Review the sociocultural trends listed in Box 8-2. What changes will need to be made in the current health care system to accommodate them?
4. Do you believe that the clinician should be of the same ethnic background as the patient to be effective? Must they be of the same age, gender, income, or educational level? Defend your response.
5. Based on the variety of experiences you have had working in the health care system, describe some of the gender biases you have observed and their consequences. Include issues related to staff as well as patients.
6. You are working with a depressed woman who tells you that she doesn't need to take the medicine prescribed by her physician because she is under the care of her "root doctor" and he has all the treatment she needs. How would you respond?
7. Some cultures have a greater tolerance for unusual behavior of certain types. Explore this issue and relate it to the diagnosis of psychiatric illness cross-culturally.
8. A classmate often talks about people with psychiatric problems as "nut cases," "crazies," "weirdos," and "half-brains." How might you go about raising this person's sensitivity to issues about stigma, stereotypes, and prejudice?
9. Use the questions identified in Box 8-4 to complete a thorough assessment of a patient's sociocultural risk factors for psychiatric illness.
10. Using your own religion or that of someone you know as an example, cite ways in which it can be either a coping resource or a stressor for someone with a psychiatric illness.
11. Describe some of the common stereotypes associated with substance abuse in this country for the various age groups. How can these interfere with a person's ability to get help?
12. Think about how we refer to patients. Why do we say patients are "schizophrenics" but not "cancers"? Why does our language convey about psychiatric versus physical illness?

CRITICAL THINKING ACTIVITIES

1. Talk with some patients and families about the sociocultural barriers they experience in obtaining mental health care. What can you as a nurse do to correct some of these problems?
2. Stigma regarding mental illness is a significant problem in this country. Watch television and read the newspaper for a week and critique the media's treatment of psychiatric illness in light of this sociocultural stressor.
3. Examine the health beliefs of two different cultural groups that live in your community. Describe how each set of beliefs could affect psychiatric treatment in both positive and negative ways.
4. Go to a health food store and examine the many products that are marketed for the relief of psychological distress. Do you believe that these can help or hurt a patient's recovery?
5. Obtain a copy of the Surgeon General's report, "Mental Health: Race, Culture, and Ethnicity." Read through the fact sheets and major recommendations. Identify implications of these for psychiatric nursing practice.

RESEARCH AGENDA FOR EVIDENCE-BASED PRACTICE

The following are some of the nursing research problems raised in Chapter 8 that merit further study by psychiatric nurses:

1. Ways in which sociocultural sensitivity by the psychiatric nurse enhances nursing care outcomes
2. Sociocultural factors that impede and enhance mental health–seeking behavior of individuals and families in distress
3. Sociocultural biases in the DSM and NANDA diagnostic systems
4. The impact of age on the course of psychiatric illness
5. The way in which ethnicity affects the patient-clinician therapeutic alliance and compliance with treatment

6. An exploration of potential gender bias in the criteria for borderline personality disorder
7. Ways in which education and income influence one's ability to access mental health care in this country
8. Degree of congruence between the health belief systems of patients and clinicians and related treatment outcomes
9. The nature and degree of sociocultural stressors experienced by the mentally ill as a result of their illness
10. The interaction of psychobiology and sociocultural factors in the assessment and treatment of psychiatric illness

ENVIRONMENTAL CONTEXT OF PSYCHIATRIC NURSING CARE

9

CRITICAL THINKING QUESTIONS

1. Describe the six forces affecting the delivery of mental health care and the vested interests of each.
2. Some people believe that health care providers are responsible for the advent of managed care because they practiced without regard to costs and were not accountable for their health care actions or outcomes. How would you respond to this?
3. In many ways managed care reflects the public health model of care rather than the traditional medical model. Discuss the problems and challenges this difference poses for health care providers who have been educated in the traditional medical model.
4. Do you believe that health care is a right? Do you think that people should have access to any and all health care services? If not, who should have access and how should access be determined?
5. Identify the six major components of a comprehensive employee-assistance program.
6. What impact do you think the three major national reports have had on the health care system?
7. Many people believe that psychiatric nursing jobs are shrinking. Disprove this faulty belief by identifying new positions for psychiatric nurses in the various levels of care identified in Table 9-3.
8. Do any of the roles for psychiatric nurses in managed care described on pages 143-144 appeal to you? Would you consider applying for these positions upon graduation? Why or why not?

CRITICAL THINKING ACTIVITIES

1. Talk to a consumer about his or her experience with the mental health care system. What changes would he or she suggest?
2. Review the advertisements of health care organizations that appear in your local newspaper next Sunday. Evaluate whether these ads are marketing services based upon reputation, facilities, quality of care, or cost. Which ads do you believe are the most effective and why?
3. Kaiser is one of the oldest managed care companies in America. Write them a letter inquiring about how they use nurses in their system of care and potential career opportunities for you as a nurse employed by them.
4. Pick a mental health problem and search for information about it on the Internet. Critique what you find.
5. There is a lively debate about how much treatment parity for mental and substance abuse disorders will cost. Review some of the most recent studies on this issue and present your findings to the class.
6. Review a recent issue of a psychiatric nursing journal. In the articles presented determine whether clinical, functional, satisfaction, or financial outcomes of nursing care were reported. Identify outcome indicators that could have been included to further strengthen the impact of nursing care.
7. Find out the ratio of registered nurses to patients in the inpatient psychiatric care facilities in your community. Evaluate the differences on the basis of patient acuity, staff safety, and service setting accountability.

RESEARCH AGENDA FOR EVIDENCE-BASED PRACTICE

The following are some of the nursing research problems raised in Chapter 9 that merit further study by psychiatric nurses:

1. Nurses' understanding of characteristics, process, and structures of managed health care
2. A comparison of the state programs in psychiatric care that arose from federal waivers
3. The degree to which psychiatric nurses work in employee assistance programs and the roles and functions they assume
4. The public's perceptions of parity of mental health care for children and adults
5. The degree to which nurse practitioners deliver mental health care, prescribe psychotropic drugs, and address psychosocial concerns of their patients
6. The nature and extent to which patient satisfaction surveys are being used in inpatient, partial-hospital, outpatient, and home psychiatric care settings
7. Quality indicators for mental health websites
8. Positions, roles, functions, and salaries of psychiatric nurses employed in managed care companies
9. Ways in which nurses help patients and families understand and make decisions in the current environment of psychiatric care
10. The impact that parity of mental health care has had on those states that have legislated it

10 LEGAL AND ETHICAL CONTEXT OF PSYCHIATRIC NURSING CARE

CRITICAL THINKING QUESTIONS

1. Describe the similarities and differences between the disciplines of psychiatry and the law.
2. Compare and contrast the following types of admission to a psychiatric hospital and considerations pertinent to each: informal, voluntary, and involuntary.
3. Explain the meaning of *police power* and *parens patriae power* in relation to involuntary commitment.
4. Commitment is usually justified on three grounds: (a) dangerousness to self or others, (b) need for treatment, and (c) inability to meet one's own basic needs. Do you believe these are necessary and appropriate? Support your position.
5. As you join your friends for lunch one day, two of them are discussing how a person can be committed. One believes that only psychiatrists can commit someone; the other maintains that only a judge can make that decision. They ask you to tell them what you know about the commitment process. How would you describe the correct procedure to them?
6. Identify the goals, process, and time limits of emergency hospitalization, temporary hospitalization, and indefinite hospitalization.
7. One of the patients on the psychiatric unit you work on has eloped (left without permission). What should the staff do, and what information will be pertinent to your decision?
8. Distinguish among conditional, absolute, and judicial discharges, and give an example of a patient situation that might best be served by each one.
9. The Wyatt court decision in 1972 defined criteria for adequate treatment in three areas. What are these areas? Evaluate to what degree the psychiatric unit on which you work meets these criteria. Do you believe psychiatric hospitalization is in itself therapeutic, or should specific treatment be mandatory? Support your position in light of current fiscal constraints.
10. Is refusal of treatment the same as noncompliance? If not, how would you differentiate between them, and what course of action would be most appropriate for each?
11. Describe what is meant by the "right to treatment in the least restrictive setting." What problems can be anticipated in the implementation of this right?
12. Lawsuits against nurses are becoming more common. Describe typical causes of malpractice suits against psychiatric nurses, criteria for malpractice claims, and preventive measures nurses should take to avoid litigation.
13. Describe the psychiatric nurse's rights and responsibilities in the roles as employee and citizen. Give specific examples of each.
14. Many well-publicized criminal cases have used the "insanity defense." Do you believe this defense best serves the interests of justice? Support your position.
15. Analyze the need, purpose, and potential impact of mental health advocacy.

CRITICAL THINKING ACTIVITIES

1. Conduct a class debate on the issue of commitment. Consider the following critical dimensions:
   A. The assessment and prediction of dangerousness
   B. Preventive detention
   C. Nonconformity and social control
   D. Freedom of choice
   E. Procedures and standards
   F. Outpatient commitment
2. Review the commitment procedure in your state. Critique it in relation to the goals of hospitalization, the quality of life, and the protection of patients' rights.
3. Determine what rights the committed patient retains in your state. Which of the rights identified in this chapter are not retained?
4. What is the law in your state regarding privileged communication? How does it affect psychiatric nurses?
5. Professional psychiatric nursing practice emerges from an interaction between patients' rights, the nurse's legal role, and the nurse's concern for quality psychiatric care. Issues are often complex and require critical judgment. To assist students in analyzing some of these issues and strengthen their decision-making skills, 15 clinical dilemmas are described. Distribute one of the situations to each student in a clinical

group and ask them to discuss it, verbally or in writing, responding to the following questions:

A. What issues are involved?
B. What information is needed to make your decision?
C. What alternative courses of action are open to you, and what are the advantages and disadvantages of each?
D. What do you decide to do?
E. What is your rationale?

1. You observe a nurse opening and reading a patient's personal mail, then resealing it and giving it to him.
2. You are summoned to appear in court to testify about a patient's testamentary capacity. The patient's son is contesting his will on the grounds that he is delusional.
3. Two hospital patients come to the staff asking to be married. The psychiatrist in charge tells them that there is a law against it because they are "diagnosed schizophrenics."
4. You have just begun to work as a staff nurse at a hospital for mentally retarded children. The parents of one of the children on your unit tell you that after waiting for 10 months for some kind of education program for their child, they have decided to sue the hospital and staff.
5. A patient comes to you and tells you he knows he is being detained in the hospital illegally. He demands that you tell him his rights.
6. You hear the receptionist at the CMHC in which you work giving information about a patient's diagnosis to someone over the telephone.
7. You have been summoned to testify at a child custody hearing regarding the issues raised in marital therapy with a couple you have been treating.
8. In the course of treating an adolescent, he reveals to you that he has been selling drugs to other students in his high school.
9. A patient is scheduled to receive electroconvulsive therapy in the morning. When you notice that the consent form is missing, you call the resident. He tells you it was omitted because signing it would have been too upsetting to the patient.
10. You observe a drug salesman, who is well known to the staff on the unit, reading some of the patients' charts.
11. The psychiatric hospital at which you work has just lost its accreditation, partly on the ground of inadequate staffing and lack of individualized care. Simultaneously the state legislature has just decreased funding for mental health by 10%, for the second time this year.
12. One of the patients on your unit has refused to take any medication. His treatment team has decided "not to engage in a power struggle" with him but to "slip" the medicine into his food, just until he is less defensive and more amenable to treatment.
13. In one of your group therapy sessions for single parents, a member says that she sometimes beats her toddler when she's under a lot of stress and tension.
14. The state legislature, in debating mental health funding, cites the right to treatment in the least restrictive setting as justification for cutting funds to state institutions. Your state nurses' association asks you to write a report analyzing this issue and making recommendations relative to it.
15. You are in private practice and are about to go on vacation. Your plane leaves in three hours. The telephone rings as you are packing your suitcase. It is one of your patients who says she is feeling suicidal.

RESEARCH AGENDA FOR EVIDENCE-BASED PRACTICE

The following are some of the nursing research problems raised in Chapter 10 that merit further study by psychiatric nurses:

1. Psychiatric nurses' knowledge of patient's legal rights at the time of admission and during psychiatric hospitalization
2. Psychiatric nurses' ability to evaluate the potential dangerousness of psychiatric patients
3. Patients' rights most commonly violated in psychiatric settings
4. Nursing interventions implemented with patients who refuse medication
5. Litigation involving psychiatric nurses, including the number of cases, basis of the lawsuit, other persons named in the suit, and outcome
6. Resolution of conflict of interest relative to the legal roles of the psychiatric nurse as provider, employee, and citizen
7. Psychiatric nurses' participation in formal and informal mental health advocacy programs
8. Mechanisms used by psychiatric nurses to affect mental health issues at the local, state, and national levels and identification of issues in which they are involved
9. The frequency and clinical outcomes associated with involuntary outpatient treatment of the mentally ill
10. Strategies for increasing awareness of advance directives in mental health
11. Providers' compliance with mental health advance directives
12. Barriers to implementing advance directives
13. Ethical dilemmas frequently encountered by psychiatric nurses and the ways in which they are resolved

11 Families as Resources, Caregivers, and Collaborators

CRITICAL THINKING QUESTIONS

1. What reasons do staff cite for not working to a greater degree with the families of patients who are mentally ill? Evaluate the validity and consequences of these reasons.
2. Evaluate the ethical issues that arise related to the patient's right to a confidential therapeutic relationship and the family caregiver's right to information.
3. Identify specific ways in which family involvement can enhance the treatment process.
4. A mother accompanies her adult son, who is agitated and delusional, to the emergency room for evaluation and disposition. What nursing actions directed to the mother would be particularly effective at this time?
5. Describe why spouses sometimes refer to their spouse's symptoms as "contagious." As a nurse, how might you reach out to help them?
6. What might aging parents with children who have mental illness worry about? How can nurses help them with these fears?
7. Discuss ways in which living with a sibling who is mentally ill may be viewed as a type of childhood trauma.
8. The father of one of your patients asks to meet with you and he tells you that his adult married daughter who suffers from serious bipolar disorder is planning on getting pregnant. He asks you to counsel her against it, given her health status. How would you respond?

CRITICAL THINKING ACTIVITIES

1. Find out the visiting hours for families in the inpatient psychiatric setting of your clinical rotation. Are the treatment team members available to talk to family members during these times? If not, how are families involved in collaborative relationships with the treatment team? Compare this to the way in which outpatient or community settings provide for the involvement of family members.
2. Interview some families who have members with psychiatric illness. Ask them which type of mental health care provider (nurse, physician, social worker, etc.) has been most helpful to them in their own experience and the specific ways in which these individuals were able to help.
3. Design a psychoeducational program for the family of a patient with bipolar disorder.
4. Describe how the nuclear family, extended family, and household may differ for immigrants, interracial couples, and step families.

RESEARCH AGENDA FOR EVIDENCE-BASED PRACTICE

The following are some of the nursing research problems raised in Chapter 11 that merit further study by psychiatric nurses:

1. The extent to which nurses include families in their work with patients, and how this differs based on treatment setting and patient characteristics
2. Boundaries of confidentiality related to patients' rights and families' need for information
3. Extent to which NAMI reaches out to family members from diverse sociocultural backgrounds
4. Helpful and detrimental ways in which staff in emergency rooms respond to patients who present with psychiatric problems and their families
5. The impact that caregiving for an adult child who is mentally ill has on the physical and emotional health of aging parents
6. Positive and negative aspects of their childhood as experienced by siblings of those who are mentally ill
7. Resiliency or protective factors that characterize well siblings of the mentally ill
8. The number and nature of programs set up to provide prenatal and postpartum care for women with severe mental illness
9. Outcomes associated with early screening and mental health promotion programs for children whose parents are mentally ill
10. The nature and outcomes associated with family psychoeducational programs conducted by nurses
11. The degree to which psychiatric nurses use the competence-empowerment model in working with families
12. Families' perceptions of the value of the genogram

12 Implementing the Nursing Process: Standards of Care and Professional Performance

CRITICAL THINKING QUESTIONS

1. How are theory, practice, and research interrelated in nursing? Clarify your explanation with a clinical example.
2. You are attending a team planning conference about your psychiatric patient. After you describe your nursing care plan, a medical student comments, "All those nursing plans are a bit premature because no medical diagnosis has been made yet." How would you respond to him?
3. Explain why the patient's participation in the problem-solving process may be more difficult and why it is also particularly important for psychiatric patients.
4. Discuss how the content, method, and process of your data collection would differ for a patient on a medical unit whom you are asked to evaluate for apparent anxiety and depression and for a newly admitted psychiatric patient to whom you are assigned as primary nurse.
5. In what way are nursing and medical diagnoses different? In what way are they complementary?
6. Describe how use of the responsive dimensions of a therapeutic relationship can help the patient develop insight and how use of the action dimensions can help the patient effect change.
7. Review the Nursing Interventions Classification (NIC) and Nursing Outcomes Classification (NOC) in relation to their usefulness in working with one of your psychiatric patients.
8. Nursing has been described as a full profession, semiprofession, subprofession, and emerging profession. Which description do you believe applies to psychiatric nursing? Support your position from both theory and practice.
9. Give examples of various mechanisms that promote accountability in psychiatric nursing.
10. Autonomy has been called the hallmark of professionalism. Critique the degree of autonomy in psychiatric nursing, and suggest ways in which it may be enhanced.
11. Describe the roles of the various members of the mental health care team, and give examples of specific functions performed by each.
12. Discuss the personal qualities and activities needed for effective interdisciplinary team functioning.
13. Give examples of ways in which nurses can participate in the research process on the basis of their education and experience.
14. As a head nurse of your psychiatric unit, you have the responsibility for conducting a comprehensive evaluation program. Describe in detail what your program would consist of and how it would be conducted.

CRITICAL THINKING ACTIVITIES

1. Read ANA's *Nursing's Social Policy Statement*. Discuss its implications for psychiatric nursing.
2. Review the work of Mager on writing behavioral objectives and identify the elements of a well-written objective. Now evaluate the expected outcomes and short-term goals you see written by nurses in clinical settings.
3. Determine how your state law defines advanced nursing practice. What acts or functions are included in this definition?
4. Ask the administrator of a psychiatric treatment facility how they evaluate the services they provide and what outcome data they make available to patients and families.
5. Determine what telecommunication technology (faxes, computers, e-mail, image transmission, interactive video sessions, etc.) are used in your psychiatric clinical setting. Ask staff about the value they do or do not provide.
6. Go to the library and examine a copy of each of the psychiatric nursing journals presented in Figure 12-3. Decide which one you would like to read on a regular basis to stay current with developments in the field.
7. Conduct an informal survey among nursing staff to identify what kind of recognition they have received and what kind they most valued.
8. Determine whether the major health care organizations in your community have clinical advancement programs for nurses and whether their positions and salaries are based on differentiated levels of nursing practice that include education and experience.

9. Use the Internet to access the home page of the American Psychiatric Nurses Association at http://www.apna.org. Review the information presented and critique the image of the specialty it projects.

RESEARCH AGENDA FOR EVIDENCE-BASED PRACTICE

The following are some of the nursing research problems raised in Chapter 12 that merit further study by psychiatric nurses:

1. The identification, classification, and validation of phenomena of concern to psychiatric nurses
2. The degree of mutuality in the nurse-patient relationship at the various phases of the nursing process, particularly in a psychiatric care context
3. The impact of cultural biases on the nursing care given to patients of different ethnic groups and social classes
4. Nursing diagnoses used by psychiatric nurses, including the extent and consistency of use, the format, their validity and reliability, and their usefulness in suggesting nursing actions that will promote adaptive coping responses
5. The content, process, structure, and outcome of health teaching conducted by psychiatric nurses
6. Outcomes of psychiatric nursing care, including levels of patient satisfaction
7. The cost-effectiveness of psychiatric nurses relative to other mental health care providers
8. The effectiveness of mechanisms to ensure accountability in psychiatric nursing practice
9. The degree to which psychiatric nurses exercise control over their nursing tasks and participate in the decision-making structure of the organizations in which they work
10. Effective methods of clinical supervision to enhance role performance of psychiatric nurses
11. Differentiation of psychiatric nursing practice based on knowledge base and clinical competencies across caregiving settings
12. Factors that influence the nurse's effective participation as a member of the mental health treatment team
13. Models of interdisciplinary collaboration in psychiatric practice, research, and education
14. Structure, process, and outcomes of effective mental health teams
15. Ways in which psychiatric nurses are utilized in hospital-based, community, and home care settings
16. Characteristics of mental health care settings that promote the full utilization of the psychiatric nursing role

MENTAL HEALTH PROMOTION AND ILLNESS PREVENTION 13

CRITICAL THINKING QUESTIONS

1. Contrast the medical and nursing models in their views of causes of mental illness, definitions of mental illness, and paradigms for primary prevention.
2. Select a particular disease or disorder that can be prevented. Show how steps of the nursing model can be used to promote its prevention.
3. What is meant by the phrase *competent community*? Give an example of one.
4. Under what three conditions is environmental change a particularly appropriate preventive strategy?
5. It has been said that supporting social systems is an important concept for all three levels of prevention—primary, secondary, and tertiary. Explain why this is true from both a theoretical and a practical perspective.
6. Identify an informal support group of which you are currently a member. Describe its goals and processes and the benefits you derive from it.
7. Evaluate the potential effect of health care reform on preventive mental health care in the United States.
8. In what settings would preventive nursing interventions directed to children and adolescents be best implemented? Justify your answer.
9. As a nurse, you wish to write a grant proposing a primary prevention program to reduce family violence. What will be your target or vulnerable population? Why?
10. Identify preventive interventions related to supporting the social systems of the elderly who are at risk for developing maladaptive responses.

CRITICAL THINKING ACTIVITIES

1. Identify a vulnerable group you are interested in working with. For this group design a prevention program that specifies the following:
   A. The risk factor or stress to which they are subject
   B. The maladaptive coping responses that might result
   C. Target areas for nursing intervention based on the components of the model of health illness phenomena used in this text
   D. Strategies of preventive intervention
   E. Social institutions and situations through which the strategies may be applied
2. Review the health care legislation currently under review in your state. Select one prevention-related issue. Study it and write a letter to your representative stating your position as a nursing professional.
3. Attend a self-help group such as Alcoholics Anonymous, Weight Watchers, Parents Without Partners, or Recovery. Identify ways in which they can promote mental health.
4. Develop a preventive health education program for adolescents under stress, incorporating the four specific aspects of competence building described in this chapter.
5. Contact the group in your community that works to prevent rape. Volunteer to work with them in one of their activities.
6. Organize an anti-stigma campaign in your school to promote knowledge and change attitudes about mental health and mental illness.

RESEARCH AGENDA FOR EVIDENCE-BASED PRACTICE

The following are some of the nursing research problems raised in Chapter 13 that merit further study by psychiatric nurses:

1. Mental health services available to women on a regional basis in relation to rape, family violence, and substance abuse
2. Study of psychiatric nurses' attitudes toward sex roles and mental health
3. Specific preventive strategies and relevant social institutions and situations through which the strategies may be applied
4. The degree, level, and type of environmental change implemented by psychiatric nurses
5. The extent of participation of nurses in mutual support groups
6. The degree, domain, and type of mental health education implemented by psychiatric nurses
7. The effectiveness of preventive nursing interventions with regard to short- and long-term outcomes, use of resources, and comparison with other prevention strategies
8. The degree and type of intervention used by psychiatric nurses in supporting social systems

9. Preventive programs implemented by nurses who work with the mental health needs of children
10. The extent to which nurses engage in the primary prevention measures identified to meet the national year 2010 objectives for the control of stress and violent behavior
11. The stigma nurses not working in psychiatry have about mental illness and psychiatric care
12. The effectiveness of public anti-stigma campaigns focused on mental health and mental illness

CRISIS INTERVENTION 14

CRITICAL THINKING QUESTIONS

1. Compare and contrast the four levels of crisis intervention. In what type of situation would you choose to use each?
2. A tornado has hit your community, and the victims are gathered in a church hall. What interventions would you institute, on both a short- and a long-term basis?
3. An 11-year-old boy has been brought to the crisis clinic by his parents. The parents tell you that their son, who has always been a "good child," was arrested yesterday for stealing. Describe the mode of crisis therapy you would plan, and provide a rationale for that plan.
4. Identify the balancing factors that influence an individual subjected to a stressful situation. Describe the effect of these balancing factors on the individual.
5. Analyze how a crisis can result in personal growth.
6. Describe a maturational crisis and possible outcomes for those who experience it.
7. Identify four basic needs of all individuals. How do you determine which of these needs is being threatened in a particular crisis patient? Include examples of questions you would ask the patient about needs during the assessment phase of crisis intervention.
8. A mother in a well baby clinic tells you she is finding it difficult to function since her mother died 3 weeks ago. You set up several crisis intervention sessions with the mother. Describe and provide a rationale for the crisis intervention techniques you would emphasize in the sessions.
9. Crisis therapy is a major technique of preventive psychiatry. Discuss implications for nursing in various settings.
10. Describe strategies for patient education in regard to crisis. Include identification of populations you would consider to be high risk for crisis development.

CRITICAL THINKING ACTIVITIES

1. Make an appointment with a local Red Cross worker. Talk to the individual about recent crises in your community and ways in which the Red Cross helped.
2. Watch one of the popular "crisis movies," such as *Volcano*, *Earthquake*, or *Twister*. For the main characters in the movie, identify the precipitating event, perception of the event, support systems, coping resources, and coping mechanisms.
3. If your community has a mobile crisis program, ask if you may spend a day with them and observe their work.
4. Seek out a telephone hotline that operates in your area. Spend an evening at the phones and evaluate the crisis intervention function performed by this service.

RESEARCH AGENDA FOR EVIDENCE-BASED PRACTICE

The following are some of the nursing research problems raised in Chapter 14 that merit further study by psychiatric nurses:

1. The conditions under which natural developmental transitions become crises
2. The relationship between the length of time for crisis resolution and individual personality factors
3. Appropriate outcome measures to use in evaluating the effectiveness of crisis theory
4. The relationship between the length of time for crisis resolution and the type of crisis
5. Empirical validation of the course of grief
6. Family functioning characteristics associated with family vulnerability to crisis
7. The relationship between characteristics of role models and the incidence of developmental crises
8. The effectiveness of debriefing for school students who experience violence
9. Ability of nurses to use the four levels of crisis intervention
10. The level of nursing education and skill needed to perform the different levels of crisis intervention

15 Psychiatric Rehabilitation and Recovery

CRITICAL THINKING QUESTIONS

1. Describe three nursing interventions that may be helpful to patients experiencing difficulty giving up the patient role.
2. Analyze rehabilitation psychiatric nursing in terms of the nursing roles described by Peplau.
3. If you were given the responsibility for developing a nursing program for outpatient psychiatric rehabilitation services, what would it be like? Describe the setting, the treatment program, its goals, and the roles of staff and patients. Explain your decisions.
4. You discover that one of the patients from your treatment program has been denied a job because he is "unreliable" and has an "unstable work history." Discuss the following questions: (a) Have his civil rights been violated? (b) What, if any, actions should he take? (c) What, if any, actions would you take? State the reasons for your responses.
5. Define the term *networking*. Discuss networking as a means of encouraging the establishment of psychiatric rehabilitation programs in the community.
6. Has deinstitutionalization improved the quality of life of the seriously mentally ill patient? Provide your evidence.
7. Discuss the concept of "strengths" and its relation to nursing care of chronically mentally ill patients.
8. Discuss the concept of recovery as it relates to nursing care of the seriously mentally ill.
9. How can nurses facilitate continuity of care as patients alternate between community and inpatient facilities?
10. In what ways can the principles of psychosocial rehabilitation be integrated into the structure of an inpatient milieu?

CRITICAL THINKING ACTIVITIES

1. Develop a proposal for a program of intervention with families of hospitalized psychiatric patients. Specify the goals and objectives, program structure, role of the nurse, and evaluation criteria.
2. Visit a community mental health center or other social agency of your choice. Ascertain what services may contribute to psychiatric rehabilitation. Discuss these services in terms of accessibility, availability, acceptability, effectiveness, and efficiency.
3. Prepare and present an educational program to a small group of consumers. Identify a learning need, write objectives, prepare and present content, and evaluate the session.
4. Talk to patients who have a mental illness. Ask them what rehabilitative services would be of help to them. Compare this to the responses of family members to this same question.

RESEARCH AGENDA FOR EVIDENCE-BASED PRACTICE

The following are some of the nursing research problems raised in Chapter 15 that merit further study by psychiatric nurses:

1. The relationship of various tertiary prevention program elements to patient outcomes
2. Description of patient behavioral profiles related to potential for success in various types of community rehabilitation programs, e.g., supported living versus supervised group housing
3. Nurses' understanding and endorsement of the recovery model
4. Testing of the ability to generalize social skills learned in a hospital or other institutional setting to a community environment
5. The relationship between student experiences in psychiatric mental health nursing and stigmatizing
6. Evaluation of the helpfulness of self-help group membership as compared to participation in other types of treatment program
7. The relationship between family burden and patient outcomes
8. The effectiveness of specific strategies used by psychiatric nurses to enhance patient medication compliance

ANXIETY RESPONSES AND ANXIETY DISORDERS 16

CRITICAL THINKING QUESTIONS

1. The twentieth century has been referred to as the age of anxiety. Discuss how this applies to current society.
2. Using your own personal experiences, give examples of the four types of conflict that can give rise to anxiety.
3. It may be said that all hospitalized patients are at risk for developing anxiety regardless of their medical or nursing diagnosis. Do you agree? Why or why not?
4. Cite a specific type of preventive health program that strives to generate mild anxiety in the public. Is this an appropriate strategy? Support your position.
5. Give examples of some precipitating stressors that have posed threats to your own self system.
6. Analyze how anxiety plays a major role in the psychogenesis of emotional illness.
7. Identify the coping mechanisms you use to relieve mild levels of anxiety.
8. For each of the four personal types of conflict you described in Question 2, describe and categorize the coping mechanism you used to resolve the situation.
9. Describe the four issues the nurse needs to consider in evaluating whether the patient's use of certain defense mechanisms is adaptive or maladaptive.
10. Neurotic health problems are described in this chapter as one type of coping mechanism related to anxiety. How have they been categorized, and what is the rationale for this conceptualization?
11. In nursing care plans you frequently see written "decrease patient's anxiety" as a nursing goal. Why is this an unacceptable goal statement?
12. Analyze the implications of the nurse's use of personal space with patients experiencing mild, moderate, severe, and panic levels of anxiety.
13. One of your friends has recurring migraine headaches. You suggest he have them evaluated at the student health services. When he returns he is very upset, saying the physician told him it was just nerves and stress and not to make such a big deal of it. He asks you what he should do now. How do you respond?
14. Examine the resistive approaches that patients may use to avoid recognizing their anxiety. Give an example of each and an appropriate nursing action for dealing with it.
15. Identify the components of a psychiatric evaluation as presented in Chapter 6. Describe how the behaviors of these components would differ for patients with mild, moderate, severe, and panic levels of anxiety.
16. Analyze how relaxation interventions can be incorporated into crisis therapy.
17. Identify types of precipitating stressors that contribute to anxiety among the elderly.

CRITICAL THINKING ACTIVITIES

1. Prepare a profile that typifies the behaviors you display when you become anxious, integrating physiological, behavioral, cognitive, and affective responses.
2. Apply the relaxation techniques to yourself to achieve a greater relaxation response. Try teaching them to a friend.
3. Observe your friends or family members when they are angry. Identify ways in which their anger may be related to anxiety. How might this influence your response to them?

RESEARCH AGENDA FOR EVIDENCE-BASED PRACTICE

The following are some of the nursing research problems raised in Chapter 16 that merit further study by psychiatric nurses:

1. Empirical validation of the four levels of anxiety and their effects on the individual
2. Exploration of the relationships between anger and anxiety and self-esteem and anxiety
3. Early life experiences that predispose the individual to high levels of anxiety later in life
4. Personality characteristics associated with use of the various types of coping mechanisms
5. The relationship between medical and nursing diagnoses associated with anxiety
6. The ability of psychiatric nurses to distinguish among anxiety, depression, and fear
7. Levels of anxiety of patients during the course of the nurse-patient relationship
8. The effectiveness of various types of supportive physical measures in decreasing a patient's anxiety
9. Effective nursing actions for dealing with the resistance of patients in recognizing anxiety and conflict
10. Evaluation of the short- and long-term effectiveness of relaxation techniques with different patient groups

17 Psychophysiological Responses and Somatoform and Sleep Disorders

CRITICAL THINKING QUESTIONS

1. Select a patient for whom you have provided nursing care. Identify and discuss the patient's stage of the general adaptation syndrome as described by Selye. Support your discussion with specific behavioral observations.
2. A co-worker says to you, "There's Ms. Jones's light again. She's such a hypochondriac." How would you respond? Provide your rationale.
3. Describe the role of secondary gain as it influences the course of a psychophysiological illness. Have you ever experienced secondary gain? Explain.
4. On the basis of your understanding of the personality types associated with cardiac disease, migraine headaches, or hypertension, construct a hypothetical situation that would be stressful to a person with one of these psychophysiological illnesses. Discuss your rationale.
5. Discuss the way in which the physical symptoms in a conversion disorder may symbolize an intrapsychic conflict. Provide an example.
6. Give an example of a psychophysiological illness that may affect each of the following body systems: integumentary, respiratory, cardiovascular, musculoskeletal, gastrointestinal, and genitourinary.
7. Mr. E, a 50-year-old patient with a complaint of diminished feeling in both hands, is referred to the psychiatric liaison nurse for evaluation. It has been determined that no organic impairment would account for his symptom. He tells you that he has no intention of seeing the liaison nurse because "My problem is real. It's not all in my head like they're trying to tell me." How would you respond to him? Support your answer.
8. List and give examples of the three types of conversion symptoms.
9. Compare and contrast hypochondriasis and malingering.
10. Identify and describe the coping mechanism that is particularly characteristic of the person with a Type A personality.
11. Discuss the potential consequences of prematurely challenging the coping mechanisms of a person with a psychophysiological illness.
12. How does hospitalization affect a person's sleep habits?
13. Ms. P, a 15-year-old patient with the conversion symptom of urinary retention, is observed to be very dependent on her mother, who in return is very protective of her daughter. During a nursing case conference, it is suggested that a limit be placed on the length of the mother's visits. Discuss your response to this recommendation.
14. What intervention would you teach parents who have a 6-year-old son who is wetting his bed?

CRITICAL THINKING ACTIVITIES

1. Read the philosophical thoughts of Plato and Aristotle, and relate the ideas of each to the interrelationship of the human mind and body. Discuss which is more closely consistent with your own point of view.
2. Read the philosophical thoughts of Descartes and Pascal, and relate the ideas of each to the interrelationship of the human mind and body. Discuss which is more closely consistent with your own point of view.
3. Ask a classmate to check your blood pressure while you are (a) studying for an examination, (b) talking, (c) watching television, and (d) lying down and listening to soft music. Discuss your observations about any changes in your blood pressure and implications for taking patients' blood pressure.
4. Make a record of your own sleep-wake cycle. Relate the nature of your sleep to your moods, energy level, and thinking processes. Change your sleep pattern and see how it affects the above.
5. Formulate a patient education plan for a 45-year-old male executive who has just experienced his second myocardial infarction. He has been observed to have characteristics of a Type A personality. His wife is supportive and willing to participate in his rehabilitation plan.

RESEARCH AGENDA FOR EVIDENCE-BASED PRACTICE

The following are some of the nursing research problems raised in Chapter 17 that merit further study by psychiatric nurses:

1. The effect of feeling states on biological parameters

2. The relationship between the stress state of the nurse and her response to patient demands
3. Nursing interventions that assist Type A patients to modify their behavior
4. Prevalence of sleep disorders among hospitalized patients
5. Behaviors that patients interpret as indicating increased stress
6. The relationship between personality characteristics and acceptance of various stress management approaches
7. Impact of having family members participate in a stress management program with the patient
8. Characteristics of activities perceived as being relaxing
9. Responses of nurses to patients with psychophysiological illnesses in medical as opposed to psychiatric settings
10. The effect of teaching good sleep hygiene strategies to patients

18 SELF-CONCEPT RESPONSES AND DISSOCIATIVE DISORDERS

CRITICAL THINKING QUESTIONS

1. Observe a preverbal child (under 1 year old) interacting with a parent. Describe parental behaviors that facilitate the development of the child's self-concept. Compare this interaction with one between a parent and a 3-year-old.
2. Identify four ways to promote a child's self-esteem. Describe one specific parenting behavior related to each.
3. Select a patient with whom you have performed a nursing assessment. Analyze the data you collected relative to the individual's self-concept, body image, self-ideal, self-esteem, role, and identity.
4. Review the "Tyranny of the Shoulds." Identify the ones that reflect your own self-ideal. Select one that you would like to change, and keep a record of your progress.
5. Identify four direct and two indirect expressions of low self-esteem. Describe nursing interventions for each type of behavior.
6. Discuss the relationship between the following behaviors demonstrated by adolescents in the process of identity formation: (a) joining a motorcycle gang, (b) trying out for the Olympic skating team, and (c) getting drunk once per week.
7. Ms. B is a 48-year-old married mother of two adult children who is hospitalized on a gynecologic unit. Her medical diagnosis is carcinoma of the cervix, necessitating a hysterectomy, a salpingectomy, and an oophorectomy. One of her nursing diagnoses is sexual dysfunction related to surgical removal of reproductive organs. Formulate one long-term goal and the contributory short-term goals. Describe your nursing interventions to accomplish these goals and your evaluation criteria.
8. You overhear a nurse and an aide discussing Mr. M, a withdrawn, isolated patient, in his presence. The aide says, "I think he's just dumb. He never even looks at you." The nurse responds, "He's not dumb. He's just stubborn. He's too lazy to care for himself." Role play or discuss in writing your response to the two staff members and your intervention with Mr. M.
9. Indicate your agreement or disagreement with the following statement: "People behave in self-defeating ways because there is a payoff involved for them." Support your position.
10. Describe nursing interventions that will assist a withdrawn patient with low self-esteem to share his thoughts and feelings with the nurse.
11. Summarize the five levels of nursing intervention for patients with alterations in self-concept. Include the major focus of the intervention at each level.
12. Discuss the influence of the mother-child relationship on the development of self-concept. Also list nursing interventions to assist the disturbed child develop a healthy self-concept.
13. The beginnings of role strain may be found in the adolescent years. Relate the conflicts and crisis of adolescence to role strain.
14. Select one of the models of family therapy presented in Chapter 33. Discuss the relationship between the selected conceptual model and the promotion of family members' self-growth.
15. Describe the ways in which alterations in self-concept can contribute to family violence. On the basis of your discussion, propose a primary prevention strategy for family violence.
16. The individual's response to aging may be influenced by self-concept. Discuss the ways in which a positive self-concept may assist the person to experience aging as a stage of continued growth. How might self-concept disturbances interfere with normal aging?

CRITICAL THINKING ACTIVITIES

1. In a small group, brainstorm personality traits associated with women and men. Discuss the influence of these perceived characteristics on work-related and family-related behavior.
2. Read a biography of a person who you believe to have a positive self-concept. Identify the life experiences that contributed to the development of the person's positive self-concept and the behaviors that reflect his or her self-concept.
3. Select a photograph of yourself that you like and one that you dislike. Analyze your preference in terms of the influence of your body image.
4. Read *The Quiet Room* by Lori Schiller. Describe a behavior that indicated Lori was experiencing depersonalization. Discuss nursing interventions you would initiate for depersonalization. Include your rationale.

RESEARCH AGENDA FOR EVIDENCE-BASED PRACTICE

The following are some of the nursing research problems raised in Chapter 18 that merit further study by psychiatric nurses:

1. Nursing interventions that enable patients to facilitate a child's development of a positive self-concept
2. The relationship between role strain and nurse burnout
3. Educational strategies that will prepare mental health clinicians to recognize role strain and intervene in a health promoting manner
4. Nursing interventions that assist the individual to recognize ego strengths and to build on existing strengths
5. Effective ways to promote positive self-esteem for individuals and groups in different life situations
6. The ability of mental health clinicians to recognize patient strengths
7. Exploration of the concept of empowerment as a self-enhancing nursing intervention
8. Nurses' awareness of role modeling as an intervention and their self-awareness relative to this concept
9. The correlation between nurses' and patients' perceptions of improvements in patients' self-concept
10. The relationship between the self-concept of the nurse and the effectiveness of interventions with patients experiencing self-concept alterations

19 EMOTIONAL RESPONSES AND MOOD DISORDERS

CRITICAL THINKING QUESTIONS

1. Identify the four adaptive functions of emotions. Give an example of each based on your own clinical nursing experience.
2. Using illustrative examples from your reading and/or your experience, describe the impact of cultural factors on the experience and expression of grief.
3. Select one theory of the cause of depression. Review the literature, and critique the theory on the basis of related research.
4. Life roles and individual response to both ascribed and assumed roles influence the probability of the occurrence of depression. Analyze this statement, including the rationale for your assertions.
5. Compare and contrast the behaviors associated with depressed and manic states.
6. Discuss the behavioral manifestations that you would assess to differentiate between an anxiety disorder and a depressive disorder.
7. The concept of hope is particularly relevant to the care of patients with disturbances of mood. Define hope in this context, and describe why it is so important to these patients.
8. Describe how you used the responsive and action communications skill dimensions in your work with a patient experiencing a severe disturbance of mood.
9. Review the mental status examination as described in Chapter 7. For each component of the examination, describe findings that would indicate the presence of depression or mania.
10. Discuss the ways in which groups may be effective for the primary prevention of major affective disorders.
11. Serious mood disturbances in elderly patients are frequently misidentified as organic mental disorders. Compare and contrast the behaviors associated with these two problems. Identify observations that the nurse can make to clarify the nature of the patient's health problem.

CRITICAL THINKING ACTIVITIES

1. Reflect on a past significant personal loss. Focus on the feelings you experienced. In writing, trace the process you went through after the loss. Identify the events that you experienced as helpful and not helpful.
2. You are the community health nurse who is assigned to care for 68-year-old Ms. G, who has diabetes mellitus, obesity, and hypertension. You have just learned that her husband has died suddenly of a myocardial infarction. Formulate a nursing care plan for this patient, including the necessary data base, nursing diagnoses, goals, and interventions based on your anticipation of an uncomplicated grief reaction.
3. Ms. G (described in Activity 2) becomes severely depressed. Modify your nursing care plan to address this disturbance.
4. Mr. P has just been informed that he has a major affective disorder, bipolar type. He asks you to explain this to him. Describe your initial response to his request. Develop a teaching plan that will provide Mr. P with the information he needs to carry out self-care activities following his discharge from the hospital.

RESEARCH AGENDA FOR EVIDENCE-BASED PRACTICE

The following are some of the nursing research problems raised in Chapter 19 that merit further study by psychiatric nurses:

1. Nursing interventions that facilitate a healthy resolution of grief reactions
2. Development and validation of an assessment instrument that will identify individuals at risk for depression
3. Comparison of the grief process when it is mediated by psychopharmacologic agents and when it is not, including behavioral outcomes
4. The relationships among various life events, the production of biogenic amines, and disturbances of mood
5. Outcomes of nursing interventions related to patients' sleep patterns
6. Identification of nursing interventions effective in primary prevention of disorders of mood
7. Description of the therapeutic characteristics of self-help groups for individuals who have experienced a loss
8. Identification of children at risk for affective disorders
9. The effect of patient education by nurses on medication compliance
10. Effectiveness of structured social interventions by nurses working with depressed and manic patients

SELF-PROTECTIVE RESPONSES AND SUICIDAL BEHAVIOR 20

CRITICAL THINKING QUESTIONS

1. Discuss the continuum of behaviors that range from self-enhancement to suicide in terms of specific behaviors that might be observed at each point on the continuum. How might this be changed in a different sociocultural context?
2. Discuss the steps you would take in response to the following situation: Mr. B is a 62-year-old man with a diagnosis of carcinoma of the bowel. He has had exploratory surgery during which the tumor was left in place but a colostomy was performed. It has been 2 weeks since his surgery, and the physician has just recommended a course of chemotherapy. As you are irrigating his colostomy, Mr. B tells you that he has considered his situation very carefully and has decided it is time for him to die. His children are grown and independent. His wife will be well provided for, and he does not want to force her to care for an invalid. He also wants to spare himself any more pain.
3. Suicide has been described as the result of society's "invitation to die." Explain this theory, and provide examples of behaviors that could be interpreted as an "invitation to die."
4. The response to health teaching partly results from the person's level of anxiety at the time the teaching takes place. Discuss the ways in which the anxiety level during health teaching could affect later compliance with the health care plan.
5. Discuss the relationship between the individual's need for self-control and the nursing care of a patient who is noncompliant with recommended health care activities.
6. Select one of the listed coping mechanisms, and discuss how it is used in indirect and self-destructive behavior:
   A. Regression
   B. Denial
   C. Rationalization
7. A 17-year-old has committed suicide. Describe the preventive interventions you would recommend in response, and identify target groups for intervention.

CRITICAL THINKING ACTIVITIES

1. Conduct a class debate around the statement: "There are times when suicide is a rational choice."
2. Watch a variety of television shows and identify the cultural expectations expressed for the behavior of a sick person. Identify whether these expectations are true for someone who is chronically ill.
3. On the basis of your knowledge of risk factors related to suicidal behavior, construct a profile of a high-risk individual.

RESEARCH AGENDA FOR EVIDENCE-BASED PRACTICE

The following are some of the nursing research problems raised in Chapter 20 that merit further study by psychiatric nurses:

1. The relationship between nurses' experiences with and attitudes toward death and their ability to intervene therapeutically with self-destructive patients
2. The prevalence of self-destructive behavior among children and adolescents
3. Health education approaches that enhance or inhibit the likelihood of compliance with a prescribed health care plan
4. The effectiveness of family therapy in decreasing the occurrence of future episodes of self-destructive behavior
5. The ability of primary care providers to identify suicidal thoughts and behaviors in their patients
6. Patient responses to one-on-one observation for the prevention of suicidal behavior
7. The relationship of various staffing patterns to the occurrence of episodes of self-destructive behavior in the hospital setting
8. Identification of behavioral responses to the physiologic condition of starvation
9. Comparison of the relative effectiveness of nursing interventions with self-destructive patients when the health care process is controlled by the nurse or patient or is collaborative
10. Identification of primary prevention nursing activities that decrease the incidence of self-destructive behavior in a community

21 NEUROBIOLOGICAL RESPONSES AND SCHIZOPHRENIA AND PSYCHOTIC DISORDERS

CRITICAL THINKING QUESTIONS

1. Assess one of the following categories of behavior of a patient who has schizophrenia: cognition, perception, emotion, movement and behavior, or relatedness. Discuss the neurobiological changes that could lead to the behavior you observed. Assess the impact on treatment.
2. A classmate tells you that she is puzzled about the behavior of her patient who has a diagnosis of paranoid schizophrenia. He repeatedly burns his fingers because he holds a cigarette until he is reminded to put it out. Based on your knowledge of maladaptive neurobiological responses, how might this behavior be explained? What nursing interventions would you advise?
3. Discuss alternative nursing approaches that might be taken with a patient who refuses all oral intake because he suspects he is being poisoned. Include rationale for each alternative.
4. The use of touch with a patient who has maladaptive neurobiological responses may be therapeutic or destructive. Compare and contrast a therapeutic and nontherapeutic use of touch, giving specific patient situations as examples.
5. Describe the phases of development of auditory hallucinations. Relate this process to the formulation of a nursing treatment plan for a patient who has hallucinations.
6. While making rounds on the nursing unit, you discover Ms. B cowering in a shower stall in the patients' bathroom. Her medical diagnosis is schizophrenia, paranoid type. She is trembling and does not respond when you speak her name. What nursing actions would you take? Why?
7. The parents of a paranoid patient approach you and ask detailed questions about the patient's behavior. Describe your responses to them and the reasons for your decision.
8. Your patient asks you if his children are at risk for schizophrenia. Describe the risk factors for schizophrenia.

CRITICAL THINKING ACTIVITIES

1. Select a patient who has had several acute hospital admissions for treatment of schizophrenia. Discuss the symptom triggers that this person has been able to identify. Plan with the patient for how to avoid or cope with the triggers in the future.
2. Identify several patients who have maladaptive neurobiological responses. Individually or in a small group, discuss their thoughts about the medications that they are receiving. What do they dislike about their medications? What do they describe as helpful? Do you think their knowledge is sufficient? Is it accurate?
3. Obtain information on the new atypical antipsychotic medications. Interview staff on their perceptions of the advantages and disadvantages of these drugs.
4. Attend a recovery or self-help group for people with severe mental illness. Describe how your attitude and beliefs about psychiatric illness have changed as a result of this experience.

RESEARCH AGENDA FOR EVIDENCE-BASED PRACTICE

The following are some of the nursing research problems raised in Chapter 21 that merit further study by psychiatric nurses:

1. Investigation and validation of cross-cultural nursing interventions with schizophrenic patients
2. Nonverbal cues that can serve as indicators of withdrawn patients' positive or negative response to a specific nursing intervention
3. Nursing interventions that will increase the schizophrenic person's tolerance for interpersonal closeness, including touch
4. Identification and validation of effective nursing approaches with delusional or hallucinating patients
5. Description of nursing interventions that patients remember as helpful during acute psychosis

Social Responses and Personality Disorders 22

CRITICAL THINKING QUESTIONS

1. Describe the developmental processes that lead to the capacity for healthy relatedness throughout the life cycle. Select one developmental stage, and describe the disruptions in relatedness likely to occur if the relevant developmental tasks are not accomplished.
2. The impersonal environment of an institution tends to discourage initiation of interpersonal relationships. Describe a nursing intervention that would personalize the environment and foster socialization.
3. Discuss the reasons for using caution when deciding whether to touch a patient who has maladaptive social responses.
4. Compare and contrast the attitudes toward closeness of the narcissistic person, the impulsive person, and the manipulative person.
5. Describe the actions you would take on becoming aware that a patient with a borderline personality disorder was setting up her family and the nursing staff to fight each other.
6. You discover that a 22-year-old manipulative male patient has been supplying drugs to and engaging in sexual behavior with two female patients, ages 14 and 16. Describe the actions you would take and why.
7. Compare and contrast situations in which narcissistic behaviors could be described as strengths or as weaknesses.
8. A young woman comes to the emergency room with a laceration of her right wrist. She reports that she received it when she smashed a mirror because "I hated the way my hair looked." On further assessment she reveals that she was getting ready to attend a dinner party at her husband's boss's house and didn't really want to go. Discuss this situation in terms of manipulativeness, impulsivity, and narcissism.

CRITICAL THINKING ACTIVITIES

1. Discuss your perspective on why there are more women than men with the diagnosis of borderline personality disorder. Include culture, stereotypes, and gender of the diagnostician. What can you do about this?
2. Observe staff members for times when they are inconsistent or demonstrate lack of team communication. Describe the impact this has on patient care.

RESEARCH AGENDA FOR EVIDENCE-BASED PRACTICE

The following are some of the nursing research problems raised in Chapter 22 that merit further study by psychiatric nurses:

1. Nursing interventions with children experiencing interpersonal stress that will assist them to continue to develop the capacity for relatedness
2. Determination of whether nurses recognize the need of patients to be alone, and the extent to which this is taken into account in planning nursing care at either the individual or the program level
3. Retrospective identification of the nursing interventions that recovered patients describe as having been helpful while experiencing maladaptive social responses
4. The personal space needs of individuals who have maladaptive social responses
5. Relationship between nurses' attitudes toward manipulative behavior, their own use of manipulation, and their ability to intervene effectively with manipulative patients
6. Characteristics of the therapeutic milieu that are effective in modifying manipulative, impulsive, or narcissistic behavior
7. Supportive nursing interventions with new parents who live in socially deprived settings that will assist them to foster healthy interpersonal relationships in their children
8. Supervisory skills that will assist staff to identify the potential for splitting and projective identification and enable them to prevent destructive consequences
9. School health nursing interventions that will assist teachers to recognize maladaptive social responses and to manage these behaviors in the classroom
10. Development of indicators of psychological accessibility in a nurse-patient relationship

23 COGNITIVE RESPONSES AND ORGANIC MENTAL DISORDERS

CRITICAL THINKING QUESTIONS

1. Although impaired cognitive functioning is often viewed as an irreversible condition, many impairments are the result of specific physiological stressors and may be reversed with appropriate treatment. Identify one such reversible condition, and discuss nursing interventions that would support its reversal. What primary prevention activities could decrease the incidence of the disruption that you selected?
2. You are a community health nurse working with an elderly patient who lives alone. You assess that this individual's diet is deficient in the B vitamins. The patient has complained of forgetfulness. He lives on a small, fixed income. His health is good. Describe the nursing actions you would take, and assign a priority to each action.
3. Describe nursing interventions that are feasible in an intensive care setting and would assist the patient to maintain optimum cognitive functioning.
4. Describe a specific observable behavioral manifestation of each of the following categories of cognitive dysfunction:
   A. Disorientation
   B. Impaired judgment
   C. Perceptual impairment
   D. Labile affect
   E. Loss of social inhibitions
5. Delirious patients often experience perceptual disturbances, such as illusions and hallucinations. Differentiate between an illusion and a hallucination. Describe nursing interventions for patients who have each of these perceptual disturbances.
6. Assign priorities to the following short-term nursing goals for the care of a delirious patient. Support your decision with rationale.
   A. The patient will accurately state the current month and year.
   B. The patient will maintain blood electrolyte values within normal limits.
   C. The patient and at least one significant other will describe the predisposing and precipitating stressors that caused delirium.
   D. The patient will remain in bed without the use of physical (mechanical) restraints.
7. A delirious patient screams that there are worms crawling all over his bed. Discuss your response to this patient.
8. Compare and contrast the criteria that you would use in evaluating the nursing care of (a) an elderly patient with memory loss, disorientation, and agitation related to progressive cerebral arteriosclerosis, and (b) a child with disorientation, hallucinations, and agitation related to accidental ingestion of barbiturates.
9. The daughter of your patient with Alzheimer's disease asks you to tell her what local services there are for families with AD. She also asks you to tell her what you know about the risk factors, protective factors, and genetic predisposition for AD in relationship to her and her four children. How do you respond?

CRITICAL THINKING ACTIVITIES

1. Cognition depends on adequate sensory inputs. Blindfold yourself and perform a routine activity, such as getting dressed. Discuss the effect of this sensory loss on your ability to make decisions. How would you need to modify the environment to enable you to function effectively?
2. Based on your understanding of the effects of aging on cognition, prepare a lesson plan for a health education class on the responsible use of medication to be presented at a senior center.
3. Visit a nursing home in your community. Identify aspects of the environment that may enhance or compromise cognitive functioning.

RESEARCH AGENDA FOR EVIDENCE-BASED PRACTICE

The following are some of the nursing research problems raised in Chapter 23 that merit further study by psychiatric nurses:

1. Validation of nursing interventions that result in improved cognitive functioning when impairment results from a specific etiology
2. The ability of nurses who work with elderly patients to identify changes in cognitive functioning
3. The ability of nurses who work with elderly patients to assess the presence of physiological stressors related to identified cognitive impairments
4. Primary prevention measures that are effective in decreasing the incidence of dementia

5. The effects on cognitive functioning of frequently used prescription and over-the-counter medications and of combinations of drugs
6. Specific stressors that lead to the occurrence of "intensive care unit psychosis"
7. Interpersonal approaches that are effective in alleviating the anxiety of delirious patients
8. The process of confabulation, including its development and the need it fulfills for the individual
9. Nonintrusive behavioral interventions that decrease the occurrence of behaviors such as wandering and falls by patients who have dementia
10. Environmental characteristics of institutions that interfere with effective cognitive functioning

24 CHEMICALLY MEDIATED RESPONSES AND SUBSTANCE-RELATED DISORDERS

CRITICAL THINKING QUESTIONS

1. Analyze the development of addictive behavior based on the following theories:
   A. Genetic transmission
   B. Learned behavior
   C. Family relationship patterns
   D. Personality

   How might the application of a specific theory of etiology affect intervention?
2. Compare and contrast the characteristic behaviors of patients who are psychotic as a result of ingesting LSD or PCP. Describe nursing interventions for each.
3. Discuss the way in which assertiveness training might be useful to an alcoholic patient and significant others.
4. Based on the understanding that co-dependent behavior is related to low self-esteem, what nursing interventions would you initiate to assist the spouse of a patient who abuses substances to overcome this behavioral pattern?
5. Substance abuse affects the entire family. Discuss the behaviors that you might observe in children of a substance-abusing parent at the following ages: 6 months, 2 years, 5 years, 12 years, 16 years, and 30 years.
6. Review the costs and benefits of the latest smoking cessation treatments.
7. Research the problem of inhalant use among children in this country. Identify potential ways to address this growing problem.
8. Select one type of substance abuse and an at-risk population, and formulate a primary prevention strategy targeted at that specific problem.

CRITICAL THINKING ACTIVITIES

1. Identify and describe the policies about addicted employees at the hospital or other health care agency where you are assigned. Critique the agency's program for dealing with this problem.
2. Prepare a patient education plan for presentation to a group of patients with a substance abuse problem of your choice. Be sure to include evaluation criteria.
3. Write an example of a behavioral contract that could be used as an element of nursing intervention with a patient who has a substance abuse problem of your choice.
4. Attend a meeting of a self-help group of substance abusers (e.g., Alcoholics Anonymous). Analyze the group's characteristics that are therapeutic, relating these to specific expected behaviors of the group members.

RESEARCH AGENDA FOR EVIDENCE-BASED PRACTICE

The following are some of the nursing research problems raised in Chapter 24 that merit further study by psychiatric nurses:

1. Effective strategies for sensitizing nurse administrators to the problems presented by and needs of addicted nurse employees
2. The application of knowledge about naturally induced euphoric states to the nursing care of people with addictions
3. The ability of nurses to identify the behaviors associated with withdrawal from commonly abused drugs
4. The long-term biopsychosocial effects of the therapeutic use of methadone
5. Identification and validation of nursing interventions that are effective during the acute and recovery phases of toxic psychosis resulting from hallucinogen or PCP use
6. Longitudinal study of physical and psychological development of children whose mothers used various types of drugs during pregnancy
7. Parenting behaviors of individuals who have been identified as drug abusers
8. The drug use habits of children of individuals who have received medical treatment or been arrested as a result of drug abuse (including alcohol)
9. Nursing interventions that are effective in overcoming the denial that is generally observed as a resistance to therapy by substance abusers
10. Identification and validation of substance abuse primary prevention strategies targeted toward specific groups of potential users, that is, middle-school students, homemakers, business people, and nurses

EATING REGULATION RESPONSES AND EATING DISORDERS

25

CRITICAL THINKING QUESTIONS

1. What do you believe is your ideal body weight and size? Compare it with a standardized height and weight table. Discuss any differences you discover.
2. Everyone has certain eating preferences and peculiarities. What are yours, and what is their impact on your health and your ability to be an effective nurse?
3. A friend tells you that after each test in school she treats herself to a gallon of ice cream and then purges herself. Do you think this is problematic, and what would you say to her, if anything?
4. You notice that another friend has not eaten a full meal in over 2 weeks. She tells you that she is dieting to fit into new jeans she bought. Do you think this is problematic and what would you say to her, if anything?
5. Some obese individuals believe that they are discriminated against by society because of their weight. Do you believe this is true? Defend your position.
6. Discuss ways in which the media contribute to women's dominant focus on their bodies. Compare this to that of men.
7. You are working with a young woman with anorexia nervosa on an outpatient basis. She has formed a contract with you related to the treatment process. Today, during your meeting, she tells you that she has broken the contract for the third time in 4 months. What are your treatment options, and what factors would influence your clinical decision making?
8. Identify cues to your own eating responses. Describe your thoughts, feelings and assumptions, eating regulation responses, and consequences for each one.
9. You are meeting with the parents of a patient with anorexia nervosa. They are extremely upset and ask if their daughter can die from her illness. How would you respond?
10. Eating disorders are frequently secretive diseases. What "clues" might you suggest that parents look for to detect the presence of an eating problem?

CRITICAL THINKING ACTIVITIES

1. Review the literature on addictive behavior and eating disorders. Note areas of overlap and divergence. Do the same comparing depression and eating disorders.
2. Ask a patient with anorexia to draw a picture of herself. Take a photograph of her and talk about what these images reveal.
3. Develop materials that can be used to educate patients and families regarding nutrition, eating patterns, and healthy behavior. Share them with nursing staff.

RESEARCH AGENDA FOR EVIDENCE-BASED PRACTICE

The following are some of the nursing research problems raised in Chapter 25 that merit further study by psychiatric nurses:

1. The incidence and prevalence of eating disorders in the nonfemale, nonwhite population
2. Degree to which nurses routinely assess for bulimia and anorexia nervosa across age groups and specialty areas
3. Early predictors for the development of eating disorders among young women
4. Biological models that explain the etiology of eating disorders
5. The interaction among environmental stressors, psychological predisposition, and biologic vulnerability in the development of eating disorders
6. Comparison of the clinical outcomes related to the treatment of anorexia nervosa in inpatient and outpatient settings
7. Specification of protocols describing nutritional stabilization strategies when working with patients with anorexia nervosa
8. Degree to which psychiatric nurses use cognitive behavioral interventions in treating patients with eating disorders
9. Description of specific body image interventions used with eating disorders and related outcomes
10. Therapeutic and psychoeducational approaches that have been demonstrated to be effective in working with families of patients

26 Sexual Responses and Sexual Disorders

CRITICAL THINKING QUESTIONS

1. Discuss how you would define "normal" sexual behavior.
2. Analyze factors that may contribute to a nurse having difficulty providing sexual health care to patients.
3. Identify precipitation stressors that may alter expressions of sexuality.
4. Several of your colleagues are discussing a new patient admitted to your unit for sex reassignment surgery. They repeatedly refer to this patient as homosexual. How would you clarify their conception?
5. Kinsey developed a seven-point rating scale to classify individuals in terms of sexual preference. Do you agree with his theory that many people are not exclusively heterosexual or exclusively homosexual? Support your opinion.
6. Before the work of Masters and Johnson, most people who experienced sexual dysfunction were referred to psychiatrists because they were believed to be severely emotionally disturbed. Does that feeling still exist today? What are your feelings about patients with dysfunctions of the sexual response cycle?
7. Identify and discuss the four phases of the nurse's growth process in developing self-awareness. Give an example of this growth process from your own experience.
8. If a sexual issue were brought up in a clinical conference, would you feel comfortable expressing your feelings and thoughts? Would you be concerned about what other members of the group were thinking about you?
9. Discuss the myth-fact table (Table 26-2) in the text. Identify one myth that you have had difficulty giving up.
10. Discuss the ineffective nursing behaviors that can result when nurses fail to resolve the anxiety phase of the growth process toward self-awareness.
11. Frequently in nursing care plans you will see the directive, "Adopt a nonjudgmental attitude." Why is this directive inadequate?
12. If an attractive patient that you have been taking care of asked you for a date, how would you respond?
13. While you are bathing a patient, he reaches up and grabs your breast. How would you respond?
14. Discuss the impact that pedophilia by priests has had on the Catholic church.

CRITICAL THINKING ACTIVITIES

1. One of the responsibilities of the nurse is referring patients for appropriate help when their concerns are beyond the scope of your practice. Identify some of the health services available in your community for individuals with sexual concerns. Where would you refer a patient who is:
   A. Requesting sex reassignment surgery?
   B. A victim of incest?
   C. A rape victim?
   D. Experiencing sexual identity confusion?
   E. Experiencing an arousal disorder?
2. Role-play the following situations:
   A. A nurse making rounds on the night shift discovers an adolescent patient masturbating.
   B. A patient reveals to the nurse that she is upset because her homosexual lover has left her.
   C. During a family meeting, a 12-year-old girl reluctantly shares that she has been upset because an uncle has made sexual advances while babysitting with her (family members present are the parents, the 12-year-old, and a 14-year-old brother). A nurse is the group leader.

   After each role-play session, discuss in a small group the feelings evoked by the situation and the nurse's response to the situation, including suggestions for alternative approaches.

RESEARCH AGENDA FOR EVIDENCE-BASED PRACTICE

The following are some of the nursing research problems raised in Chapter 26 that merit further study by psychiatric nurses:

1. The specific nursing behaviors that promote or inhibit the expression of sexual concerns by patients
2. The effectiveness of nursing interventions in the sexual acting-out behaviors of patients
3. The validity of various sexual assessment tools in sexual history taking

4. The effects of nurses' feelings, attitudes, and values on therapeutic interventions with patients with sexual concerns
5. The ability of psychiatric nurses to diagnose maladaptive sexual responses in physical and emotional illness
6. The long-term effect of alcohol abuse on male and female sexual functioning
7. The relationship between levels of self-esteem and adaptive sexual behavior
8. Effective strategies for sensitizing nurses to the sexual needs of the institutionalized elderly
9. The impact of HIV/AIDS and STDs on sexual behavior of psychiatric patients
10. Nursing interventions related to sexual side effects of patients taking psychiatric medications

27 PSYCHOPHARMACOLOGY

CRITICAL THINKING QUESTIONS

1. A paranoid patient refuses to take his prescribed chlorpromazine, 100 mg PO. Outline your approach to this patient, and describe the alternatives.
2. Describe the precautions that you would take when giving oral medication to a seriously suicidal patient.
3. Identify and describe each of the four types of extrapyramidal effects that may result from the use of antipsychotic medications. Include treatment and nursing implications.
4. Discuss the elements of a premedication patient workup.
5. The following two patients have been admitted to your ward: Ms. J, a 63-year-old woman with depression, and Mr. S, a 24-year-old man with schizophrenia. They are in relapse and admit that they were noncompliant with their outpatient medication regimens. Discuss the possible reasons for their nonadherence from the perspective of each patient, and suggest problem-solving approaches for their discharge care plans.
6. Describe the application of group theory to the education of psychiatric patients about their medications. Identify the advantages and disadvantages of a group approach.
7. Controversy surrounds the administration of psychotropic medications to children. State your position on this issue, and support with rationale.
8. Discuss the ways in which the long-term use of typical antipsychotic medication may contribute to the development of behaviors associated with chronic mental illness. Would the atypicals make a difference? How?
9. Analyze the special considerations that apply to the administration of psychotropic medications to elderly patients. How would you alter your nursing actions to respond to the special needs of these patients?
10. Why does an understanding of neurotransmission and central nervous system drug effects have an impact on patient education, choice of drug, and nursing care planning?
11. Discuss the ethics of withholding psychiatric medications from patients diagnosed with a severe mental illness.
12. A patient with a past history of substance abuse requests a benzodiazepine PRN until the antidepressant prescribed for his social phobia begins to work. What would you tell this patient?

CRITICAL THINKING ACTIVITIES

1. Design a patient education plan for each of the following drugs:
   A. Venlafaxine
   B. Lithium
   C. Alprazolam
   D. Imipramine
   E. Fluoxetine
   F. Phenelzine
   G. Depakote
   H. Clozaril

   Include dosages, possible routes of administration, dosing schedule, side effects and treatment profiles, blood levels if appropriate, short- and long-term considerations, and drug alternatives.
2. Hold a class debate on the following statement: "Psychotropic drugs are biochemical replacements. With the right drug for the right patient, pharmacotherapy alone will be sufficient treatment in the future." Include its potential impact on the following: (a) therapeutic alliance, (b) holistic care, (c) nursing practice, (d) research directions, (e) health care costs, and (f) nurses' role in the future mental health system.
3. Find out the cost of treatment for depression with traditional tricyclic medication compared to the SSRIs. Then do a literature review on current cost-effectiveness studies on treatment for depression. Report your findings to your class.

RESEARCH AGENDA FOR EVIDENCE-BASED PRACTICE

The following are some of the nursing research problems raised in Chapter 27 that merit further study by psychiatric nurses:

1. Identification of people at risk for particular side effects and adverse reactions to psychopharmacological drugs
2. Predictors of factors related to patient nonadherence with medication treatment regimens

3. Effective nursing interventions that maximize patient adherence with medication treatment regimens
4. Nonpharmacological interventions that enhance drug effectiveness and treat residual target symptoms
5. Development of behavioral rating scales that are specific in assessing nursing care effectiveness in the psychopharmacological treatment of mental disorders
6. Outcomes associated with the nurse's role in the long-term psychiatric treatment of patients on drug maintenance regimens
7. Patient education strategies associated with drug therapy effectiveness, compliance, and safety
8. Ways to maximize nurse-patient collaboration in medication treatment regimens and related outcomes
9. Evaluation of the effectiveness of involving the patient's social support system in short-term and long-term medication regimens
10. Knowledge level of nurses of the biological basis, mechanisms of action, clinical uses, and adverse effects of psychopharmacological drugs and its correlation with the effectiveness of nursing care

28 Somatic Therapies

CRITICAL THINKING QUESTIONS

1. How does the nursing care given to patients undergoing ECT compare with those of other brief surgical procedures?
2. A patient who is to receive ECT tells you that he is worried that he will suffer permanent brain damage. How would you respond?
3. What biological, psychological, and environmental nursing measures post-ECT might enhance the patient's recovery?
4. If phototherapy is an effective somatic treatment, why do people who live in warm, sunny climates also experience seasonal affective disorder?
5. How does the cost of a light box ($180 to $500) compare with the cost of other treatment options for depression?
6. Little is known about the precise relationship between sleep and illness. Describe the impact that lack of sleep has on your physical and psychological health and well-being. What changes do you observe when you are sleep deprived? How do these compare when your sleep is disturbed or your usual sleep patterns are disrupted? How might your experiences generalize to patients?
7. How might the new somatic therapies of transcranial magnetic stimulation and vagal nerve stimulation advance our understanding of the etiology of various psychiatric illnesses?

CRITICAL THINKING ACTIVITIES

1. Poll your nursing colleagues about their knowledge of ECT as a contemporary somatic treatment. Do you think their responses reflect those of the general public?
2. You are the primary nurse for Ms. W, a 58-year-old woman who has consented to treatment with ECT. During visiting hours her husband and two grown daughters ask you for information about ECT. The only information they have was acquired from watching *One Flew Over the Cuckoo's Nest*, so they are unaware of modern treatment practices. Formulate a teaching plan to provide Ms. W's relatives with information about ECT.
3. Before observing ECT, record your expectations, including anticipated feelings. Following your observational experience, compare the real events and feelings with those anticipated. Compare reactions with those of other students.
4. Design an inservice presentation for nursing staff related to ECT. Include indications, mechanism of action, adverse effects, and nursing care.

RESEARCH AGENDA FOR EVIDENCE-BASED PRACTICE

The following are some of the nursing research problems raised in Chapter 28 that merit further study by psychiatric nurses:

1. Nurses' awareness of the legal and ethical issues related to the use of somatic therapies
2. Nurses' perceptions of the effectiveness of ECT
3. Information about ECT that is helpful to patients and families who are deciding whether to agree to this treatment
4. Identification of patterns of cognitive responses to ECT and pretreatment predictors of cognitive responses
5. Predictors of the occurrence of agitation during the early ECT and pretreatment predictors of cognitive responses
6. Geriatric nurses' knowledge of the indications for and outcomes associated with ECT for depressed elderly patients
7. Implementation of the informed consent process with ECT patients
8. The short- and long-term effectiveness of phototherapy
9. The mechanism of action for vagal nerve stimulation
10. The relationship between sleep patterns and emotional responsiveness

29 Complementary and Alternative Therapies

CRITICAL THINKING QUESTIONS

1. Why are there relatively few scientific studies of CAM in patients with psychiatric illnesses? What strategies could be used to overcome this problem?
2. Analyze the reasons why it is dangerous for patients not to let their primary health care provider know whether or not they are using CAM.
3. Why is it difficult to conduct a double-blind study using acupuncture?
4. Describe the physiology and neurobiology that may account for the antidepressant effect of exercise.
5. Why might the intervention of therapeutic touch be distressing to psychotic patients?

CRITICAL THINKING ACTIVITIES

1. Examine the nursing assessment form you use. Does it ask patients about their use of complementary and alternative therapies? If not, how would you revise it?
2. Look in your local phone book and find the range of complementary and alternative therapies offered in your community.
3. Begin asking the patients you care for whether or not they use alternative therapies. Keep a tally of the numbers of patients who answer yes and the therapies they use.
4. Review the conditions for which acupuncture has been used over the centuries. Which of these is supported by current research?
5. Review the physiological changes that have been associated with therapeutic touch. What implications do they have for psychiatric patients?
6. Join a yoga class and describe your own physiological and psychological response to it.

RESEARCH AGENDA FOR EVIDENCE-BASED PRACTICE

The following are some of the nursing research problems raised in Chapter 29 that merit further study by psychiatric nurses:

1. The extent to which psychiatric nurses endorse and/or practice complementary and alternative therapies
2. Ways in which nurses who use CAM evaluate the efficacy of their interventions
3. Specific ethical issues posed by the use of CAM and how they are resolved
4. The types of research designs most frequently and least frequently used in the study of alternative therapies in general and in the research conducted by nurses
5. The efficacy of herbal products versus the SSRIs in treating depression
6. Ways in which relaxation can enhance other conventional interventions in the treatment of anxiety
7. The efficacy of acupuncture in treating addictive disorders such as gambling and smoking
8. Ways in which CAM can enhance hospital-based treatment programs
9. Biases nurses hold for and against CAM and ways this affects their care
10. Nurses' knowledge of potential side effects and drug interactions of herbal products and other medical treatments

30 Preventing and Managing Aggressive Behavior

CRITICAL THINKING QUESTIONS

1. Discuss your reaction to the statement, "When anger is accompanied by a clear communication, it is a sign of basic respect for a loved person."
2. Identify and describe positive functions of anger. Include examples.
3. You observe that another member of the nursing staff is using unnecessary roughness when turning an elderly debilitated patient. What action would you take in this situation? Would you behave differently if the other staff member was observed hitting the patient?
4. Existential therapists emphasize the individual's responsibility for his or her behavior. Could an existentialist accept the theory that aggression is biologically determined? Support your position.
5. Personal space in an institutional setting may be limited, leading to outbursts of aggression. Recommend nursing interventions that could alleviate this problem.
6. You are late for an appointment and are waiting in line at the supermarket when another shopper approaches you and says, "I just have a few items and I'm in a hurry. You wouldn't mind if I went ahead of you, would you?" Describe the response that you would usually make to this person. Classify it as passive, assertive, or aggressive. Describe responses that represent the other two categories.
7. Discuss the relationship between passive, assertive, and aggressive behaviors and recognition of the rights and responsibilities of oneself and others.
8. Define passive-aggressive behavior, and give an example.
9. Describe the body language associated with passive, aggressive, and assertive behavior.
10. Compare and contrast the levels of self-esteem expected in individuals who respond to anger passively and those who respond aggressively.
11. You are alone in an office with a patient who is showing signs of agitation. This person has a history of violent behavior. Describe and provide rationale for the steps you would take at this point.
12. A nurse's aide informs you that one of the patients on your unit is standing on a chair and threatening to attack anyone who comes near him. Discuss your steps to intervene in this situation and your criteria to evaluate your intervention.
13. There are several reasons for the use of restraints. Select one of these; discuss alternative approaches to the selected situation that might avoid the need for restraint.
14. It has been stated that physical restraint is the most therapeutic intervention in selected circumstances. Do you agree or disagree with this statement? Provide rationale to justify your position.
15. A patient on your nursing unit has just been placed in wrist and ankle restraints because he is experiencing alcohol withdrawal delirium. Formulate the section of the nursing care plan relative to the nursing care needs resulting from the use of these restraints.
16. Discuss the legal issues related to the use of seclusion with regard to "treatment in the least restrictive setting."
17. Outline the key points to be considered in providing nursing care to a patient in seclusion. Begin with the decision that seclusion is necessary, and end with the decision to terminate seclusion.
18. Provide clinical examples for the use of seclusion as (a) containment, (b) isolation, and (c) reduction of stimuli.

CRITICAL THINKING ACTIVITIES

1. Under faculty supervision, allow a small group of students to experience the various types of mechanical restraint. Follow with a discussion of feelings related to the experience of being restrained.
2. Select a personal behavior related to the expression of anger that you would like to change. Formulate a long-term goal, and develop a hierarchy of related short-term goals that will lead to the desired behavioral change.
3. Select a situation in which you would like to be more assertive. Describe the steps you would take to train yourself to be more assertive.

RESEARCH AGENDA FOR EVIDENCE-BASED PRACTICE

The following are some of the nursing research problems raised in Chapter 30 that merit further study by psychiatric nurses:

1. Nursing interventions that are effective alternatives to the use of seclusion or restraints

2. The relationship between nurse attitudes about the use of restraints and the effective use of this therapeutic intervention
3. Indicator behaviors that can be used as a guide for terminating the use of seclusion or restraints
4. The impact of reduced length of stay and stricter hospitalization criteria on the level of aggressive behavior by patients in the inpatient, day treatment, and home settings
5. The occurrence of aggressive responses related to the amount of personal space allotted to the individual
6. The relationship between intrastaff conflict and the incidence of aggressive behavior by patients
7. The effectiveness of limit-setting interventions by nurses in response to selected aggressive behaviors
8. The relationship between a nurse's comfort with assertive behavior and one's effectiveness in setting limits with patients
9. Interventions with aggressive patients that minimize the risk of injury to the patient and the involved staff members
10. Strategies to assist staff members to recover after having been assaulted by a patient

31 Cognitive Behavioral Treatment Strategies

CRITICAL THINKING QUESTIONS

1. In an intensive care unit, a patient's spouse interrupts life-support nursing care at least seven times per shift. Develop a plan of care for this problem using principles of cognitive behavioral therapy.
2. Define concerns that must be considered when one is planning a reinforcement schedule.
3. You observe that the treatment plan meeting for a psychiatric patient focuses primarily on strategies for the patient's delusions and hallucinations. What concerns from a cognitive behavioral perspective would you have about the treatment being given?
4. An acutely suicidal patient is receiving constant one-to-one care. A team member objects, stating that this level of care is reinforcing the patient's suicidal behaviors. Provide a behaviorally sound response to this concern.
5. Identify an ethical dilemma that arises from the application of behavior therapy principles.
6. Contrast nursing interventions in anxiety on the basis of behavioral and cognitive conceptual models.
7. Identify cognitive therapy interventions that can be used with depressed patients.
8. How does a cognitive behavioral assessment compare and contrast with a nursing assessment?

CRITICAL THINKING ACTIVITIES

1. Teach a friend relaxation training and then implement this intervention with a patient.
2. Ask a patient with whom you are working to complete a daily record of dysfunctional thoughts. Work with the patient to distinguish between thoughts and feelings and to identify adaptive responses that would be alternatives to the current situation.
3. Develop a health education plan using principles of cognitive behavioral therapy for a patient you have been working with in the clinical setting.

RESEARCH AGENDA FOR EVIDENCE-BASED PRACTICE

The following are some of the nursing research problems raised in Chapter 31 that merit further study by psychiatric nurses:

1. The degree to which cognitive and behavioral principles are taught in nursing programs
2. The use of cognitive behavioral interventions by nurses in various health care settings
3. Treatment outcomes associated with behaviorally oriented psychiatric milieus compared with psychodynamically oriented milieus
4. The effectiveness of patient determined reinforcers versus staff-determined reinforcers
5. Clinical outcomes associated with teaching patient cognitive and behavioral principles
6. Reinforcers that staff inadvertently provide for maladaptive coping responses by patients
7. Effects of nurse-monitored, but patient-initiated and patient-implemented cognitive behavioral therapies
8. Cognitive and behavioral strategies that are incorporated in parent effectiveness training programs
9. The stage of treatment (crisis, acute, maintenance, or health promotion) in which anxiety reduction strategies are most useful to patients
10. The extent to which nurses use modeling, shaping, role playing, and social skills training with patients and the outcomes associated with each

Therapeutic Groups 32

CRITICAL THINKING QUESTIONS

1. Based on your understanding of group dynamics and group process, describe two patient situations in which group intervention is likely to be more effective than an individual approach.
2. Compare and contrast the characteristics of a task group and peer support group.
3. Compare and contrast leadership behaviors observed in two different types of groups, e.g., a staff team meeting and a patient-staff community meeting.
4. Some say that group therapy is less effective than individual therapy because each member of the group has to share the therapist's attention. Do you agree or disagree with this statement? Give the rationale for your position.
5. Think about all of the clinical areas in which you have had experience as a nursing student. Identify an opportunity for the development of a nursing group related to each area.

CRITICAL THINKING ACTIVITIES

1. Obtain permission to observe an ongoing therapy group. If this cannot be arranged in a way that is not disruptive to the group, view a videotape of a group therapy session. Identify the developmental stage of the group, using examples of group interaction to support your conclusion.
2. Observe an informal patient-staff group interaction. List all of Yalom's curative factors that you can identify during this experience.
3. Observe a task-oriented group. Identify and describe the primary group role taken by each member. Did each member facilitate or obstruct the group process?
4. Develop a plan for a group. Define a purpose and group goals, describe membership criteria, identify an appropriate setting, develop interview questions for prospective members, and formulate evaluation criteria.

RESEARCH AGENDA FOR EVIDENCE-BASED PRACTICE

The following are some of the nursing research problems raised in Chapter 32 that merit further study by psychiatric nurses:

1. Comparison of the relative effectiveness of multifamily groups and traditional family therapy
2. Comparison of the effectiveness and comfort of nurses who are co-leading groups with other nurses as opposed to with colleagues from other disciplines
3. Effect on length of hospital stay of inpatient participation in group counseling sessions led by consultation liaison psychiatric nurses
4. Cost effectiveness of group counseling or group therapy as a nursing intervention
5. Effectiveness of groups for medical patients (e.g., post–myocardial infarction patients in coping with disease process and its implications)
6. Identification of the relative effectiveness of various approaches of the supervision of training groups (e.g., direct observation, videotaping, audiotaping, or review of written notes)
7. Utilization of groups for staff team building, skill acquisition, and support
8. Effectiveness of patient/family peer support groups
9. Measurement of the group leadership skills of nurses who are in middle management positions
10. Effects of cross-cultural differences on nurse therapist/group interaction

33 FAMILY INTERVENTIONS

CRITICAL THINKING QUESTIONS

1. Summarize the major differences between functional and dysfunctional families.
2. Describe how the pathology paradigm may serve to stigmatize and alienate families. Compare it to the competence or empowerment paradigm of family work.
3. Review the indications for family therapy described in the chapter. Would any of them apply to you or your family?
4. A 20-year-old woman comes to a mental health center depressed (though not psychotic or suicidal) almost 3 weeks after the complicated delivery of her first baby. Her husband of 1 year is about to return to work after a 2-week leave that he spent at home helping her when she and the baby came home. She wants to move back with her family, who live only a mile away, at least until the baby seems stronger. "He seems too frail and helpless," she says. What theoretical concepts seem most relevant in guiding the nurse therapist's initial understanding and interventions?
5. A wife complains to her husband's nurse that since the husband's heart attack 6 months ago, her husband has become depressed. He has not complied with the dietary and exercise regimen prescribed, saying, "What's the use? I'm going to die from my next heart attack." The wife tearfully proclaims she has tried every way she knows to cheer him up and to force him to eat and exercise properly, but he angrily rejects her efforts. In fact, he seems worse. How might the nurse intervene with the wife for the cardiac patient?
6. A 39-year-old divorced woman who has had sole custody of her four children for 2 years comes to the mental health center because her 12-year-old daughter is depressed. Her oldest daughter, 14 years old, is in charge of the three younger siblings, aged 12, 10, and 6. The mother gets home at 7 PM and is told by her eldest about misbehavior of the children and other problems. If there are major problems, her oldest knows she can tell her grandmother, who lives two blocks away, but the mother hates for her daughter to do this because the grandmother has a bad heart and tends to get "too upset." What problems confront the nurse therapist? How does the nurse therapist restructure this single-parent family within the financial realities of such a household? What are the generational subsystem and power hierarchy considerations?

CRITICAL THINKING ACTIVITIES

1. Design a psychoeducational program for the family of a patient with bipolar illness.
2. Describe how the nuclear family, extended family, and household may differ for gays, immigrants, interracial couples, and step families.

RESEARCH AGENDA FOR EVIDENCE-BASED PRACTICE

The following are some of the nursing research problems raised in Chapter 33 that merit further study by psychiatric nurses:

1. Nature and outcomes associated with family psychoeducational programs conducted by nurses
2. The degree to which psychiatric nurses use the competence-empowerment paradigm in working with families
3. Comparison of the effectiveness of individual family therapy versus multiple family therapy with a specified presenting problem
4. Comparison of nurse-run multiple family therapy groups to non–nurse-run groups, measuring comparable effectiveness and cost
5. The effectiveness of doing therapy with the single-generation sibling group when the parental dyad or single parent refuses to participate in the target child's treatment
6. Outcomes associated with creating a ritual with a family suffering unresolved grief from loss through death, miscarriage, or abortion, to promote freer affect or grieving
7. The effect of nurse-run multiple-family support groups for families suffering from chronic medical illness on measures of quality of life and family coping
8. Outcomes of a group composed of nursing staff and family caregivers (of chronically medically ill family members) on the quality of care and use of services of respite care in a hospital or nursing home setting
9. Family outcome measures most commonly used by nurse family therapists
10. Extent to which family interventions are currently provided in schools throughout the United States

HOSPITAL-BASED PSYCHIATRIC NURSING CARE 34

CRITICAL THINKING QUESTIONS

1. What influence have historical developments in inpatient psychiatric nursing had on current practice?
2. Discuss the relationship between the nursing process and the practice of inpatient psychiatric nursing.
3. What do you predict will be the average length of stay of patients in psychiatric hospitals 2 years, 5 years, and 10 years from today? What impact will this have on inpatient psychiatric nursing care?
4. Compare the patients admitted to your unit based on the current indications for inpatient hospital use. Do they meet the criteria? If not, why were they admitted to the hospital for treatment and could they have been treated in a different setting?
5. Do you believe that the principles of Maxwell Jones' therapeutic community still have value in today's psychiatric hospitals? Defend your answer.
6. Describe how the five functional components of the therapeutic milieu as defined by Gunderson can also be implemented in a community setting.
7. Discuss some of the difficulties experienced in inpatient psychiatric nursing related to nursing autonomy and professional identity.
8. Distinguish between the independent and dependent functions of the inpatient psychiatric nurse.
9. Compare Delaney's Four S Model with Gunderson's components of the therapeutic milieu. What are the unique features of each?
10. On the basis of your readings, describe and discuss one future change that you would predict related to hospital-based psychiatric nursing practice.

CRITICAL THINKING ACTIVITIES

1. Ask the head nurse or nurse manager of an inpatient unit how nursing staff assignments are made each day. Analyze this on the basis of staff education and experience as well as patient acuity.
2. Design and implement a therapeutic group or program for psychiatric inpatients or their families. Include ways in which you will measure whether or not the intervention was successful.
3. Critique the discharge process used in your clinical setting.

RESEARCH AGENDA FOR EVIDENCE-BASED PRACTICE

The following are some of the nursing research problems raised in Chapter 34 that merit further study by psychiatric nurses:

1. Clinical, functional, perceptual, and financial outcomes that are associated with inpatient psychiatric nursing interventions
2. Evaluation of the Masters-prepared nurse's role in inpatient settings
3. The nature and extent of nursing involvement in implementing and ensuring professional and regulatory standards
4. The effectiveness of nurse-led transitional groups, the goal of which is to keep patients out of the hospital
5. The degree to which the five functional components of the therapeutic milieu as described by Gunderson are implemented by nurses in inpatient settings
6. Outcomes related to implementing the therapeutic elements of the milieu in the inpatient setting
7. The nature and extent of nursing involvement in the discharge planning process in the various hospital-based settings
8. Types of hospital-based groups conducted by nurses and the impact they have on patients and families
9. The outcomes associated with implementing Delaney's Four S model of inpatient nursing care
10. Strategies to increase nursing satisfaction and quality of care provided in state mental hospitals

35 Community-Based Psychiatric Nursing Care

CRITICAL THINKING QUESTIONS

1. Trace the historical development of community mental health.
2. Evaluate whether governmental involvement in community mental health has helped or hindered the achievement of its goals.
3. Determine how your community is attempting to meet the needs of the homeless mentally ill.
4. Design a prevention and wellness program that targets a population at risk for developing mental illness.
5. Analyze whether managed care has increased or decreased services to the mentally ill in your community.
6. Compare psychiatric home nursing with the early role of public health nurses in terms of activities, scope of practice, and autonomy.
7. Do you think that the slow development of psychiatric home care is related to the stigma that is associated with psychiatric illness?
8. One of your colleagues tells you that she would never visit the home of someone who is mentally ill because "those kinds of people do violent and crazy things." How would you respond?
9. You are visiting a patient during your community health experience, and you realize that he would benefit from psychiatric home care. Detail the steps you would take with the patient, agency, and other health care providers to implement this intervention.
10. Do you think that a suicidal patient can ever be cared for in the home without hospitalization? Defend your position based on the issues of safety, treatment options, compassion, and costs.
11. Review Box 35-8. Are there other conditions that might also make a patient homebound and therefore eligible for psychiatric home care?
12. How does case management by a psychiatric nurse differ in an inpatient setting, outpatient setting, and home setting?
13. Identify three boundary issues that you think may arise in the home setting and therapeutic ways in which you could handle each one.

CRITICAL THINKING ACTIVITIES

1. Hold a class debate on whether nurses are better suited to the role of case manager than are other mental health providers.
2. Devise a format for completing a community assessment using a systems approach to problem identification and care provision.
3. Using the format from above, select a community and gather sufficient data to complete a community assessment. Identify three community mental health problems and, using existing resources, plan a method to intervene in each problem.
4. Using a case management approach, critique the discharge planning process of a local state psychiatric facility. Compare it with that of a private psychiatric facility.
5. Spend a day with a psychiatric home care nurse, and evaluate whether this role is one that you would like to pursue in your own nursing career.
6. Obtain a copy of your own or your family's health insurance policy. Check to see if home care is reimbursed. Determine if this includes psychiatric home care. If it is not included, write a letter to the company addressing this issue.
7. Write your local NAMI chapter and ask if they have an official position on reimbursement for psychiatric home care.
8. Call the home care agencies in your community and find out if they provide psychiatric home care. If not, ask them about this omission.

RESEARCH AGENDA FOR EVIDENCE-BASED PRACTICE

The following are some of the nursing research problems raised in Chapter 35 that merit further study by psychiatric nurses:

1. Exploration of factors present in successful community mental health outreach programs
2. The roles and functions of nurses in community-based psychiatric care
3. Systematic analysis of the various types and preparations of ace managers related to efficiency, effectiveness, and cost
4. Predictor variables for patients who do not receive follow-up and do not benefit from community psychiatric care

5. Development of a valid and reliable evaluation method for psychiatric home care
6. Models of successful nurse-physician collaborative practices in community psychiatric care
7. The cost-effectiveness of psychiatric home care
8. Quality-of-life outcomes reported by patient and families who receive psychiatric home care
9. Areas of conflict and complementarity among mental health providers
10. The needs and interventions provided patients in forensic psychiatric settings

36 CHILD PSYCHIATRIC NURSING

CRITICAL THINKING QUESTIONS

1. You are assessing the nursing needs of an 8-year-old girl. She adamantly refuses to use play materials and asks to be returned to her mother. What would you do?
2. Describe the behaviors of a child with deficits in ego competency skills.
3. A 7-year-old boy sleeps with his mother since her separation from the father. Is this normal or harmful to the child's development? Defend your answer.
4. In planning a child's nursing care, what are the nurse's responsibilities with administering psychotropic medications?
5. A parent complains that "talking doesn't work with our children." What advice might the nurse offer?
6. A child greets you at each shift change with the comment, "Oh no! Not you again!" What meaning might her message have? How would you best respond?
7. A 10-year-old boy in an acute care setting is confronted by his peer for stealing. As you see him become anxious and frightened, what ego supportive technique might be indicated?
8. A mother reports that her child is not able to get to bed without a struggle. He dawdles with his bedtime routine and repeatedly gets out of bed. What interventions could be used to handle this problem?
9. What is the goal of setting limits on the behavior of children?
10. What might be included in a child's care plan for facilitating a successful termination from a partial hospitalization program?
11. How would you evaluate the success of a child's treatment program?
12. List the benefits of therapeutic home visits.
13. What concerns might arise when medicating child psychiatric patients with psychotropic drugs?
14. How can you help parents use play time with their children to promote the building of ego competency skills?
15. There is a shortage of child psychiatric nurses. Why do you think that is, and what can be done about it?
16. Children are underserved in this country. Discuss reasons for this and potential solutions.

CRITICAL THINKING ACTIVITIES

1. Spend a day in a psychiatric treatment setting for children. Share your observations and impressions with your class.
2. Determine what mental health services are available to children in your community. Compare these to the types and amount of resources available to mentally ill adults.
3. Hold a class debate regarding the nature versus nurture etiology of psychiatric illness in children.

RESEARCH AGENDA FOR EVIDENCE-BASED PRACTICE

The following are some of the nursing research problems raised in Chapter 36 that merit further study by psychiatric nurses:

1. The number, settings, and scope of practice of child psychiatric nurses throughout the United States
2. Curative factors of the milieu of child psychiatric inpatients
3. Attitude change of parents toward their child following psychiatric nursing intervention
4. Methods for establishing relationships with children who have difficulty trusting adults
5. Prospective studies of child patients to identify factors associated with the development of adult psychiatric disorders
6. Retrospective studies of the childhood environment of adults with psychiatric disorders
7. The use of PRN medication for behavioral management of children
8. Frequency and type of family interventions provided by child psychiatric nurses
9. The effect of seclusion on child psychiatric patients
10. The nature and extent of community-based child psychiatric nursing interventions

ADOLESCENT PSYCHIATRIC NURSING 37

CRITICAL THINKING QUESTIONS

1. Compare the different theoretical views on adolescence and describe their relevancy to adolescents in today's world.
2. Describe adolescence as a developmental task. Explain it as the second stage of individualization.
3. Discuss treatment strategies and their indications for use with the adolescent. Describe how these treatments differ from those for the adult.
4. Analyze the different stages in the individual treatment of the adolescent.
5. Choose two maladaptive responses seen in adolescents, and describe the possible underlying causes.
6. List and discuss special considerations in talking to an adolescent.
7. Describe in detail how one evaluates a suicidal adolescent. Identify a course of action.
8. Using your own personal experiences, describe an area of conflict for the adolescent. Include possible actions by others that may help. How can personal experience help or hinder the nurse's ability to help the adolescent?
9. Select one adolescent disorder that interests you. Review the literature on it, and describe appropriate nursing actions.
10. You observe another member of the nursing staff overidentifying with an adolescent patient on the unit. What action would you take in this situation?
11. Choose a theorist's position on defining and describing adolescence. Defend its validity using references from the literature.
12. After making a serious suicidal attempt, an adolescent is admitted to the psychiatric unit where you are a staff nurse. Describe the nursing actions you would take with this patient.

CRITICAL THINKING ACTIVITIES

1. Watch a movie or read a novel that depicts an adolescent's struggle. What are the main issues? How are they resolved?
2. Poll a group of adolescents about their primary worries, sources of gratification, and future goals. Analyze their answers based on the sociocultural factors identified in Chapter 8 of this text.
3. Create a case study to show the use of the nursing process with an adolescent including assessment, diagnosis, care plan, treatment strategy, and rationale.

RESEARCH AGENDA FOR EVIDENCE-BASED PRACTICE

The following are some of the nursing research problems raised in Chapter 37 that merit further study by psychiatric nurses:

1. The relationship between coping skills in early life and later adolescent adjustment
2. The implications of new and blurred sexual roles for adolescent development
3. Evidence of an extended adolescence as a result of prolonged economic dependence
4. Indicators of increased depression associated with body image in girls during middle adolescence as compared with older adolescents
5. The effect of the AIDS epidemic on sexual exploration in adolescence
6. Exploration of the relationships between depressed and conduct-disordered adolescents and problems with moral and superego development
7. Effective nursing actions for dealing with resistance and negative transference in treatment of the adolescent
8. The effectiveness of limit-setting interventions by nurses in response to selected acting-out behavior in adolescents
9. The relationship between a nurse's comfort with assertive behavior and her effectiveness in setting limits with adolescents
10. The effect of the nurse's own adolescent experiences in creating countertransference problems when working with adolescents

38 Geropsychiatric Nursing

CRITICAL THINKING QUESTIONS

1. What examples can you give for stress being a positive force in aging; a negative force?
2. What implications for nursing does the activity theory of psychosocial aging have in relation to: (a) assessment of older adults and (b) planning nursing interventions?
3. What are some of the positive implications of the life review?
4. What are some limitations of Erikson's stage of ego integrity in explaining the behavior of older adults?
5. You are conducting an admission interview with an 80-year-old woman complaining of feeling nervous and being unable to sleep. She sits slumped in her chair, facing you, and mumbles. Describe your approach to the nurse-patient interview, including verbal responses and nonverbal behavior.
6. Discuss ways in which the physical environment would influence the responses of an older patient to the nurse-patient interview.
7. How and when is touch used with older patients?
8. During an admission interview, a patient suddenly stands up and shouts, "I want to go home," and begins to cry. What would be your initial response? How would you proceed with the interview?
9. Describe nursing actions for a confused patient. What type of assessment would be conducted? Describe overt behaviors indicative of confusion. What is the relationship between confusion and disorientation?
10. Discuss nursing actions for a depressed elderly patient. What family teaching would be done for this patient?

CRITICAL THINKING ACTIVITIES

1. Spend a couple of hours with an elderly person and engage them in a review of important aspects of their life.
2. Determine what resources are available for the elderly in your community and evaluate them based on adequacy and effectiveness.

RESEARCH AGENDA FOR EVIDENCE-BASED PRACTICE

The following are some of the nursing research problems raised in Chapter 38 that merit further study by psychiatric nurses:

1. The relationship between personality factors and coping with loss as individuals age
2. Factors contributing to sundown and sunrise syndromes
3. The effectiveness of nursing actions with agitated elderly people
4. The relationship between family stress and elder self-esteem
5. The effectiveness of reminiscence with moderately depressed elderly people
6. The relationship between functional ability and cognitive function
7. Supportive measures to reduce anxiety in the dementia patient
8. The relationship between relocation of an elderly person and changes in recent memory
9. Factors that contribute to abuse of the elderly
10. Effects of crime and victimization on the emotional well-being and quality of life of older people

CARE OF SURVIVORS OF ABUSE AND VIOLENCE 39

CRITICAL THINKING QUESTIONS

1. Do you agree with the premise that the root cause of family violence is the use and abuse of power? Explain your reasons.
2. Some people learn to be abusive from growing up in a violent home. What factors do you think are influential in preventing future violence when a person has been raised in a violent home?
3. What attitudes of health professionals have you observed toward survivors of violence? Were they helpful or supportive to the survivor? Why or why not?
4. Describe the paternalistic model of working with survivors of violence. Why do you think nurses use this approach?
5. How would you approach a family in which there was suspected child abuse? What information would you want to know before the interview?
6. Why do you think elderly people are reluctant to report abuse? What would you do if you suspected abuse of an elderly person, but the patient denied it?
7. Why do you think people have a tendency to "blame the victim" in cases of sexual assault? Have you ever observed this phenomenon?
8. How would you respond to the mother of a 6-month-old infant who tells you that she frequently disciplines her son by spanking him? What if the child was 4 years old? Develop a health teaching plan for this situation.
9. Discuss your personal feelings regarding the acceptability of a man forcing a woman into sexual activity in the following situations:
   A. He has spent a lot of money entertaining her.
   B. She has been sexually active with him in the past.
   C. He is so excited he cannot control himself.
   D. She appears to be interested in sex but then changes her mind.
   E. He believes that women do not really mean "no" and want to be overpowered sexually.
   F. He believes she is frigid and is trying to help her overcome her aversion to sex.

CRITICAL THINKING ACTIVITIES

1. Interview a staff member at a shelter for abused women or rape crisis center. Focus on the adequacy of available services and the strong and weak aspects of current laws. Develop a plan for addressing one identified area of need.
2. Find out what services in your community are available to help women who have been raped, spouses who have been abused, and children who have been abused or neglected. Evaluate whether they are adequate and effective for the scope of the problem.

RESEARCH AGENDA FOR EVIDENCE-BASED PRACTICE

The following are some of the nursing research problems raised in Chapter 39 that merit further study by psychiatric nurses:

1. The effect of violence during pregnancy on the health of the mother and infant, including the relationship with low birth weight
2. The effects of different cultural groups' values and beliefs regarding women, children, and elderly persons on specific forms of family violence
3. The effective coping strategies of survivors of family violence and specific nursing interventions to support effective coping
4. Testing the effectiveness of various nursing interventions for survivors of violence, including group interventions
5. The most effective nursing assessment strategies for survivors and perpetrators of violence
6. Differing responses to rape and sexual assault and the most effective nursing strategies to assist in recovery
7. Short-term and especially the long-term effects of family violence on those not directly victimized (e.g., children of battered women, siblings of abused children, witnesses of violence)
8. Testing of nursing interventions for primary and secondary prevention of violence in families
9. Developing and testing various strategies for changing attitudes within the health care system toward survivors of violence
10. Ways to enhance identification of victims and perpetrators of violence in the health care system, especially in settings other than the emergency room

40 Psychological Care of Patients with Life-Threatening Illness

CRITICAL THINKING QUESTIONS

1. You are a pediatric ICU nurse taking care of a 6-month-old infant who received a severe brainstem injury 3 months ago. The attending doctor feels the child has a poor prognosis for recovery of meaningful cognition and feels further treatment should not be offered. The parents confide in you that they are praying for a miracle. How do you respond?
2. Your patient with a new diagnosis of congestive heart failure tells you she will not take her heart medications when she gets home because she knew someone who died slowly of this condition and she doesn't want to be a burden to her family. How would you intervene?
3. The dialysis patient you have known for 3 years is admitted for emergency dialysis for the fourth time in 4 months. He has not kept dialysis or clinic appointments but denies that he wants to die. How would you approach him about his behavior?
4. A member of your church is admitted with jaundice and hepatitis C. Your sister has hepatitis C and has been waiting for a transplant. Do you talk with the patient about your sister's situation? Why or why not?
5. This is your first day taking care of a patient who is awaiting the results of a breast cancer biopsy. She says, "I don't know what I'll do if it comes back positive. My aunt died a terrible death with breast cancer." What do you tell her to reassure her?
6. You notice that the patient with multiple sclerosis you have been assigned to for several days now keeps his room dark, mumbles, and is refusing physical therapy. How will you approach him about his withdrawal? What will you suggest to the team?
7. A patient with colorectal cancer has had two complete cycles of chemotherapy treatment and has been in remission for the past 2 years. You see him in an outpatient clinic and he tells you excitedly that he is trying a new therapy that has been successful in Europe but not approved in this country. He does not want you to tell his doctor because he is afraid the doctor will ridicule his choice. Do you mention the alternative treatment to the physician? Why or why not?
8. Your brother has been diagnosed with cancer and is depressed. He asked his oncologist for an antidepressant but was told he did not need one because "Of course you're depressed . . . you have cancer." How would you advise your brother?

CRITICAL THINKING ACTIVITIES

1. Talk with patients from different ethnic groups about their views on end-of-life care. How might these insights influence your nursing practice?
2. Attend an ethics consultation in your hospital. Evaluate the role of each participant, the nature of the discussion, and the ultimate outcome.
3. Visit a hospice in your community and evaluate the quality of care received by the patients.
4. Talk with your family about the importance of advance directives. Encourage them to begin the process of planning their end-of-life health care decisions.

RESEARCH AGENDA FOR EVIDENCE-BASED PRACTICE

The following are some of the nursing research problems raised in Chapter 40 that merit further study by psychiatric nurses:

1. The familiarity of nurses with advance directives and their comfort in discussing them with patients and families
2. The percentage of nurses who have prepared their own living wills and durable powers of attorney
3. The number of hospitals across the country that employ psychiatric consultation liaison nurses and their varying roles and functions
4. Nurses' attitudes and behaviors in treating anxiety, depression, and pain in the terminally ill
5. Ways in which nurses deal with withholding or withdrawing life-sustaining treatment
6. Referral patterns of nurses to hospice care
7. Nurses' beliefs about euthanasia and assisted suicide
8. Nursing outcomes in working with patients who have life-threatening illness

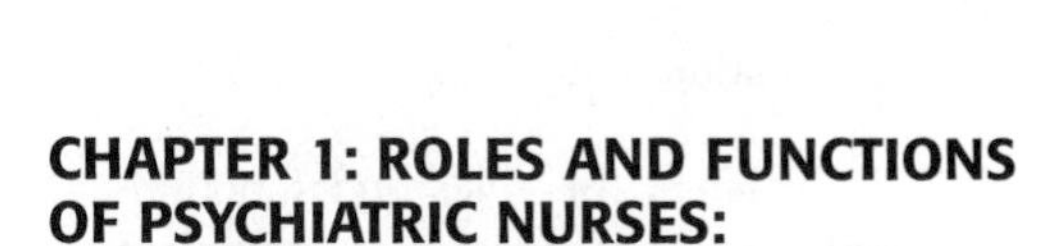

TEST BANK

CHAPTER 1: ROLES AND FUNCTIONS OF PSYCHIATRIC NURSES: COMPETENT CARING

1. Hildegard Peplau, in 1952, defined the psychiatric nurse's role as:
   1. a professional who helps patients with attitude adjustment needs.
   2. a nurse who is trained to care for psychiatric patients.
   3. a resource person, a teacher, a leader, and a counselor.
   4. a nurturer, a provider of psychiatric care, and a leader in nursing.

2. The contribution of Linda Richards that remains a part of contemporary psychiatric nursing practice is the idea that:
   1. psychiatric nurses should have advanced preparation.
   2. nurses should assess both the physical and the emotional needs of patients.
   3. psychotic behavior must be controlled before psychotherapy begins.
   4. basic physical needs must be met before emotional needs are addressed.

3. Nurse K. states, "I plan ways for patients assigned to me to participate in their own care and to be actively involved in all of the activities on the unit." Her approach demonstrates the concept of:
   1. social accountability.
   2. therapeutic community.
   3. nurse-patient relationship.
   4. multidisciplinary mental health team.

4. Peplau's classic article, "Interpersonal Techniques: The Crux of Psychiatric Nursing," directed psychiatric nursing future growth by stating that the primary role of the psychiatric nurse was that of:
   1. leader.
   2. teacher.
   3. counselor.
   4. surrogate parent.

5. During the orientation portion of a psychiatric nursing course, which would the instructor be most likely to tell students?
   1. "There is one approved theoretical framework for psychiatric nursing practice."
   2. "Psychiatric nursing has yet to be recognized as a core mental health discipline."
   3. "Contemporary practice of psychiatric nursing is primarily focused on inpatient care."
   4. "The psychiatric nursing patient may be an individual, a family, a group, an organization, or a community."

6. For psychiatric nurses in the early 1980s and 1990s, the scope of practice began to change to include:
   1. psychiatric care and medical care given by the home care nurse.
   2. psychoanalytical therapy provided by the psychiatric nurse in the outpatient setting.
   3. new advances in psychobiology and technology.
   4. new advances in the psychodynamic model of therapy employed by the psychiatric nurse in the inpatient setting.

7. During orientation to the inpatient psychiatric unit, new staff members are told, "Address all patients by their title and surname, for example, Ms. Jones or Mr. Rodriguez, until you are directed by the patient to do otherwise." The philosophical belief underlying this directive is the idea that:
   1. every individual has the potential to change.
   2. the goal of the individual is one of growth, health, autonomy, and self-actualization.
   3. the individual has intrinsic worth and dignity, and each person is worthy of respect.
   4. the person functions as a holistic being who acts on, interacts with, and reacts to the environment as a whole person.

8. The psychiatric aide says, "I don't know why Ms. R. does all that silly giggling and posturing. It's senseless!" The best reply to her comment would make reference to the psychiatric nursing principle that:
   1. every individual has the potential to change.
   2. illness can be a growth-producing experience for the individual.
   3. all behavior is meaningful; it arises from personal needs and goals and can be understood only from the internal frame of reference of the person performing the behavior and within the context in which it occurs.
   4. the individual has the right to self-determination, including the decision to pursue health or illness.

9. The role of the psychiatric nurse in today's contemporary practice settings is:
   1. centered on the nurse-patient partnership.
   2. caring for chronically ill psychiatric patients in acute-care settings.
   3. concentrated on psychosomatic therapies.
   4. centered on management of the patient's daily needs.

10. An advanced practice psychiatric nurse muses, "Our specialty is vulnerable." Which fact supports this statement?
    1. More nurses are attracted to psychiatric nursing than other specialties.
    2. Psychiatric nursing content in nursing education has increased during the past decade.
    3. The biopsychosocial skills and expertise of psychiatric nurses often are underused in mental health systems.
    4. Role differentiation on the basis of education and experience is clearly spelled out in job descriptions and rewards.

11. Clinical rotations for nursing students include a psychiatric mental health rotation to give the student an opportunity to:
    1. become familiar with patients who have chronic psychiatric mental health issues.
    2. work with patients who have psychiatric as well as physical health issues.
    3. learn to care for patients who have emotional disorders.
    4. learn to work with patients with psychiatric mental health issues and to become familiar with new information in the behavioral and psychiatric fields.

12. When considering psychiatric nursing roles and functions, one could suggest that to perform delegation, the nurse must have knowledge of the domains of:
    1. communication and management.
    2. management and direct care.
    3. direct care and communication.
    4. direct care, communication, and management.

13. Case management is a psychiatric nursing activity that falls within the nursing practice domain of:
    1. communication.
    2. management.
    3. direct care.
    4. community education.

14. When one considers the roles and functions of psychiatric nursing, the overlap of communication and management roles is seen in the function of:
    1. teaching.
    2. delegation.
    3. collaboration.
    4. direct care.

15. The major determinants of the roles in which a psychiatric nurse engages are:
    1. personal preference and age.
    2. local custom and physician support.
    3. state law and personal qualifications.
    4. work setting and personal preference.

16. In a reformed health care system that places emphasis on efficient patient care, which of the following are most important responsibilities for the psychiatric nurse?
    1. Clinical case conferences and leadership
    2. Telehealth and research
    3. Patient care and leadership
    4. Patient triage and management

17. There are two levels of certification for psychiatric mental health registered nurse—basic and advanced levels. Registered nurses become certified by which of the following?
    1. American Psychiatric Nurses Association
    2. National League for Nursing
    3. The American Nurses Association
    4. National Council of State Boards of Nursing

18. We need to advocate the funding of outcome studies because they:
    1. increase patient compliance with therapeutic regimens.
    2. document quality, cost, and effectiveness of psychiatric nursing.
    3. update psychiatric nursing specialists on new practice developments.
    4. lead to the implementation of untried interventions and practice guidelines.

19. New opportunities for psychiatric nursing practice have emerged as psychiatric hospitals have changed from large institutions providing custodial care to:
    1. small units providing acute inpatient care.
    2. integrated clinical systems providing a full continuum of care.
    3. community-based home care systems focused on the persistently mentally ill.
    4. agencies more concerned with mental health promotion than in providing direct care.

20. A psychiatric nurse utilizes leadership skills to strengthen the profession by:
    1. working as a change agent in psychiatric nursing and in multidisciplinary groups who advocates for patients, families, and communities.
    2. voting for candidates in local elections who will advocate for nurses.
    3. volunteering time each week to outpatient clinics in poor neighborhoods.
    4. working for state government representatives at local voting sites.

21. In the 1960s the psychiatric nurse began to shift to primary prevention and psychiatric nursing practice began to focus more on community care. This focus was initiated by which of the following?
    1. The Therapeutic Community Act of 1962
    2. The Primary Prevention Act of 1960
    3. The Deinstitutionalization Act of 1961
    4. The Community Mental Health Centers Act of 1963

22. The premise for psychiatric nursing is based on knowledge from nursing and which of the other sciences to derive a theoretical framework?
    1. Psychodynamic, psychobiological, and personality theories
    2. Psychosocial, biophysical, and theories of personality and human behavior
    3. Behavioral science, psychodynamic, and psychobiological sciences
    4. Psychiatry, psychodynamic principles, and biophysical theories

23. Psychiatric nurses work in a variety of settings. A nurse is contemplating a change from a medical surgical nursing unit to a psychiatric nursing unit in a community hospital. What would you, as a psychiatric nurse, suggest she seek in the unit as indicators that the unit has a supportive environment for the new psychiatric nurse?
    1. Team meetings for all nurses each shift to discuss patients' conditions and unit census and an orientation schedule to include the nurses' responsibilities for each day
    2. Orientation to last at least 2 weeks with the charge nurse of the day and a scheduled daily task assignment
    3. A daily patient assignment during the second week of employment to help the nurse become more autonomous and daily reading assignments to be discussed with a preceptor daily
    4. A mentor for the first 6 weeks in the unit and a schedule for progression of learning throughout the orientation phase into the unit

24. A psychiatric nurses' support group would include which of the following?
    1. Improvement of medical education materials for patients and families
    2. Development of nursing practice guidelines for the unit
    3. Discussion of interdisciplinary information found on the internet
    4. Incorporation of occupational therapy projects that could be used for patients with schizophrenia

25. It is essential that psychiatric nurses become aware of their ability in the area of political action. Of the following, which would be considered the important contribution the nurse could make toward positive political action?
    1. Raising donations for a local community health center
    2. Becoming involved in an election campaign for a local sheriff
    3. Becoming an active volunteer at a crisis center
    4. Working on a city committee to help register voters in that locale

CHAPTER 2: THERAPEUTIC NURSE-PATIENT RELATIONSHIP

1. A novice nurse states, "Psychiatric nursing can't be very difficult. After all, I believe in showing caring and in mutual exchange with my friends." The experienced nurse formulates a reply based on knowledge of the difference between a social and a therapeutic relationship with emphasis on:
    1. the kind of information given.
    2. the amount of emotion invested.
    3 the degree of satisfaction obtained.
    4. the type of responsibility involved.

Use the following to answer question 2.

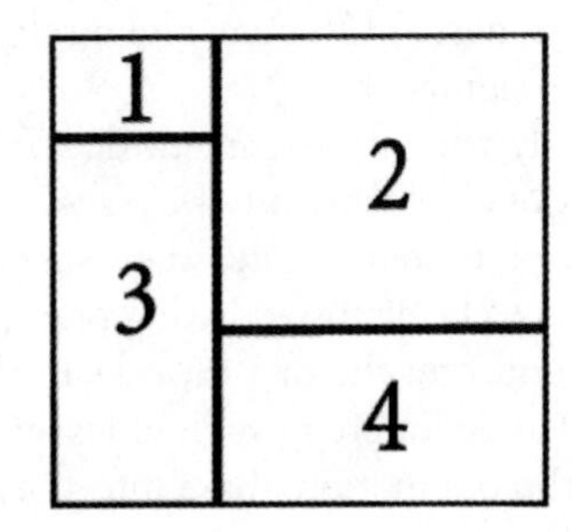

2. The diagram above is a Johari window that a nurse thinks accurately represents her. If she wishes to be more successful in psychiatric nursing, the nurse should make it her initial goal to increase the size of:
   1. quadrant 1.
   2. quadrant 2.
   3. quadrant 3.
   4. quadrant 4.

3. Which of the following strategies can the student nurse use to foster authenticity in therapeutic relationships with clients?
   1. Reading and discussing textbook assignments with a study group
   2. Modeling behaviors with patients on those of a clinically competent staff nurse
   3. Analyzing feelings associated with psychiatric clinical experience with the help of instructors and peers
   4. Attending patient-centered clinical conferences on the assigned psychiatric inpatient unit

4. Ms. C., who has always wished to share her love with "special children," adopts a biracial son and a daughter who has spina bifida. What is the highest step of the value clarification process that Ms. C. has achieved?
   1. Doing something with the choice in a pattern of life
   2. Choosing freely from alternatives
   3. Being happy with the choice
   4. Affirming the choice publicly

5. A nurse who is working with a patient diagnosed with major depression remarks, "My patient seems to be affectively brighter and to have more energy, yet I am struck by a sense of hopelessness and despair about her." The best advice to give this nurse would be:
   1. "Sometimes it's best to ignore perceptions like that and focus on the objective signs."
   2. "Pay attention to your feelings. They are a valuable clue about the patient's feelings."
   3. "You should share your perceptions with the patient and seek an explanation."
   4. "Confrontation is a useful tool in situations like this."

6. A new nurse has these thoughts run through her mind: "How will I handle things if my patient walks away from me? How will I react if the patient is sexually provocative? How will I cope with a patient who cries?" These thoughts indicate that the nurse is engaged in:
   1. role modeling.
   2. self-exploration.
   3. altruistic thinking.
   4. value clarification.

7. The nurse's most appropriate initial action during the preinteraction phase of a relationship with Stan, a gay male patient, should be to:
   1. examine his or her own feelings about homosexuality.
   2. focus on a method to assist the patient with changing his sexual values.
   3. review the literature that pertains to the human sexual response.
   4. attempt to identify the underlying reasons for the patient's values.

8. A nurse who has considered what he or she has to offer the patient, reviewed the general goals of a therapeutic relationship, and planned for the first interaction with the patient has engaged in the tasks appropriate to which phase of the nurse-patient relationship?
   1. Working phase
   2. Orientation phase
   3. Termination phase
   4. Preinteraction phase

9. When asked to contrast social superficiality with therapeutic intimacy, the experienced nurse mentor explains to the new nurse that the termination component in therapeutic intimacy is:
   1. unknown.
   2. open-ended.
   3. specified and agreed upon.
   4. closed to negotiation or agreement.

10. Which task would be most appropriate to focus on during the introductory phase of work with Anthony, a teenage patient with low self-esteem?
    1. Mutual formulation of a contract
    2. Nurse's analysis of his or her own strengths
    3. Promotion of patient use of constructive coping mechanisms
    4. Review of progress of therapy and goal attainment with patient

11. A patient who is admitted with a diagnosis of schizophrenia, paranoid type, coldly tells the nurse, "I am here because my family brought me here and locked me up." The best nursing response to use in the introductory session with the patient would be:
    1. "How has hospitalization affected your life?"
    2. "Do you feel angry or resentful about being hospitalized?"
    3. "I see you are angry about being here. I hope that after we talk you may feel differently."
    4. "We are here to protect you and see that, in your anger, you do not harm yourself or others."

12. Mr. D. is admitted to your unit and complains of "being depressed." He "wants to feel like his old self again." Which nursing response will be most therapeutic?
    1. "How long have you felt this way?"
    2. "We're all here to help you get better."
    3. "What do you think the hospital can do for you?"
    4. "Tell me more about how things are so that I can better understand."

13. In the initial sessions, a patient frequently asks the nurse for cigarettes and money and expresses doubt about the nurse's ability to be of help. Which principle provides guidance for the nurse in this situation?
    1. This behavior is typical of transference reactions.
    2. All patients have feelings of insecurity and low self-esteem.
    3. Manipulative behavior is part of this patient's psychopathology.
    4. Testing behavior is common during the introductory phase of a relationship.

14. The nurse and Mr. R. have had eight sessions. Mr. R. tells the nurse, "I got to the point that I was feeling pretty good, but now I'm beginning to get anxious again. I don't know if I'll be able to handle things on my own. Things feel uncertain, like they did when I left home to go to college." The nurse and Mr. R. most likely are entering which phase of the relationship?
    1. Working
    2. Termination
    3. Introductory
    4. Preinteraction

15. The new nurse is pleased that the patient, Ms. S., has been making steady progress during their sessions and mentions this to her supervisor. The supervisor smiles and says, "That's great, but be prepared for resistance." What resistance behaviors are most easily identified as such by the novice nurse?
    1. Acting-out behaviors
    2. Forced flight into health
    3. Intensification of psychiatric symptoms
    4. Superficial talk and suppression of pertinent information

16. During the working phase of the relationship, the nurse assesses that Ms. S. may be demonstrating resistance. The most appropriate way to deal with this would be to:
    1. assist Ms. S. in exploring her past for uncovered issues and conflicts.
    2. clarify, share observations, and reflect content and feelings with the patient.
    3. confront the patient with the behavior and state that she will be expected to work harder.
    4. avoid mentioning the therapeutic impasse and wait until the patient again indicates readiness.

17. A patient sees a hideous face on the wall of his room. The nurse attempting to calm him says that shadows have been created on the wall by the sun coming through the leaves of a tree near the window. This can be assessed as the patient having made an error in:
    1. feedback.
    2. perception.
    3. experience.
    4. transmission.

18. A patient says to a nurse, "My husband and I get along just fine. We usually agree on everything." As the patient speaks, her foot is moving and she continuously twirls a button on her blouse. The nurse can assess this communication as:
    1. inefficient.
    2. inadequate.
    3. incongruent.
    4. inappropriate.

19. The nurse tells a patient who is feeling guilty about an infidelity to call his wife and beg her forgiveness. According to the transactional model of communication, the nurse's response originated from the:
    1. adult ego state.
    2. child ego state.
    3. parent ego state.
    4. complementary transaction state.

20. Nurse: "I understand that you stopped taking your medications after you left the hospital." Patient: "I didn't want to rely on medications to solve my problems, but I see now that not taking them only made things worse." According to transactional analysis theory, the type of transaction recorded above can be assessed as a(n):
    1. ulterior transaction.
    2. crossed transaction.
    3. incongruent transaction.
    4. complementary transaction.

21. A patient seeks the nurse's help with feelings of anxiety that overwhelm him at work. When the nurse suggests he try to communicate his feelings to his boss, the patient responds, "Yes, but I'll get fired if I do that." According to transactional analysis theory, this is an example of a(n):
    1. ulterior transaction.
    2. crossed transaction.
    3. congruous transaction.
    4. complementary transaction.

22. Patient: "Some days I think it's just not worth it. I'd be better off alone. Maybe things would be calmer and simpler without him." Nurse: "Are you saying that things might be better if you left your husband?" Which therapeutic communication technique is used in this interaction between patient and nurse?
    1. Focusing
    2. Restating
    3. Reflection
    4. Clarification

23. Patient: "Sorry I'm late. I didn't realize what time it was." Nurse: "This is the third time we've met, and you've been late for each of our sessions. You say how important they are to you, but you can't seem to get here on time. Could it be that you aren't ready to work on your problems?" Which therapeutic communication technique is the nurse using?
    1. Informing
    2. Suggesting
    3. Identifying themes
    4. Sharing perceptions

24. The therapeutic communication technique of suggesting is appropriate to use when it:
    1. meets the patient's unmet dependency needs.
    2. shifts responsibility from the patient to the health care professional.
    3. is used during the working stage to present alternative coping strategies.
    4. is used early in the relationship to provide everyday "common sense" advice.

25. Patient: "I wish my parents would stop treating me like an irresponsible child." Nurse: "You say you want your parents to treat you like an adult, but you skip school, stay out after your curfew, and come home stoned. How does that fit?" Which action dimension does the nurse use in this interaction?
    1. Immediacy
    2. Confrontation
    3. Emotional catharsis
    4. Nurse self-disclosure

26. Which statement is true of planning the timing for the use of confrontation?
    1. Confrontation should never be used during the orientation phase of the relationship.
    2. Confrontation is useful during the working phase to focus on specific patient discrepancies.
    3. Confront patients with their limitations early in the relationship and with their assets later in therapy.
    4. Confront patients when other therapeutic action dimensions have proved to be ineffective.

27. Patient: "You can't tell people very much about yourself: it gives them too much power over you." Nurse: "I wonder if you're concerned about talking to me about your problems. I think I may need to earn your trust with a little more time." This interaction best represents an example of the action dimension called:
    1. immediacy.
    2. confrontation.
    3. emotional catharsis.
    4. nurse self-disclosure.

28. The patient writes to the nurse, "Over the weeks that we've been meeting I've come to feel as though you are a very special person sent from heaven to guide me out of this darkness of the soul. I know I can count on you to chart my course back to health. I will do whatever you advise and will be forever in your debt." The nurse can assess this as indicating:
    1. a boundary violation.
    2. emotional catharsis.
    3. positive countertransference.
    4. dependent reaction transference.

29. The nurse tells her supervisor, "I'm having a difficult time empathizing with my patient, Sally Clarke. I just can't understand her perspective and her unwillingness to change. Sometimes I find myself wanting to argue with her. After sessions with her I feel both frustrated and kind of depressed." Self-analysis will probably reveal:
    1. countertransference.
    2. that Sally is a difficult patient.
    3. a boundary violation by the nurse.
    4. poor use of therapeutic communication techniques.

CHAPTER 3: CONCEPTUAL MODELS OF PSYCHIATRIC TREATMENT

1. The nurse using Peplau's model for therapy will focus assessment on:
   1. identifying interpersonal problems.
   2. making interpretations about patient behavior.
   3. considering the way the social environment has affected the patient.
   4. comparing patient symptoms with DSM-IV descriptions.

2. Which model is employed when, during the course of therapy, the nurse consciously conveys empathy, concern, and nonjudgmental acceptance to the patient while focusing on the reduction of the patient's subjective distress and maladaptive coping behaviors?
   1. Medical model
   2. Existential model
   3. Supportive model
   4. Psychoanalytic model

3. The nurse states, "The patient, who is gay, has problems relating to his family. Presently he is experiencing a high level of anxiety related to fear of rejection when he reveals his sexual orientation." This statement reveals that the nurse views the patient's problem from the viewpoint of:
   1. the medical model.
   2. the existential model.
   3. the interpersonal model.
   4. the supportive therapy model.

4. The nurse using the supportive therapy model is caring for a patient who is assessed as having a high level of anxiety. The nurse's immediate goal would be to:
   1. reduce patient self-criticism.
   2. increase patient self-awareness.
   3. reduce symptoms of anxiety to a moderate to low level.
   4. accept the patient unconditionally in a relationship that satisfies patient needs.

5. According to the medical model, which interventions would be most important to include in the plan of care of a patient who is admitted with the diagnosis of acute alcohol withdrawal and who is taking prescribed benzodiazepines?
   1. Assess influences of society on the development of alcohol abuse
   2. Explore influences of early relationships within the family of origin
   3. Institute seizure precautions, monitor vital signs, and provide nutrition and fluids
   4. Counsel to help the patient integrate this episode of illness into total life experience

6. Which nursing intervention would be most consistent with the basic intent of the psychoanalytical model of therapy?
   1. Emphasizing the patient's strengths and assets
   2. Giving the patient psychoeducational materials to read
   3. Emphasizing the importance of medication compliance
   4. Focusing on positive or negative feelings developed by the patient toward the nurse

7. The nurse uses the psychoanalytical conceptual model when treating patients with an anxiety disorder. As the nurse treats a patient, she will focus on:
   1. correcting inappropriate learning patterns.
   2. changing a dysfunctional social environment.
   3. here-and-now encounters with the patient and family.
   4. freeing psychological energy bound by fixation at an early age.

8. The nurse who uses the psychoanalytical conceptual model when treating patients with anxiety disorders will most likely use an intervention called:
   1. interpretation.
   2. self-revelation.
   3. positive reinforcement.
   4. therapeutic double-bind.

9. The therapist tells the patient, "I believe that you are unconsciously casting me in the role of your mother and that your antagonistic behavior relates to feelings you have toward her." On the basis of this statement, one can correctly hypothesize that the therapist is using the:
   1. medical model.
   2. existential model.
   3. interpersonal model.
   4. psychoanalytical model.

10. The patient's goal is to improve self-esteem and self-awareness. He states, "I don't want to hear any mumbo jumbo from a therapist about my childhood. I'm self-alienated, and I want to deal with what's going on in my life right now." The nurse hearing this should think in terms of referring the patient to therapists who use the:
    1. medical model.
    2. existential model.
    3. psychoanalytical model.
    4. supportive-therapy model.

11. A nurse using Peplau's interpersonal approach will use interventions that focus on:
    1. a pleasant personality and a good sense of humor.
    2. changing social conditions to make conformity easier.
    3. a repertoire of encounters to increase self-awareness.
    4. unconditional acceptance and corrective interpersonal experiences.

12. A nurse mentions: "Thomas Szasz is my hero. His work coincides with my beliefs." In this nurse's work with patients, one can expect to see:
    1. liberal use of psychotropic medications.
    2. interest in exploring developmental relationships.
    3. advocacy for freedom of choice for psychiatric patients.
    4. strong reliance on groups to provide authentic relationships.

13. Which statement is most likely to be made by a therapist who uses the social model?
    1. "We need to examine your interpersonal games."
    2. "You must take the medication that is prescribed for you."
    3. "Tell me about the feelings you have toward your mother."
    4. "Describe the problem that you would most like to change."

14. The patient is going to undergo psychoanalysis as part of his training as a therapist. What roles can he expect the psychoanalyst with whom he works to demonstrate?
    1. Active and directive
    2. Passive and interpretive
    3. Nonexistent, because the therapy is self-administered
    4. Directive and autocratic with the patient taking a passive role

15. The patient is going to see a therapist who practices supportive therapy. When she asks what to expect of the therapist, the best reply would be, "The therapist will most likely:
    1. be warm and active and give you suggestions for behavioral change."
    2. be cool and passive and say very little as you tell him or her your thoughts."
    3. support whatever decisions you decide to make in relation to your problems."
    4. expect you to do as he or she tells you to do and not allow much input from you."

16. The emotional responsiveness shown by therapists as part of therapy will be most similar during:
    1. interpersonal therapy and supportive therapy.
    2. social model therapy and medical model therapy.
    3. existential model therapy and psychoanalytical model therapy.
    4. social model therapy and psychoanalytical model therapy.

17. The role of the patient in interpersonal therapy is to participate:
    1. with the therapist in discussion and open dialogue for the purpose of the patient becoming more verbal and better able to participate in social settings.
    2. in a therapy group where there is an opportunity to speak with others who are in situations similar to those of the patient.
    3. as actively as possible to share concerns with the therapist and to participate as fully as possible in the relationship.
    4. to observe the therapist and model the behavior learned in therapy in the family situation.

18. Szasz (1961) writes of the "myth of mental illness." He believes that society must find a way to manage "undesirables," so it labels them as:
    1. social misfits
    2. mentally ill
    3. aggressive deviants
    4. angry social outcasts

19. Existential therapists help patients by helping them to find meaning in:
    1. life experiences.
    2. the ability to see beyond the here and now.
    3. looking back at their past.
    4. their family heritage.

20. The patient is hospitalized after a suicide attempt. The medical model of psychiatric care is implemented, which indicates that the caregiver will:
    1. base therapy on the principle of the physician-patient relationship.
    2. help the patient identify the reason for his suicide attempt and then utilize medical regimes to treat the patient with medication and hospitalization.
    3. become the patient's primary physician because of the hospitalization for the suicide attempt.
    4. discharge the patient as soon as possible with a prescription for outpatient therapy.

21 The patient states, "I don't want just anyone to help me with this problem. I want the best." The patient would probably be referred to a therapist who utilizes the:
   1. supportive model.
   2. psychodynamic model.
   3. existential model.
   4. medical model.

22. According to the medical model of psychiatric care, even the most complex psychological processes derive from operations of the brain. Therefore, for patients to be treated effectively for psychological problems, the treatment is directed to:
   1. treating excesses or deficits in chemical transmission.
   2. using appropriate medications, as all psychological disorders usually are treated.
   3. using scientific treatments, as all psychological disorders must be treated.
   4. treating the psychiatric problem with medication and individual therapy.

23. According to the medical model, treatment for the psychiatric patient is the formulation of the treatment plan by:
   1. the psychiatrist.
   2. the psychiatrist and the patient.
   3. a psychiatric nurse and the patient.
   4. the psychiatrist and multidisciplinary team.

24. Each psychiatric diagnosis listed in the DSM-IV TR is based on:
   1. the psychiatric model
   2. the eclectic model
   3. Freud's psychodynamic model
   4. the medical model

25. According to Peplau, two interacting components of health are necessary. Which of the following indicates a healthy individual, according to Peplau's components of health?
   1. An individual who exercises at the gym three times per week for 1 hour each time and has been married for 24 years, with two school-age children with whom he spends time at least three times per week
   2. An individual who is employed as a psychiatric nurse in an inpatient unit and who spends two to three evenings a week in school earning a nursing degree and spends one or two evenings a week socializing with other nurse colleagues
   3. An individual who is a member of a gym and is married with two school-age children
   4. An individual who is employed as a salesperson, exercises three times per week at the gym, and socializes with friends at least two times per week

CHAPTER 4: THE STUART STRESS ADAPTATION MODEL OF PSYCHIATRIC NURSING CARE

1. Which statement can a nurse use to describe the Stuart Stress Adaptation Model to someone who is unfamiliar with it?
   1. "The model recognizes the obsolescence of the nursing process and organizes treatment along critical pathways."
   2. "The model bases psychiatric nursing practice on principles solely derived from nursing science and establishes generic goals for each discrete stage of psychiatric treatment."
   3. "The model integrates biopsychosociocultural, environmental, and legal-ethical aspects of psychiatric nursing care into a unified framework for practice throughout the care continuum."
   4. "The model is based primarily on the medical model and organizes psychiatric nursing practice according to discrete treatment stages, selected treatment settings, and legal mandates."

2. A nurse talking about the Stuart Stress Adaptation Model states, "I don't understand why the model uses both the health/illness continuum and the adaptation/maladaptation continuum." The best reply to this would be:
   1. "The more that's in the model, the more it represents life."
   2. "The model recognizes that nature is ordered as a social hierarchy from simplest to most complex. The health/illness continuum is a simple concept; the adaptation/maladaptation continuum is more complex."
   3. "To also integrate the theory of the levels of prevention and the four stages of psychiatric treatment, Stuart had to have a health/illness frame of reference. The adaptation/maladaptation continuum was necessary to complement the holistic framework."
   4. "The health/illness continuum derives from a medical worldview, whereas the adaptation/maladaptation continuum derives from a nursing worldview. The two reflect the complementary nature of the nursing and medical models of practice."

3. A patient is in the emergency room of a local community hospital. The patient's vital signs are within normal range but she is crying uncontrollably and repeating over and over, "He will hurt me if I don't get away from him. You have to help me, please." Based on the fifth assumption of Stuart's Stress Adaptation Model, you will begin caring for this patient by:
   1. getting a physician to order a sedative for the patient.
   2. calling the lab to have her necessary blood specimen drawn immediately.
   3. beginning your nursing assessment.
   4. putting the patient in a quiet room and having someone sit with her until she calms down.

4. An adolescent who belongs to a neighborhood gang has been discovered by his parents to lie and steal. His worried parents bring him to the mental health center where it is determined that he is able to adequately test reality and has no symptoms of a major psychiatric disorder. The psychiatric nurse clinical specialist decides to assess his behavior using the health/illness continuum and the conformity/deviance continuum. The most likely finding will be:
   1. healthy deviant.
   2. healthy conformist.
   3. unhealthy deviant.
   4. unhealthy conformist.

5. Which criterion of mental health is the nurse assessing when he or she explores the patient's sense of self-determination, balance between dependence and independence, and acceptance of the consequences of behavior?
   1. Autonomy
   2. Integration
   3. Reality perception
   4. Environmental mastery

6. A patient states, "Sometimes I hear voices when no one else is in the room. This makes me wonder who is plotting against me to drive me crazy." Which criterion of mental health can the nurse assess as lacking?
   1. Autonomy
   2. Integration
   3. Reality perception
   4. Environmental mastery

7. The nurse documents that the patient is appropriately emotionally responsive and in control and expresses a unified philosophy of life. This implies that the patient has met the mental health criterion of:
   1. autonomy.
   2. integration.
   3. reality perception.
   4. environmental mastery.

8. A patient mentions, "I must be some kind of a freak. I'm mentally ill. No one else I know is mentally ill." What reply would help the patient understand the extent of mental illness?
   1. "You are not unique, nor are you a freak."
   2. "Let's concern ourselves with you; never mind other people."
   3. "Mental illness affects 60% of the adult population each year."
   4. "Nearly 50% of all people between the ages of 15 and 54 have had a psychiatric or substance abuse disorder."

9. On the basis of predictions from the Global Burden of Disease Study, mental health professionals should be most concerned with increasing primary prevention efforts for:
   1. alcohol abuse.
   2. schizophrenia.
   3. bipolar disorder.
   4. unipolar major depressive disorder.

10. The spouse of a patient with unipolar major depressive disorder tells the nurse, "I feel pretty hopeless about my wife's condition. Treating mental illness isn't the science that treating people with physical illness is, so results probably aren't as good." The reply that would help the spouse understand comparative treatment efficacy would be:
    1. "The truth is that people with mental illness get well more than 90% of the time."
    2. "New studies show that treatment of depression is effective 65% to 80% of the time, whereas treatments for heart disease and cancer are often only 40% effective."
    3. "You're right that treatment of mental illness is less effective, but we're making great strides with the use of new antidepressants."
    4. "It's not right to try to make comparisons between the effectiveness of treatment of mental and physical illnesses. It's like comparing apples and oranges."

11. At a meeting of a professional association, a speaker announced, "To be effective advocates for those with mental illness, nurses should be prepared to address the major barrier to treatment for the mentally ill." The speaker identified this barrier as:
    1. inadequate insurance coverage.
    2. ineffective treatment modalities.
    3. a shortage of mental health practitioners.
    4. a lack of accurate assessment tools for diagnosis.

12. Which of the following best describes the nurse's understanding of predisposing factors that influence mental illness? They are:
    1. risk factors that influence a person's vulnerabilities and the type and amount of resources used to handle stress.
    2. biological factors such as genetic background, general health, nutritional status, and exposure to toxins.
    3. psychological factors such as intelligence, morale, self-concept, motivation, and past experiences.
    4. sociocultural characteristics such as education, income, occupation, culture, religion, and relatedness.

13. The nurse who is to perform a patient assessment identifies precipitating stressors by using the hallmark criterion that precipitating stressors are stimuli that:
    1. society views as deviant.
    2. the family views as disruptive or burdensome.
    3. the patient views as challenging, threatening, or demanding.
    4. the nurse views as noxious, overwhelming, or culturally unacceptable.

14. Which individual would a nurse consider to be at the highest risk for the onset of stress-related problems?
    1. A 42-year-old patient whose father (to whom he was devoted) died 3 months ago and who is losing his job because of corporate restructuring. He states, "Living with loss and the threat of loss makes me feel helpless."
    2. A 24-year-old patient who is graduating from college and being married in a month's time. She states, "I'm anticipating the changes these events will make in my life."
    3. A 36-year-old patient whose new business is growing slowly and who plans to adopt a child with his wife. He says, "I think I'm in control of my destiny."
    4. A 50-year-old patient who was passed over for promotion and quit to start her own business. She states, "This is just one of a series of challenges I've faced in my life."

15. The nurse taking the history of a depressed patient discovers that the patient has a number of life strains, all of which contribute to daily hassles. She and her husband argue frequently, the teenage children in the family are rebellious, and there is seldom enough money to meet all the bills. In what way is this information relevant?
    1. Negative life events are more likely to affect physical health than mental health.
    2. Daily hassles are a source of considerable stress and affect mood more than major misfortunes.
    3. Life strains associated with the work role are most predictive of the development of major depression.
    4. Stressful life events are largely overrated as precipitating stressors that lead to the onset of symptoms.

16. The nurse assessing a patient is interested in the patient's appraisal of her divorce as a stressor. To obtain this information, it is important for the nurse to gather data about the patient's:
    1. affective responses.
    2. behavioral and social responses.
    3. physiological, affective, and social responses.
    4. cognitive, affective, physiological, behavioral, and social responses.

17. A patient has decided to resign from a job that embroiled him in many daily hassles. Using Caplan's theory of response to stress, the patient can be seen to be using:
    1. behavior that adjusts his appraisal of the stress.
    2. behavior that allows him to escape from the stressful environment.
    3. intrapsychic behavior to defend against unpleasant emotional arousal.
    4. intrapsychic behavior to come to terms with the event and its sequelae by internal readjustment.

18. At her last clinic visit, the patient was diagnosed with fibromyalgia. At this visit she tells the nurse that she spends several hours each week on the internet seeking information about her illness. The nurse can correctly hypothesize that Ms. Smith is:
    1. engaged in a search for meaning.
    2. devising a new coping strategy.
    3. making a social attribution.
    4. making a social comparison.

19. Of the four individuals who have been diagnosed as having cancer, which person's social attribution is most likely to lead to an active, successful coping response?
    1. Jim: "I was dealt a hand that included bad genes."
    2. Sam: "I never led a healthy lifestyle, and it caught up with me."
    3. Hank: "I was negligent when I didn't go for my yearly checkup."
    4. Joe: "I thought ignorance was bliss, but now I'm paying for that ignorance."

20. A major difference between coping resources and coping mechanisms is that:
    1. coping resources are adaptive, whereas coping mechanisms are maladaptive.
    2. coping resources are assets, whereas coping mechanisms can be assets or liabilities.
    3. individuals have multiple coping resources, but coping mechanisms are limited in number.
    4. available coping resources are more predictive of outcome than are the coping mechanisms used.

21. A comparison of the nursing and medical models of care will yield the finding that:
    1. nurses assess disease states and causes.
    2. physicians assess risk factors and vulnerability.
    3. nursing intervention consists of curative treatments.
    4. nursing diagnoses focus on the adaptive/maladaptive continuum of coping responses.

22. A physician mentions, "I don't see the benefit of using nursing diagnosis when the patient already has a medical diagnosis." The best reply for the nurse to make would be that Nursing diagnoses:
    1. "provide a way for all health professionals to view a patient holistically and to combat the problem of mind-body dualism."
    2. "complement medical diagnoses and are best described as the patient's behavioral response to stress."
    3. "offer an alternative to health professionals who wish to use complementary treatment modalities in lieu of traditional medical treatment."
    4. "contribute little in the everyday clinical setting, but do provide nurses with a common language to use for research on outcomes of standard nursing interventions."

23. The spouse of a patient displaying symptoms of schizophrenia asks the nurse, "How do the doctors know that my husband is psychotic and not neurotic?" The best reply would be:
    1. "Patients with neuroses are not bothered by their symptoms of illness."
    2. "Patients with neuroses suffer the severest forms of personality disorganization."
    3. "Patients with psychoses display more social deviance than those with psychiatric symptomatology."
    4. "Patients with psychoses incorrectly evaluate external reality and have great difficulty functioning."

24. Under what condition may the nurse implement the nursing process for a patient with a maladaptive stress response?
    1. Only after obtaining a physician's order
    2. Only after diagnostic tests rule out organic pathology
    3. Regardless of whether a physician has diagnosed a psychiatric disorder
    4. After case discussion with the mental health treatment team

25. A patient became acutely anxious and hysterical in response to the stress of her home being destroyed by fire the previous evening. The nurse assesses the patient's treatment stage as:
    1. crisis.
    2. acute.
    3. maintenance.
    4. health promotion.

26. A patient became acutely anxious and hysterical in response to the stress of her home being destroyed by fire the previous evening. The immediate nursing goal for the patient is:
    1. the patient will be stabilized.
    2. the illness will go into remission.
    3. the patient will completely recover.
    4. the patient will achieve optimal wellness.

27. A patient who became delusional after the accidental death of his son believes that his son was killed by the CIA and thinks that the CIA is now plotting to kill him. During the acute stage of treatment, the expected outcome of nursing care is:
    1. the patient will experience symptom relief.
    2. the nurse will validate the patient's strengths.
    3. the patient will identify vulnerabilities that led to the symptoms.
    4. the nurse will focus on the patient's quality of life and well-being.

28. A patient is diagnosed with bipolar disorder and hospitalized. According to the Stuart Stress Adaptation Model, nursing interventions for this stage of treatment will focus on
    1. inspiring and validating the patient.
    2. managing the environment to provide safety.
    3. mutual treatment planning, modeling, and teaching adaptive responses.
    4. reinforcement of the patient's adaptive coping responses and advocacy.

29. The patient was diagnosed with bipolar disorder and had been hospitalized. Her symptoms remit and she is now living in the community. During this stage of treatment, the expected outcome will be that the patient will:
    1. be safe from harm.
    2. experience symptom relief.
    3. demonstrate improved functioning.
    4. attain an optimal quality of life in the community.

30. The nurse caring for a patient suspects that the patient has a personality disorder in addition to the presenting symptoms of a maladaptive stress response. To confirm this, the nurse would look in the patient's medical record on the DSM-IV Axis:
    1. I.
    2. II.
    3. IV.
    4. V.

31. The nurse caring for a patient wonders how the patient's functioning has been evaluated in the past. To learn this, the nurse would look in the medical record on the DSM-IV Axis:
    1. I.
    2. II.
    3. IV.
    4. V.

32. The nurse caring for a client would look at DSM-IV Axis III to obtain information about the patient's:
    1. clinical syndromes.
    2. general medical conditions.
    3. global assessment of functioning.
    4. psychosocial and environmental problems.

CHAPTER 5: EVIDENCE-BASED PSYCHIATRIC NURSING PRACTICE

1. To plan effective responses to the 1999 Surgeon General's Report, psychiatric nursing clinicians and researchers must act on the information that:
    1. mental health treatment efficacy is well-documented.
    2. satisfaction of consumers of psychiatric nursing services with service delivery is largely unknown.
    3. psychiatric nurses are to be commended for documenting the nature and outcomes of the care they provide.
    4. schools of nursing are doing an excellent job in teaching clinicians to use evidence-based psychiatric nursing practice.

2. Which statement could a nurse use in an argument to support evidence-based psychiatric nursing practice?
    1. "Licensing helps ensure effective clinicians."
    2. "Clinical supervision results in more effective clinicians."
    3. "It is risky to generalize from a small sample of patients to the universe of patients."
    4. "Information gathered by clinical means tends to be in the form of systematic observations."

3. Which activities on the part of nurses are necessary to provide evidence-based psychiatric nursing care?
    1. Obtaining advanced degrees and providing clinical supervision for peers
    2. Seeking sound opinion-based processes and maintaining self-directed practice
    3. Critically synthesizing research findings and applying relevant evidence to practice
    4. Attending continuing education programs and supporting advanced practice licensure

4. The base for nursing practice upon which a psychiatric nurse should place the greatest reliance to substantiate clinical practice is the:
    1. traditional basis.
    2. regulatory basis.
    3. evidence basis.
    4. philosophical/conceptual basis.

5. Which activity will be most useful to a nurse wishing to provide evidence-based psychiatric nursing care?
    1. Relying on findings of a properly designed, randomized, controlled trial
    2. Using a protocol from a well-designed, cohort, quasi-experimental study
    3. Seeking sound opinion-based processes and maintaining self-directed practice
    4. Applying findings from a meta-analysis of relevant randomized, controlled trials

6. You are one of the nurses developing a set of practice guidelines for your clinical unit. You begin the process of a literature review to search for examples of criteria that will be relevant to your patient-care goals. Of the following, which criteria for your search will be the most relevant?
    1. Guidelines that include reduced costs as a major criterion for use
    2. Guidelines that can assure a design to provide methods and procedures that ensure safe and effective treatment for your patients
    3. Guidelines that document preferred practices among other mental health professionals
    4. Guidelines that explain their complexity in detail

7. A nurse working at a facility that has just introduced the use of clinical pathways must understand that they:
   1. do not require quality monitoring.
   2. are more specific than clinical algorithms.
   3. fail to reflect an interdisciplinary approach.
   4. are maps with timetables for care delivery.

8. Nurses are easily oriented to the use of algorithms because they are familiar with the format of:
   1. tables.
   2. free text.
   3. flow charts.
   4. SOAPIE notes.

9. To what extent is outcome measurement important to psychiatric nursing?
   1. It is more "nice" than necessary.
   2. It will give information about the most appropriate settings for treatment.
   3. It will promote descriptive and correlational nursing research.
   4. It will ensure the legitimacy of psychiatric nursing practice and safeguard nursing positions in mental health services.

10. For psychiatric nurses, an essential part of outcome measurement is the:
    1. development of practice guidelines.
    2. systematic review of research literature.
    3. systematic use of reliable patient-rating scales.
    4. identification of the core knowledge and skills of psychiatric nurses.

11. The patient is being seen today in an outpatient facility for follow-up care after treatment for addiction to alcohol and marijuana. The psychiatric nurse who will be his case manager will formulate a nursing-care plan based on evidence-based practice. Which of the following will be a part of the patient's care plan?
    1. The client will try to abstain from alcohol and will assure that he will not take any illegal drugs.
    2. The client is willing to participate in a psychoeducational group every Tuesday for 8 weeks to learn about the disease process of addiction.
    3. The client will find a job within 2 weeks.
    4. The client will live with his parents until he is able to secure employment and find an apartment of his own so that he can move out of his parents' home.

12. As a psychiatric nurse working with patients with schizophrenia, you would like to learn more about evidence-based practice in nursing and how you can better meet the patient's needs. You want to begin examining research for the most current and significant data therefore you will begin your search using:
    1. nursing textbooks
    2. nursing journal articles
    3. DSM-IV-TR
    4. electronic databases

13. As the psychiatric nurse in a community health clinic, you are assigned a new patient. The patient is going to be discharged from an inpatient setting where he has experienced his first admission to an inpatient facility. He has a diagnosis of schizophrenia and will be discharged home where he lives with his elderly parents. You want to develop evidence-based care for the patient. You will first:
    1. identify the major support person for the patient.
    2. define the patient's clinical problems.
    3. help the patient to be reoriented to living outside of a locked psychiatric unit.
    4. help the patient to find employment.

14. As the admission and discharge nurse today, you find that a nursing care plan for a patient indicates that he is scheduled to be discharged from the locked inpatient psychiatric unit tomorrow. To evaluate the outcome of care for this patient, you will:
    1. gather evidence from the patient's chart that shows changes in his medical condition from admission to the present to prepare the evaluation of the outcomes.
    2. bring the evidence-based plan and ongoing documentation for the patient to an interdisciplinary team meeting, where you will discuss the progression of the evidence indicating the patient's current condition and prognosis for discharge.
    3. ask the patient's family members how they feel the patient will do after discharge because they have visited him daily since his admission.
    4. ask the patient to meet with you today to discuss his feelings about discharge and returning home after his hospitalization.

15. In formulating practice guidelines for patients with mental health disorders, the nurse ensures that the guidelines:
    1. have been formulated in the correct format.
    2. are designed by appropriate teams of psychiatric nurses.
    3. are updated regularly to ensure currency.
    4. list detailed specifications of methods and procedures.

16. Most often clinical pathways are used in:
    1. outpatient community mental health centers.
    2. inpatient units.
    3. mental health clinics.
    4. home-care settings.

17. To focus a patient's treatment or medication regime in a very specific format, which of the following would be used?
    1. Clinical pathway
    2. Algorithm
    3. Patient satisfaction survey
    4. Graph

18. Outcome measurement can focus on a practitioner's clinical intervention, on a patient's condition, or on a process utilized by the caregiver. The categories of outcome indicators include:
    1. process and reliability
    2. clinical and functional
    3. process and evaluation
    4. measurement and evaluation

19. An outcome measurement tool which psychiatric nurses should be familiar is quality report cards. Like academic counterparts, report cards for mental health and substance abuse services are intended to provide feedback on achievements and problems of the organization. A dimension of the quality report cards include:
    1. performance appraisal of the institution
    2. outcome of patient care
    3. nurses' system evaluation
    4. content, point of view, and intended audience

20. Which of the following best describes the evidence-based model for psychiatric nursing practice?
    1. Proof that the psychiatric nurse in a home-care setting really does care for assigned patients
    2. What the psychiatric nurse does and how the nurse adds value to the health care organization
    3. How psychiatric nurses prove to their employer that they do what they are required to do for patient care
    4. How the psychiatric nurse documents nursing care on the psychiatric nursing unit

21. You are a psychiatric nurse caring for a patient with a DSM-IV-TR diagnosis of schizoaffective disorder. You are formulating a care plan for the patient and want to be sure you are using the best practice guidelines for the patient. You know that practice guidelines are formulated to:
    1. establish evidence of appropriate psychiatric care based on anecdotal data collected only on the unit where you are using the practice guidelines.
    2. promote consistency of patient care for all patients with a particular need regardless of age or DSM-IV-TR diagnosis.
    3. identify treatments that are safe and effective for a particular psychiatric disorder based on scientific data.
    4. eliminate the need for nurses to continuously update the guidelines after they have been established.

22. The American College of Mental Health Administration (ACMHA) has created a classification of "building blocks" for informed decision making in behavioral health assessment and treatment. Of the following prevention and treatment options, which is the most specific set of treatment decisions based on the strongest evidence base?
    1. Standards
    2. Algorithms
    3. Best practices
    4. Practice guidelines

23. You are a psychiatric nurse working in an inpatient unit. You and two other colleagues have formulated a task force to identify a process to set up clinical pathways for patient care. The task force members have identified the first step as:
    1. reviewing patient records to identify why most patients on the unit are admitted.
    2. reviewing for efficiency and necessity the many activities that take place from the time the patient is admitted through discharge and aftercare.
    3. identifying the nursing skills used while patients are hospitalized.
    4. identifying the number of patients who are admitted with the same diagnosis more than once within a calendar year.

24. The nursing unit supervisor has asked you to be responsible today for admitting a new patient to the unit. She also asks that you be sure with this patient that you complete a behavioral rating scale commonly used on the unit. You understand that the reason for using the behavioral rating scale is:
    1. to gather data to have in the patient's record indicating how the patient behaved during the admission assessment.
    2. to assess the patient's state at the beginning of treatment, as the patient progresses in treatment, and at the conclusion of treatment.
    3. to satisfy requirements for hospital accreditation.
    4. because the unit supervisor asks that patient behavior scales be done routinely on the unit.

25. For theory to be useful in practice, nurses need to validate the theory by:
    1. learning the theory.
    2. performing research.
    3. formulating a theoretical paradigm.
    4. informing other clinicians of the theoretical frameworks.

CHAPTER 6: BIOLOGICAL CONTEXT OF PSYCHIATRIC NURSING CARE

1. A patient tells the nurse, "My doctor thinks my problem may lie with the neurotransmitters in my brain. What are neurotransmitters?" The reply that will give the patient the best understanding of neurotransmitters is, "Neurotransmitters are:
    1. the chemical messengers that cause brain cells to turn on or off."
    2. small clumps of cells that alert the other brain cells to receive messages."
    3. tiny areas of the brain that are responsible for controlling our emotions."
    4. weblike structures that provide connections among various parts of the brain."

2. A patient tells the nurse, "My doctor thinks my problem may lie with the neurotransmitters in my brain. What are neurotransmitters?" The best reply would be:
    1. "Let's explore what your doctor has told you about your problem."
    2. "What concerns do you have about having a serious mental disorder?"
    3. "Neurotransmitter problems can be handled with medication therapy."
    4. "Neurotransmitters are chemical messengers in the brain responsible for brain communication."

3. The nurse explains to a patient with a mental health disorder that the following parts of the brain is responsible for fine motor coordination?
    1. Cerebellum
    2. Medulla
    3. Temporal lobe
    4. Thalamus

4. Which neurotransmitter is located only in the brain, particularly in the raphe nuclei of the brainstem, and is implicated in depression?
    1. Acetylcholine
    2. Dopamine
    3. Norepinephrine
    4. Serotonin

5. What part of the brain is responsible for regulating pituitary hormones and is known to regulate the body's temperature?
    1. Cerebellum
    2. Hypothalamus
    3. Limbic system
    4. Thalamus

6. Which neurotransmitter is involved in the movement disorders seen in Parkinson's disease and in the deficits seen in schizophrenia and other psychoses?
    1. Dopamine
    2. Melatonin
    3. Norepinephrine
    4. Serotonin

7. The nurse explains to a patient undergoing diagnostic testing that the following brain imaging technique measures brain structure?
    1. Brain electrical activity mapping (BEAM)
    2. Computed tomography (CT)
    3. Positron emission tomography (PET)
    4. Single photon emission computed tomography (SPECT)

8. The objective information that has helped mental health professionals understand that schizophrenia has a biological component has been obtained primarily from which of the following?
    1. Magnetic resonance imaging (MRI) studies
    2. Genetic studies
    3. Patient histories
    4. Comparisons of blood chemistries

9. A genetic counselor is called by the hospital to see patients with genetic questions or concerns. Which of the following patients should be asked whether they would like to speak with the counselor?
    1. A patient who has made a recent suicide attempt
    2. A pregnant patient with multiple sclerosis
    3. A man with schizophrenia who has multiple hospital admissions
    4. A patient prescribed the most drugs on the treatment Kardex

10. A patient, Ms. L., tells the nurse that her daughter is pregnant with her first grandchild. Her son-in-law has a sister with cystic fibrosis. She asks the nurse if there is a chance the baby might have this disease. Which of the following responses is best?
    1. "This is not an inherited disorder."
    2. "Science has not yet developed gene testing for this disease."
    3. "You probably should speak to a genetic counselor."
    4. "There are new treatments for this illness that are readily available."

11. Pharmacogenetics will eventually allow researchers to do which of the following?
    1. Remove the genes that cause illness
    2. Allow the design of custom drugs
    3. Develop foods that fight disease
    4. Splice genes to improve health

12. A patient tells the nurse, "My doctor thinks my problem may lie with the neurotransmitters in my brain. Does that mean I have a serious problem?" How should the nurse reply to the patient's question about the seriousness of the problem?
    1. "Let's explore what your doctor has told you about your problem."
    2. "What concerns do you have about having a serious mental disorder?"
    3. "Neurotransmitter problems usually can be handled with medication therapy."
    4. "The fact that you're seeing a psychiatrist suggests that you think there is a serious problem."

13. The physician reviewing Mr. T.'s medical record states, "This patient's behavior leads me to wonder if he may have a limbic system problem." If this is true, the nurse would be most likely to observe the patient having difficulty:
    1. regulating emotional behavior.
    2. performing abstract reasoning and higher-order thinking.
    3. with critical decision making, weighing alternatives, and planning.
    4. with coordinating stress-related responses and complex movements.

14. A patient states, "I'm going to have a positron emission tomography (PET) scan. What are they going to learn from it?" The best reply would be:
    1. "They will be looking for tumors and scars."
    2. "They will learn about the activity in the various portions of your brain."
    3. "They will be able to outline the structures of your brain more clearly."
    4. "Probably nothing clinically useful—scans are primarily research tools."

15. A patient mentions, "My doctor told me I was going to have a PET scan that would make my brain light up. Does that mean I'm getting an electrical jolt?" The best reply would be:
    1. "No, PET scans and electroconvulsive therapy are entirely different."
    2. "No, a PET scan is a diagnostic test, and electroconvulsive therapy is a treatment."
    3. "PET scans involve an injected substance that travels to the brain. Wherever brain activity is high, a bright spot shows on the scan."
    4. "PET scans show us the electrical activity that occurs throughout the brain in the form of light bands that glow in measurable degrees of brightness on a computer screen."

16. A patient tells the nurse that she is scheduled for an MRI the next day. She asks the purpose of the test and whether it will hurt. The best response would be:
    1. "This test is used to diagnose mental illness and no, it won't hurt."
    2. "This test is painful, but it's important to determine which mental illness you have."
    3. "It might be somewhat painful because it assesses electrical activity in different parts of the brain."
    4. "The MRI takes a picture of the brain. It doesn't hurt, but you will have to lie still, and that can be uncomfortable."

17. A depressed patient tells the nurse, "I don't feel rested. It's as though I didn't sleep at all." However, comments by night shift staff show that the patient slept through most of the night. How can these two observations be reconciled?
    1. The patient is considered the more accurate reporter.
    2. The staff observations are more objective that the patient's statement.
    3. Studies show that depressed people have disturbed sleep cycles that can result in sleep deprivation.
    4. Depressed individuals characteristically underreport sleep satisfaction because of cognition flaws.

18. The husband of a patient who has just been diagnosed with breast cancer asks, "What do you think about the relationship of stress and the development of cancer? My wife has been under a huge amount of stress at work and now they've diagnosed cancer." The answer that best reflects the current thinking about psychoneuroimmunology is:
    1. "It's thought that the immune system is negatively affected by high stress."
    2. "The literature doesn't say much, but it is believed that the mental state and the physical state affect each other to some degree."
    3. "Your wife's situation may reflect a coincidence. There's little evidence that stress makes one prone to physical illness."
    4. "Grief and depression are known to cause physical illness, but other types of stress have not been implicated as illness producers."

19. A patient's husband asks the nurse, "Why are they wasting money doing all these tests on my wife? It's obvious that she's mentally ill. She's hallucinating and delusional!" The best reply would be:
    1. "Don't be upset. We are using the most modern approach to caring for your wife."
    2. "I know you must be worried about costs, but having these tests is very necessary."
    3. "Physical illnesses can cause psychiatric symptoms. We must be sure of what we are treating."
    4. "I think that you are upset about your wife's illness and not thinking clearly. To avoid harming her, physical illness must be ruled out before we can give psychiatric medications."

20. Mr. and Ms. J. tell the nurse that they are concerned about having children because there is bipolar disorder in first-degree relatives of both of them. What advice should the nurse give?
    1. "Do not have children."
    2. "Seek genetic counseling."
    3. "Do as your conscience dictates."
    4. "Bipolar disorder is not hereditary."

21. Mr. T. demonstrates disoriented thinking and irrational ideas. The nurse can anticipate that a PET scan would most likely show dysfunction of the part of the brain called the:
    1. frontal lobe.
    2. parietal lobe.
    3. occipital lobe.
    4. temporal lobe.

22. A family member asks the mental health nurse, "I am reading a lot of information about gene therapy in the news lately. Will gene therapy be able to help my wife, who has schizophrenia?" Which of the following responses by the nurse is best?
    1. "Gene therapy has already shown promise in treating schizophrenia but not enough large-scale studies have been carried out to date."
    2. "Gene therapy for schizophrenia is common in Europe but has not become popular yet in the United States."
    3. "Gene therapy for schizophrenia is available but the high cost prohibits most people from taking advantage of it."
    4. "Gene therapy is still an experimental field and is not likely to be used to treat mental health disorders in the near future."

23. A patient with a history of depression reports not feeling well rested in recent weeks. Before making the assumption that the complaint is related to depression, the nurse should investigate whether the patient has had any recent changes in:
    1. work schedule that affect the hours of sleep.
    2. vacations taken within the same time zone.
    3. fluid intake with reduced overall intake of water.
    4. food intake with decreased intake of heavy foods before bedtime.

CHAPTER 7: PSYCHOLOGICAL CONTEXT OF PSYCHIATRIC NURSING CARE

1. A patient is admitted for treatment of uncontrolled diabetes mellitus. During the admission assessment, you notice that she is withdrawn and tearful. She tells you she has gained excessive weight because she hates her diet and hates taking insulin. She says she just wants to be normal again. What primary purpose would a psychiatric evaluation of the patient serve?
    1. Assisting the patient in verbalizing her distress about her disease
    2. Assessing the emotional factors affecting the patient's present condition
    3. Assessing priorities to be set for the patient's overall nursing care plan
    4. Assisting the patient in emotionally accepting the chronicity of her disease

2. Success in obtaining sufficient data in the initial psychiatric interview depends largely on the:
    1. patient's ability to communicate effectively.
    2. interviewer's ability to establish good rapport.
    3. number of psychiatric interviews the nurse has performed.
    4. interviewer's ability to organize and systematically record data.

3. A nurse plans to engage in participant observation as he conducts a mental status examination. This will require him to
    1. increase verbalization with the patient.
    2. listen attentively to the patient's response.
    3. engage in communication and observation simultaneously.
    4. advise the patient on what to do about the data that is obtained during the interview.

4. The nurse conducting a mental status examination should plan to:
    1. compare results with at least one other nurse.
    2. perform the examination without the patient knowing.
    3. integrate the examination into the nursing assessment.
    4. perform the examination as the first communication with the patient.

5. The admitting nurse is to conduct a mental status examination with Ms. G., a visitor from Puerto Rico, who has become psychotic while on a visit to her daughter's home in the United States. When completing the mental status examination, the nurse should remember that:
   1. sociocultural factors may greatly affect the examination.
   2. liking the patient as a person is very important to the outcome.
   3. agreeing with the life choices the patient has made is important.
   4. biological expressions of psychiatric illness are not usually significant factors.

6. A patient is 68 and suffering from cognitive impairment. She has been hospitalized for 3 days. Today, when the nurse asks her how her evening was, she replied, "I had the best time. My husband took me out to dinner and then to a concert. The music was wonderful." The nurse knows that the patient's husband died several months ago. The patient's remarks can be assessed as:
   1. delusions.
   2. confabulation.
   3. concretization.
   4. circumstantiality.

7. A depressed patient tells the nurse during the admission interview, "If I hadn't been admitted, I would have carried out my plan, and everyone would have been better off without me." The most appropriate response would be:
   1. "It's frustrating when plans are interrupted."
   2. "Things can still turn out all right for you while you're here."
   3. "What specifically did you plan to do before you were admitted?"
   4. "I know you're feeling bad now, but if you talk, things will be better."

8. A student nurse asks the nurse, "What can you really expect a mental status examination to reveal about the patient?" The best response would be:
   1. "It reflects the patient's current state."
   2. "It gives us a complete family history."
   3. "It reveals a lot about the patient's past experiences."
   4. "It helps us determine the patient's future prognosis."

9. The nurse who is admitting a patient will perform a mental status examination. The data most pertinent for determining the patient's affective response will be the patient's:
   1. judgment and insight.
   2. sensorium and memory.
   3. appearance and thought content.
   4. statements of mood and the nurse's empathic responses.

10. Which clinical skills used in the interview process to conduct a mental status examination are most relevant to establishing rapport?
    1. Clarification and restatement
    2. Information giving and feedback
    3. Systematic inquiry and organization of data
    4. Attentive listening, observation, and focused questions

11. The physician describes a female patient as being dressed like a "typical manic." From this statement, the nurse can assume that the patient's mode of dress was:
    1. drab.
    2. slovenly.
    3. flamboyant.
    4. The nurse cannot assume anything about the patient's appearance.

12. The nurse generally can expect the motor activity of a profoundly depressed patient and the motor activity of a manic patient to:
    1. be similar.
    2. show many tics and grimaces.
    3. be at opposite ends of the continuum.
    4. show unusual bizarre gestures or posturing.

13. The nurse observes the patient during the mental status examination. The patient believes that the CIA is plotting to kill him but he exhibits little emotional response to the situation. The nurse thinks that an individual dealing with such a situation normally would exhibit strong emotions such as fear or anger. The nurse should document the patient's affect as:
    1. labile
    2. elated.
    3. flat.
    4. congruent.

14. During the mental status examination, the patient is happily telling the nurse her past history and then shouts angrily at the nurse, "You are too nosy for your own good!" But then, almost immediately, she happily says, "Well, let's let bygones be bygones and be buddies." The nurse can assess this as:
    1. labile affect.
    2. magical thinking.
    3. ideas of reference.
    4. hallucinations.

15. To assess for the presence of hallucinations, during the mental status examination the nurse should ask:
    1. "Can you tell me what the name of this building is?"
    2. "Do you ever see or hear things that others don't see or hear?"
    3. "Do you think your moods shift more often that other people's do?"
    4. "Tell me the meaning of the saying, 'Don't count your chickens before they hatch.'"

16. A patient tells the nurse, "I am an exalted person. God has given me special powers to heal the sick and raise the dead. I can cast out demons and cure cancer, but the doctors had me arrested when I went into the operating room." The nurse can assess the patient's statements as indicating:
    1. a phobia.
    2. depersonalization.
    3. grandiose delusions.
    4. an idea of reference.

17. Which question would not be used to assess a patient's orientation?
    1. "What is your name?"
    2. "How long have you been here?"
    3. "What is the name of the building we're in?"
    4. "If you won $10,000, what would you do with it?"

18. The nurse who is assessing a patient's emotional intelligence will focus on the patient's:
    1. linguistic and musical abilities.
    2. bodily kinesthetic and spatial abilities.
    3. interpersonal and intrapersonal skills.
    4. logical mathematics and linguistic abilities.

19. The nurse asks the patient to remember the following object, color, and address: pencil, red, and 15 Maple Street. After 15 minutes, the nurse asks the patient to repeat the object, color, and address. The nurse is assessing:
    1. judgment.
    2. recent memory.
    3. ability to abstract.
    4. immediate recall.

20. While interviewing a patient, the nurse notes that the patient uses several words that he has invented and that his thoughts do not seem to flow logically. These observations are most consistent with a DSM-IV diagnosis of:
    1. depression.
    2. panic disorder.
    3. schizophrenia.
    4. defensive coping.

21. To gather data about a patient's judgment, which question would be most appropriate?
    1. "What brought you to the hospital?"
    2. "On a scale of 1 to 100, what would you consider your stress level to be?"
    3. "What problem would you like to work on while you are hospitalized?"
    4. "If you found a stamped, addressed envelope lying in the street, what would you do with it?"

22. The Mini-Mental State Examination would be used by the nurse who is interested in obtaining information about:
    1. affect changes.
    2. cognitive processes.
    3. thought content and processes.
    4. abnormal psychological experiences.

23. Asking a patient to give the meaning of the proverb "People who live in glass houses shouldn't throw stones" will assist the nurse in assessing the patient's:
    1. short-term memory.
    2. orientation to reality.
    3. ability to think abstractly.
    4. emotional intelligence.

24. During the mental status examination, the patient sits looking tense and suspicious. His shirt is torn and he has a reddened scar on his left cheek. He is married, has three children, and is a police officer currently taking a leave of absence. Which observation about appearance should be documented?
    1. He is a police officer on leave.
    2. He is married and has three children.
    3. He may possibly be on the wrong medication.
    4. He has a scar, looks tense and suspicious, and his shirt is torn.

25. During an interview of a manic patient, the patient demonstrates very rapid speech and talks continuously and loudly. His speech pattern is best documented as:
    1. tangential.
    2. pressured.
    3. inappropriate.
    4. circumlocution.

26. While being interviewed, the patient expresses that he believes that other people can place thoughts in his mind. This statement can be assessed as evidence of:
    1. thought insertion.
    2. nihilistic delusions.
    3. somatic delusions.
    4. ideas of reference.

27. During a mental status evaluation, the nurse's gut feelings may indicate:
    1. clues about the patient's physical well-being.
    2. subtle emotions being expressed by the patient.
    3. areas to be explored in the predischarge interview.
    4. potential nursing diagnoses that relate to a patient knowledge deficit.

28. The nurse who is assigned to admit a patient will follow the patient during her hospitalization for depression. The nurse plans to use the Beck Depression Inventory Scale at admission and during the course of treatment. What purpose will not be served by this plan?
    1. Confirming the diagnosis
    2. Measuring the extent of the patient's problem
    3. Tracking the patient's progress over time
    4. Replacing nursing documentation in the medical record

CHAPTER 8: SOCIAL, CULTURAL, AND SPIRITUAL CONTEXT OF PSYCHIATRIC NURSING CARE

1. To be most successful intervening with Mr. R., a Muslim patient from Iran, the nurse must have which of the following characteristics?
    1. Cultural awareness
    2. Specific knowledge of his cultural practices
    3. Cultural sensitivity to differences in belief systems
    4. Cultural awareness, knowledge, and intervention skills

2. The mental health nurse who is assessing a patient for sociocultural risk factors would assess which of the following patient characteristics?
    1. Family history of drug allergies
    2. Daily habits
    3. Belief system
    4. Restfulness of the home environment

3. Which of these statements by a nurse suggests that the nurse will display cultural competency when interviewing a patient from a different culture?
    1. "The patient's cultural background is very different from my own."
    2. "I think I'll try telling an ethnic joke as a way of establishing rapport."
    3. "I have to remember to document the patient's ethnic origin and religion in the record."
    4. "Before the interview I will take a few minutes to review actions that might offend a patient of his culture."

4. Which of the following statements will be most important to planning future community mental health services?
    1. The population over age 65 will decrease.
    2. More people will move out of cities and into rural areas.
    3. The U.S. population will decrease drastically by the year 2050.
    4. The U.S. population will become more diverse with regard to race and ethnicity.

5. Based on an understanding of current sociocultural risk factors for mental illness, the nurse assesses that which of the following patients is at highest risk for depression?
    1. A 26-year-old female
    2. A 72-year-old female
    3. A 33-year-old male
    4. A 57-year-old male

6. The mental health nurse is screening a group of older adult women for depression. The nurse concludes that the person at lowest risk based on sociocultural risk factor identification would be the one who:
    1. has high socioeconomic status.
    2. has a large number of children for support.
    3. attends church services a few times per year.
    4. belongs to a book club and plays cards each week.

7. The nurse beginning employment in an urban mental health center keeps which of the following in mind when working with individuals from ethnic minority groups?
    1. They delay seeking help until problems become intense or chronic.
    2. They tend to dislike utilizing community support systems.
    3. They tend to avoid utilizing family support systems.
    4. They characteristically do not engage in early termination from care.

8. When conducting an admission interview, the mental health nurse asks Ms. J. a series of questions related to her personal beliefs. When Ms. J. asks why these questions are being asked of her, which reply by the nurse would be best?
   1. "These questions are routine and are a mandatory part of the admission process."
   2. "The prime reason is that these questions help the staff to identify any specific health care practices that would conflict with your religious beliefs."
   3. "Mental health can be positively or negatively affected by personal belief systems, so it is important that your treatment plan be developed to be compatible with your beliefs."
   4. "These questions are necessary to give holistic nursing care, and they also help provide data that shows unit efforts at continuous quality improvement."

9. The nurse working in a mental health center would refer which of the following patients as the best candidate for a spirituality-based 12-step intervention program?
   1. A 58-year-old who has generalized anxiety disorder
   2. A 29-year-old who has an addiction to alcohol
   3. A 42-year-old who has agoraphobia
   4. A 35-year-old with a personality disorder

10. The student nurse mentions to the instructor, "The patients on the unit are mostly female. Does that mean that women suffer more mental illness than men?" The reply that shows the best understanding of the prevalence of mental illness is:
    1. "That's a very astute observation. You're right."
    2. "The prevalence is relatively the same for men and women."
    3. "As a matter of fact, mental illness is more prevalent among men."
    4. "That would be a good question for you to research and report back to the class."

11. During a team conference about a patient in the psychiatric unit at the local state hospital, the patient's wife states, "He's Irish, so I should have expected him to have a drinking problem." This statement is an example of:
    1. racism.
    2. intolerance.
    3. stereotyping.
    4. discrimination.

12. A task of an administrator of a culturally sensitive mental health system would be to:
    1. eliminate all staff bias.
    2. hire only minority health care providers.
    3. incorporate the value of culture into all levels of care.
    4. keep access to care open for the dominant ethnic, social, and religious groups.

13. While monitoring patient medications in an outpatient psychiatric setting, the nurse should keep in mind that Asian patients:
    1. experience fewer side effects when taking anticholinergic medications than do white patients taking the same dose.
    2. have less tendency to abuse alcohol with their medications than do whites.
    3. have extrapyramidal side effects at lower dosage levels than do other ethnic groups.
    4. exhibit better response to antidepressants and phenothiazine than do blacks.

14. The nurse working in a mental health center is beginning a therapeutic relationship with an elderly black patient. Which of the following should the nurse consider to be a central responsibility when planning for culturally competent treatment?
    1. Learn what the illness means to the patient and how the patient's beliefs can help mediate the stressors.
    2. Learn as much as possible about the beliefs of the patient and those of the extended family.
    3. Ask the patient about beliefs in a formal organized religion and daily or weekly religious practices that can be factored into treatment.
    4. Tell the patient that it will be important to examine together the belief systems of both the nurse and patient to be sure that they are congruent.

15. With regard to sociocultural risk factors, nursing care should be based on the premise that:
    1. risk for individual development of psychiatric disorder remains constant over time.
    2. all members of ethnic groups have the same risk for developing psychiatric disorder.
    3. risk factors interact constantly, so different factors become important at different times.
    4. sociocultural risk factors affect assessment and nursing-care planning more than implementation of care.

16. An elderly Hispanic woman has become depressed after the death of her husband. In applying knowledge of sociocultural risk factors, the nurse would anticipate that this patient is most likely to:
    1. be less able to adapt than before.
    2. recover and return to her pre-illness state.
    3. remain depressed, believing her husband's death is a punishment for past acts.
    4. suffer recurrences of depression because of cultural strain.

17. As a nurse assesses sociocultural risk factors for Ms. X., age 34, who is a single, poorly educated Mexican immigrant with three young children and who receives support from social services, he or she should be most concerned about the negative effects of:
    1. age.
    2. gender.
    3. disadvantagement.
    4. immigration.

18. Ms. T., a 32-year-old college graduate who weighs 150 pounds, is heavily sedated by the amount of lorazepam (Ativan) prescribed for anxiety reduction. Mr. H., a heavy laborer who is the same age and weight as Ms. T. and who has taken the same dose of Ativan, states that his anxiety is barely under control. What factor most likely accounts for this difference?
    1. Mr. H. is Hispanic, while Ms. T. is white.
    2. Social stratification and poverty make treatment more difficult.
    3. Men more often underrate the efficacy of antianxiety medication.
    4. Women more readily absorb benzodiazepines because they secrete less stomach acid.

19. Both Mr. S., a black man, and Ms. B., a white woman, are diagnosed as having schizophrenia, paranoid type. Both of these people are 42 years old and live at the poverty level. The age of onset of Mr. S.'s illness was 21, whereas Ms. B. was diagnosed at age 41. Mr. S. is an agnostic; Ms. B. is a Baptist. Mr. S.'s prognosis is listed as poor, while Ms. B.'s prognosis is given as favorable. What sociocultural factor accounts for Mr. S.'s less favorable prognosis?
    1. His religious belief system
    2. Ethnic Americans are less amenable to treatment.
    3. Males living in poverty receive less social support than women living in poverty.
    4. Mr. S. had an earlier onset of illness and has had a longer course of illness.

20. Minorities often delay seeking mental health treatment until problems are intense, chronic, and difficult to treat. What factor is not causative of the delay and therefore does not need to be addressed by community intervention efforts?
    1. Lack of medical insurance
    2. Lack of primary physicians for referrals
    3. Better support from family and ethnic community
    4. Language barrier and inability to negotiate an unfamiliar system

CHAPTER 9: ENVIRONMENTAL CONTEXT OF PSYCHIATRIC NURSING CARE

1. A review of the literature suggests that health professionals who are planning treatment initiatives should be most concerned at the national level with the burden of disease created by:
    1. violence and injury.
    2. environmental quality.
    3. behavioral health problems.
    4. irresponsible sexual behavior.

2. The psychiatric nurse who is conducting mental health screenings is aware that a patient with which of the following disorders is most likely to have a psychiatric disability based on current worldwide statistical data?
    1. Depression
    2. Obsessive-compulsive disorder
    3. Bipolar disorder
    4. Schizophrenia

3. To work effectively within the health care system, the nurse must understand the current interface between mental health care and the environment. Which statement accurately reflects this interface?
    1. The once simple system has grown from two to six parts, which has significantly complicated the interface.
    2. Biases on the part of providers have largely been abolished.
    3. Reimbursers and insurers are primarily concerned with protecting the patient's constitutional rights regarding access to care and treatment received.
    4. Families are becoming less concerned with education and empowerment for patients.

4. A nurse states, "I work in a managed behavioral health care setting." From this information, the listener understands that the nurse is involved in:
    1. health care reform.
    2. universal health care.
    3. health care for the underserved.
    4. treating mental and substance abuse disorders.

5. The psychiatric nurse working on an inpatient unit has volunteered for an institutional committee to address goal 1 for a transformed mental health system: Americans understand that mental health is essential to overall health. The nurse would expect that the focus of this group's work would be to:
   1. collaborate with the emergency department to treat mental health problems with the same urgency as physical health problems.
   2. protect and enhance the rights of people with mental illness.
   3. improve access to quality care that is culturally competent.
   4. develop and implement integrated electronic health record and personal health information systems.

6. A patient receiving mental health services complains that he doesn't like having to get a referral from his primary care physician in order to obtain mental health services. The nurse explains to the patient that this is a cost-control practice used in managed care that is described as:
   1. case management.
   2. utilization review.
   3. preadmission certification.
   4. gatekeeping.

7. A patient asks the nurse, "How do managed care systems control costs?" The best reply would be:
   1. "HMOs offer only inexpensive plans."
   2. "HMOs enroll only healthy populations."
   3. "HMOs insure Medicare and Medicaid patients exclusively to facilitate payment."
   4. "HMOs use preadmission certification, utilization review, and case management."

8. The patient tells the nurse, "I belong to an HMO that advertises being a capitated system. What does that mean?" The nurse should reply:
   1. "As a nurse, I know very little about health care finance."
   2. "You pay a sliding fee for each illness, and this fee is based on your monthly income."
   3. "You pay a fixed fee per month, and the HMO provides all medically necessary care."
   4. "It means the HMO will pay your physician or the hospital caring for you a flat fee for a particular episode of illness regardless of the number of days you are hospitalized or the number of office visits you make."

9. The nurse is responsible for surveying patients with respect to access to care. He or she will need to explain to patients that access means:
   1. the availability of health care.
   2. the degree to which services are comprehensive.
   3. the overall use of mental health services in a community.
   4. the convenience and ease of obtaining service and information.

10. In many rural communities, the ratio of consumers to doctors is higher than it is in cities. This is an example of:
    1. a health access problem in rural areas.
    2. a lack of compassion among physicians.
    3. reimbursement barriers in rural states.
    4. appropriate distribution of health care providers.

11. The facility administrator mentions to the mental health liaison nurse, "We may have to do away with our employee assistance program (EAP) because of its expense." The response by the nurse that shows the best understanding of the actual value of EAPs is:
    1. "That might be okay, because EAP screenings do duplicate the annual physical examinations our employees receive."
    2. "Most of our employees do not use the EAP because they fear confidentiality issues."
    3. "The EAP is actually cost-effective because of the prevention contributions, early detection, education, and skill training it provides."
    4. "Because EAPs focus primarily on substance abuse, their focus is very narrow. Broader programs should be funded first."

12. What effect has recent federal and state legislation had on treatment parity for physical and behavioral health problems?
    1. There is equal coverage or absolute parity.
    2. Physical health problems have stricter cost controls applied.
    3. Fewer patients are covered for behavioral health problems and stricter cost controls are applied to these problems.
    4. Because there are so many different state laws, few accurate conclusions about parity can be drawn.

13. A psychiatric nurse is considering becoming more active as an advocate for behavioral health system changes. Which topic should be considered?
    1. Abolishing HMOs
    2. Limiting consumer empowerment based on lack of expert knowledge
    3. Strengthening utilization review guidelines
    4. Providing more resources for preventive, rehabilitative, and chronic care mental health services

14. A case manager at the local mental health center is asked to evaluate the clinical appropriateness of a patient's current level of care. To do this, the case manager will try to assess:
    1. the type of service currently provided.
    2. the fitness of the client to whom the service is provided.
    3. the type, amount, and level of care needed to achieve positive outcomes.
    4. whether the level of client care is currently considered cost-effective.

15. The nurse works in an organization that provides an integrated behavioral continuum of care. This month she is assigned to the crisis clinic. The goal of treatment at this stage of the continuum is:
    1. remission.
    2. recovery.
    3. stabilization.
    4. optimal level of wellness.

16. The nurse working in an integrated behavioral continuum of care as an assignment officer decides that Mr. J., who has stopped taking his medication and has begun hearing voices, should be admitted for a short-term stay. Which is a suitable goal and expected outcome for Mr. J.?
    1. Goal, rehabilitation; outcome, attain optimal quality of life
    2. Goal, remission; outcome, symptom relief
    3. Goal, recovery; outcome, improved functioning
    4. Goal, safety; outcome, no risk for violence

17. Mr. G. tells the mental health nurse that he will soon be changing jobs and will need to choose a new health insurance plan. He asks the nurse what type of managed care plan will allow him the most flexibility in choosing health services and providers. Which type of plan will be most likely recommended by the nurse?
    1. Health maintenance organization (HMO)
    2. Independent practice organization (IPO)
    3. Point of service plan (POS)
    4. Preferred provider organization (PPO)

18. The nurse who advocates for consumer empowerment will seek to help psychiatric patients do which of the following?
    1. Achieve a sense of self-responsibility
    2. Comply with treatment programs determined by health professionals
    3. Understand that their viewpoints are largely the product of mental illness
    4. Utilize resources predominantly from the formal mental health system

19. Which nurse in a managed care setting has the greatest responsibility for allocating resources to an individual patient?
    1. Clinician
    2. Case manager
    3. Risk manager
    4. Patient educator

20. An emerging trend in psychiatric nursing related to cost controls imposed in the managed care environment is:
    1. reduced emphasis on utilization review.
    2. a marked increase in the use of risk managers.
    3. reduced use of patient and family educators to promote compliance.
    4. a shift from acute inpatient care positions to community-based positions.

21. A psychiatric nurse working in a rural area is serving on a committee that is studying how to better provide access to mental health services to people living at some distance from the agency. Using the recommendations from the Department of Health and Human Services report, *Achieving the promise: transforming mental health care in America*, the group should explore which of the following options as a means to improve access to care?
    1. An increased number of satellite centers
    2. Telehealth services
    3. Mobile mental health clinics
    4. Federal grants to supplement the agency budget for personnel

22. The psychiatric nurse reads in a patient's chart that the expected outcome of treatment is relief of symptoms. The nurse concludes that this patient is in which of the following stages of treatment in an integrated behavioral continuum of care?
    1. Crisis
    2. Acute
    3. Maintenance
    4. Health promotion

23. The psychiatric nurse hears in a patient-care conference that the goal of treatment is stabilization. The nurse concludes that this patient is in which of the following stages of treatment in an integrated behavioral continuum of care?
    1. Crisis
    2. Acute
    3. Maintenance
    4. Health promotion

24. A patient is being scheduled for transfer to a rehabilitation-oriented residential mental health program. The expected outcome to be formulated for the patient after transfer to the new care setting will be which of the following?
    1. No harm to self or others
    2. Symptom relief
    3. Improved functioning
    4. Attain optimal quality of life

CHAPTER 10: LEGAL AND ETHICAL CONTEXT OF PSYCHIATRIC NURSING CARE

1. A patient with severe depression was given all the facts about the risks, benefits, alternatives, and expected outcomes of ECT. She conferred privately with her family and then signed permission for ECT. Later she told the nurse, "I signed permission for treatment after my husband told me they could deport me if they can't cure my depression." The nurse should make the assessment that
    1. all the elements of informed consent were met.
    2. the patient's consent may have been coerced.
    3. the patient may not fully understand the risks and benefits.
    4. the patient is not competent to sign permission for treatment.

2. When the nurse is told by the patient that she consented to ECT out of fear of being deported, what nursing action is required?
    1. Reassure the patient that the decision is sound.
    2. Reprimand the husband for coercing his wife.
    3. Explain that consenting to treatment will not stop deportation.
    4. Document the comment and notify the physician immediately.

3. A voluntary patient mutilates herself whenever she leaves the unit. The nurse suggests use of four-point restraint to prevent the patient from further harming herself. What question should be considered before this measure is undertaken?
    1. Is this the least restrictive measure possible?
    2. Can four-point restraint be used for voluntary patients?
    3. What litigation is likely to follow from this action?
    4. What documentation will be necessary after restraint application?

4. At report, the nurse learns that a patient was admitted involuntarily on the previous shift. What assumption can the nurse make about the patient?
    1. He can leave the unit upon demand.
    2. For the first 48 hours, he can be given medication despite his objections.
    3. He has, through informed consent, agreed to accept treatment and participate fully in care planning.
    4. At the time of admission, he was considered to be an imminent danger to himself or to others or was deemed unable to provide for his own basic needs.

5. What is the staff nurse's duty when the patient tells the nurse that he plans to kill his spouse and her lover as soon as he is released from the hospital?
    1. Keep this information confidential.
    2. Immediately contact the spouse and the lover.
    3. File oral and written reports with the local police department.
    4. Document the information in the record and seek guidance from the supervisor.

6. A patient was admitted voluntarily to the psychiatric unit. To provide effective care, the nurse must understand that voluntary status confers the right of the patient to:
    1. have visitors at any time she wishes.
    2. come and go from the unit as she chooses.
    3. choose the nursing staff to be assigned to care for her.
    4. accept or refuse recommended treatment modalities.

7. The patient was admitted voluntarily to the psychiatric unit. To provide effective care, the nurse must understand that, if asked, she must tell the patient that she may:
    1. leave at any time by simply walking out the door.
    2. be retained in the hospital against her wishes.
    3. leave after giving written notice of intent to the staff.
    4. be discharged if evaluated through administrative hearings.

8. The patient's private psychiatrist has advised the patient that she needs psychiatric hospitalization. In the admitting department of a private psychiatric hospital, the patient fills out a standard admission form and agrees to receive treatment and abide by hospital rules. When the nurse reads the medical record, it will be apparent that this type of admission is known as:
    1. legal.
    2. informal.
    3. voluntary.
    4. involuntary.

9. The patient arrives at a state psychiatric hospital escorted by the police. They report that he was "disturbing the peace" by running naked in the street, striking out at others, and smashing car windows. He was hyperactive and belligerent when they took him into custody. The staff members on call are considering committing the patient to the hospital. Which is not a criterion for commitment that they should consider as they make their decision?
   1. He is dangerous to others.
   2. He was disruptive in the community.
   3. He is mentally ill and in need of treatment.
   4. He is unable to provide for his own basic needs.

10. The patient was admitted via emergency commitment after a serious suicide attempt. The nurse establishing the patient's plan of care knows that arrangements must be made to provide for diagnostic interviews and tests within the first:
   1. 96 hours of hospitalization.
   2. 36 hours of hospitalization.
   3. 7 days of hospitalization.
   4. 10 days of hospitalization.

11. Which of the following is the right upon which the nurse must be prepared to act for any patient, regardless of the type of commitment under which the patient is hospitalized?
   1. The right to consult a lawyer
   2. The right to release after 72 hours
   3. The right to choose agency caregivers
   4. The right to keep any and all personal effects at all times

12. A patient who is court-committed for an indefinite amount of time elopes from the hospital. The staff members notify the police, who then return the patient to the hospital. What is the most appropriate action for the staff to take?
   1. Discuss alternatives with the patient.
   2. Ask the patient to sign an "against medical advice" release.
   3. Request the patient to give written notice of his intent to leave.
   4. Readmit the patient, because the original commitment is still effective.

13. Two nurses are discussing the rights of hospitalized psychiatric patients. Which of their beliefs is erroneous and should not be the basis for nursing action?
   1. The hospital is responsible for the patient's safety.
   2. If a committed patient is judged to be incompetent, he retains the right of habeas corpus.
   3. Privileged communication does not apply to hospital charts, so they can be used in court.
   4. Confidentiality allows for disclosure of information about a psychiatric patient to insurers and law enforcement agencies without signed permission of the patient.

14. Which action by a nurse violates a right of a psychiatric patient?
   1. The nurse pays a patient minimum wage for working in the hospital kitchen.
   2. The nurse confiscates letters to the local newspaper written by a committed patient.
   3. A nurse takes an expensive watch from a patient's room and places it in the hospital safe.
   4. A patient with paranoid delusions about his family is told that if he makes a will, it would not be valid.

15. A patient tells the nurse, "My daughter had me ruled incompetent. I'm going to ask the doctor to reverse that ruling." The nurse's reply should be predicated on the fact that:
   1. a separate court hearing is required to reverse the ruling.
   2. incompetence is associated with specific medical diagnoses.
   3. competency is automatically restored on discharge from the hospital.
   4. competency is not a major issue, because someone who has been ruled incompetent retains the right to vote, marry, and divorce.

16. A psychiatric nurse working in a community health center receives a call asking whether a Ms. J. has been a patient in the facility. How should the nurse respond?
   1. The nurse should ask why the information is being sought.
   2. The nurse should suggest that the caller speak to Ms. J.'s therapist.
   3. The nurse should state that he or she is unable to give any information to the caller.
   4. The nurse should state that Ms. J. has been seen at the center but should give no further information.

17. While making a home visit, a community health nurse sees evidence that the 8-year-old daughter of her patient has been abused. What rationale should be the basis for his or her nursing action?
   1. Privileged communication prevents the nurse from reporting it.
   2. Documenting the evidence in the medical record is sufficient.
   3. A federal ruling requires that she report the suspected abuse.
   4. A signed release from the patient is needed before action can be taken.

18. A patient is about to receive electroconvulsive therapy (ECT) when the nurse sees that the patient has not signed a consent form for treatment. Which fact should determine the action the nurse takes?
    1. Verbal consent by the patient is sufficient.
    2. A patient is needed to witness the consent form.
    3. Failure to obtain the patient's written consent can result in a lawsuit.
    4. Permission has already been granted because the patient signed the hospital's standard admission form.

19. A 22-year-old female patient with a diagnosis of borderline personality disorder is manipulative and very disruptive to the hospital staff. Although she is not assessed to be dangerous to herself or others, she has created many problems on the unit and is clearly not making any therapeutic progress. Staff members want her to accept medication, but she consistently refuses. Nursing actions must be guided by the realization that legally this patient can:
    1. refuse treatment.
    2. receive forced treatment if the treatment team concurs.
    3. be medicated if her family signs permission for treatment.
    4. be coerced to accept treatment recommendations by threatening loss of privileges.

20. A nurse was sued for malpractice but proven not liable. Which fact from the case was decisive in determining its outcome?
    1. Negligence was implied.
    2. The nurse had a duty to the patient.
    3. The nurse failed to give competent care.
    4. No harm was actually suffered by the patient.

21. A patient was tried for the murder of his wife and child. He was found guilty but mentally ill (GBMI). A psychiatric nurse is asked, "Does that mean he'll be walking the streets after a short hospitalization?" Which reply shows the best understanding of GBMI?
    1. "You sound as though you are angry with the way our criminal justice system works."
    2. "A person found guilty but mentally ill will be treated but will serve his sentence."
    3. "He will be hospitalized and released when he is no longer mentally ill."
    4. "It will depend on whether the American Law Institute's Test was applied or whether the Irresistible Impulse Test was used."

22. The parents of a young man with schizophrenia ask whether he is likely to become violent. The best answer the nurse can give is that the vast majority of mentally ill individuals are:
    1. somewhat more dangerous than ordinary people.
    2. definitely more violence-prone than others on the street.
    3. no more dangerous than other individuals in the population.
    4. unpredictable and therefore considerably more dangerous than others in the population.

23. The nurse can identify all but one of the patients described below as having a higher-than-normal potential for violence directed at others. Which patient is least apt to display violent behavior directed at others?
    1. The patient who is severely depressed after the loss of his job
    2. The patient who has a history of assaulting people when "the voices" command him to do so
    3. The patient who has been noncompliant with his psychotropic medication and whose manic behavior has escalated
    4. The patient who has an antisocial personality disorder and who has been using amphetamines

24. The patient signed a sales contract to purchase a new home and a week later she was voluntarily hospitalized for treatment of depression. Her sales contract is now most likely:
    1. invalid.
    2. still valid.
    3. in litigation.
    4. not something for which she can be held responsible.

25. Ms. M. is in the process of being involuntarily committed and demands to be evaluated by her own private psychiatrist. To preserve the patient's rights, the treatment team must:
    1. proceed with the commitment.
    2. have her seen by the unit psychiatrist.
    3. allow her access to her own private psychiatrist.
    4. not release her, even if her psychiatrist disagrees with the proceedings.

CHAPTER 11: FAMILIES AS RESOURCES, CAREGIVERS, AND COLLABORATORS

1. A female patient reports during a mental health assessment that she lives with her two children, her sister, and her sister's three children. To use the most precise documentation, the nurse documents that the patient is part of a(n):
    1. nuclear family.
    2. extended family.
    3. traditional family.
    4. household.

2. The nurse determines during an assessment interview with a female patient that which of the following patient data is a positive indicator of family functioning?
   1. The 12-year-old daughter occasionally has an asthma attack when the patient and her husband argue.
   2. The husband leaves for a few days and gambles when he and the patient have a serious fight.
   3. The 12-year-old daughter has one daily and one weekly household chore to complete.
   4. The patient calls her mother often to get her input on daily decisions such as what to purchase at the market for family meals.

3. The nurse notes during a patient interview that which of the following patient data could indicate a potential problem with the functioning of the patient's family and warrants further assessment?
   1. The patient and spouse resolve an argument on their own, although it often takes a few hours.
   2. The patient visits her aging mother and father who live an hour away every other week.
   3. The patient takes weekly art class and a weekly dance class.
   4. The patient often "grounds" the children for misbehavior in an attempt to raise them "the right way."

4. The nurse anticipates that which of the following aspects of a family is least likely to be determined or influenced by cultural or ethnic differences?
   1. Beliefs governing family relationships
   2. Educational level its members are allowed to achieve
   3. How outside events are perceived and interpreted
   4. Family norms regarding what is right and wrong

5. The nurse constructing a family genogram for an adult patient would not necessarily include which of the following family members mentioned by the patient?
   1. 28-year-old brother
   2. 4-year-old stepson
   3. 43-year-old aunt
   4. 91-year-old great grandmother

6. Which item would not be included by the nurse when utilizing the family APGAR tool as an assessment measure of family roles and relationships?
   1. Decisions
   2. Nurturing
   3. Recreational activities
   4. Emotional experiences

7. The psychiatric nurse working within a competence paradigm would emphasize which of the following when working with a 33-year-old patient with an anxiety disorder?
   1. Use of natural family support networks
   2. Prevention of negative outcomes
   3. The view of anxiety disorder as a disease
   4. Treatment of family dysfunction

8. A nurse would conclude that another nurse working on the psychiatric unit approaches working with mentally ill patients from a pathology paradigm after hearing the nurse make which of the following statements?
   1. "It's understandable that Ms. J. keeps getting readmitted. The family dysfunction that she has to cope with must be such a burden after each discharge."
   2. "Ms. J. made some important gains during the group session today. She was able to identify two strategies for coping with stressors to use after discharge."
   3. "During our session today, I hope to be able to get Ms. J. to share more about the cultural background of her and her family."
   4. "Ms. J. has not yet fully grasped that she is a full partner in her care and in setting goals for functioning after discharge."

9. The psychiatric nurse is sharing information with a patient and family about psychoeducational programs offered by the National Alliance for the Mentally Ill (NAMI). The nurse explains that which of the following is the overarching primary purpose of such programs?
   1. Reducing hospital readmission rates
   2. Enhancing compliance with medication therapy
   3. Evaluating effectiveness of therapy
   4. Providing education and support

10. The psychiatric nurse is helping to plan an educational program for families of mentally ill patients. The title of the program is *Enhancing Personal and Family Effectiveness*. Which of the following topics should the nurse include in developing this program?
    1. Hygiene and appearance
    2. Legal issues
    3. Conflict resolution
    4. Medications

11. Which of the following components would not be part of a comprehensive program for working with families of mentally ill patients?
    1. Skill
    2. Social
    3. Family process
    4. Debate

12. The nurse working with the mentally ill self-assesses for which of the following beliefs that is a barrier to educating patients' families about becoming directly involved in the patients' treatment?
    1. The family system perpetuates the patient's illness.
    2. Alliance with the family will not interfere with patient confidentiality.
    3. An alliance with the family will not threaten the nurse's relationship with the patient.
    4. Services provided to families are as important as the services provided to patients.

13. The clinician mentions to a staff nurse working with mentally ill patients, "I think you should be aware of the symbolic interactionism theoretical model. It will help explain:
    1. why schizophrenic patients hear voices."
    2. why bipolar clients have interpersonal relationship difficulties."
    3. the meaning that the experience of living with a mentally ill person has for families."
    4. the relative lack of support for mentally ill patients of certain American sub-cultures."

14. Which of the following would be the lowest priority resource utilized by the nurse looking to provide education and involvement for families of mentally ill patients?
    1. Literature from the National Alliance for the Mentally Ill
    2. Policies and procedures of the managed care agency
    3. Accreditation criteria for the Joint Commission on Accreditation of Healthcare Organizations
    4. American Psychiatric Nurses Association Position Papers on Collaboration

15. Which of the following questions would be best if the nurse is seeking to understand the experiences of the family of Ms. Y., a patient with schizophrenia, using symbolic interactionism?
    1. "What situations create stress in your family at this time?"
    2. "What are the transportation costs of traveling to and from therapy sessions?"
    3. "Is there enough money to pay the family bills and pay for therapy also?"
    4. "Have things become better at home since Y. was discharged this last time?"

16. Ms. R. has frequent recurring bouts of bipolar illness. She is separated from her husband and lives in an apartment with her 4-year-old daughter. Her mother and her sister are living and well. Which member of Ms. R.'s family is likely to be most profoundly and negatively affected?
    1. Her mother
    2. Her daughter
    3. Her husband
    4. Her adult sister

17. Nurse C. is in the process of hospitalizing a patient who was brought to the unit by his family. When dealing with the family, Nurse C. should keep in mind that the family:
    1. may also be in need of support.
    2. may be relieved that someone else is responsible.
    3. will soon forget how the staff communicated with them.
    4. must be informed that confidentiality prevents the sharing of information.

18. During an outpatient clinic interview with K, a persistently mentally ill patient who has schizophrenia and who is accompanied by his mother, Nurse G. should keep in mind that:
    1. K's mother is part of his problem.
    2. K's mother is a potential source of valid information.
    3. the interview should focus on medication compliance.
    4. K's secondary symptoms make obtaining valid information difficult.

19. To plan and budget for preventive services, the nurse in charge of the community mental health center has reviewed the records to discern how many families received services in the current year. To estimate the need for the coming year, the nurse should:
    1. increase the allocation, because most eligible families are underserved.
    2. decrease the allocation, because most eligible families are overserved.
    3. keep the allocation the same and place an emphasis on inpatient care.
    4. ask for a consultant to ascertain community interest in preventive services.

20. L. is being returned to the hospital for a recurrence of bipolar disorder. Nurse W. notes that the well sibling who lives with and currently accompanies the patient doesn't say much. The nurse should act on the thought that the sibling:
    1. may be quiet by nature.
    2. is probably thankful that he's well.
    3. may be feeling hurt, anger, or resentment.
    4. may not have very much to be concerned about.

21. The nursing action for nurse H. that is critical in engaging in effective collaboration with the family of Ms. K., a mentally ill patient, is:
    1. utilizing skills in the area of family dynamics.
    2. teaching problem-solving strategies.
    3. addressing the issue of patient confidentiality.
    4. helping the family access entitlements and rehabilitation.

22. Nurse A. has established a helping relationship with the family of a mentally ill patient. This relationship should focus
    1. only on the patient and his needs.
    2. exclusively on educational sessions.
    3. on maximizing family concerns with burden and grief.
    4. on helping the family members meet their own needs.

23. When a family is having particular difficulty adjusting to the burden of having a mentally ill family member, which of the following is the best resource the nurse can suggest to the family?
    1. AMA
    2. NAMI
    3. APNA
    4. A family therapist

CHAPTER 12: IMPLEMENTING THE NURSING PROCESS: STANDARDS OF CARE AND PROFESSIONAL PERFORMANCE

1. A nurse who is planning to teach a patient about the effects and side effects of his medication should base her plan on the knowledge that learning is more effective when:
    1. patients are actively included in the process.
    2. topics are introduced without relating them to need.
    3. nurses establish goals for learning on behalf of the patient.
    4. patients have responsibility for directing the teaching-learning process.

2. The nurse has interviewed Ms. W., who was a reluctant participant in the interview and who answered questions with minimal responses and rarely looked at the nurse. When documenting baseline data collected in the interview, the nurse should include:
    1. interview content only.
    2. a description of the process of the interview.
    3. both the content and the process of the interview.
    4. both factual data about the patient and the nurse's emotional reaction.

3. While gathering a baseline history about a patient, the nurse is told by a team social worker that the patient "acts weird and has bad hygiene." The nurse's responsibility is to:
    1. accept the data without question.
    2. form an impression based on his or her own data.
    3. document the impression of the team social worker.
    4. discuss the social worker's impression with the patient during the interview.

4. To obtain the clearest clinical information about a patient, the nurse who has used several secondary sources including the patient's spouse and the report of the admitting psychiatrist, will seek validation from:
    1. the patient.
    2. psychiatric nursing textbooks.
    3. the patient's extended family.
    4. the use of psychiatric behavioral rating scales.

5. Nurses understand DSM-IV. If physicians wish to understand a comparable aspect of nursing, they should seek understanding of:
    1. nursing diagnoses.
    2. the nursing process.
    3. behavioral rating scales.
    4. computerized medical records.

6. Goals for Ms. W. are listed below. Which goal should be given the highest priority?
    1. Reduction of anxiety
    2. Alleviation of depression
    3. Enhancement of self-esteem
    4. Protection from self-destructive impulses

7. Ms. B., a nurse who is new to the mental health setting, is having difficulty writing meaningful outcome criteria. Her mentor could suggest that she look at which of the following sources?
    1. NIC
    2. NOC
    3. DSM-IV
    4. NANDA Classification of Nursing Diagnoses

8. Which of the following is a well-written short-term goal for a socially withdrawn patient who tells the nurse he wishes to reduce his social isolation?
    1. Patient will be more outgoing.
    2. Patient will become more independent.
    3. Patient will express desire to go shopping.
    4. By day 3, patient will participate in one unit activity.

9. As the nurse formulates expected outcomes for a patient who will be taking an antidepressant after discharge, consideration should be given to including the three domains of:
   1. content, affect, and process.
   2. cognitive, affective, and psychomotor.
   3. conscious, unconscious, and preconscious.
   4. conscious, actualized, and psychological.

10. A patient is admitted with a diagnosis of bipolar disorder, manic phase. He is extremely hyperactive, agitated, talkative, and emotionally labile. Which of the following would be a high priority nursing diagnosis?
    1. Risk for injury related to extreme hyperactivity
    2. Disturbed thought processes related to manic state
    3. Impaired social interaction related to excessive verbalization
    4. Impaired sensory-perception related to biochemical alterations

11. If a patient-centered goal answers the question of "What?" the nursing care plan answers the questions:
    1. "How and why?"
    2. "Where and when?"
    3. "How and to whom?"
    4. "Where and to whom?"

12. Nurse J. is working with a depressed patient. To help the patient translate insight into action, a major challenge for Nurse J. will be to:
    1. promote self-care activities.
    2. consult appropriate resources.
    3. build adequate incentives to change.
    4. identify ineffective behavior patterns.

13. Nursing interventions that have the greatest validity are those that:
    1. are used by nurse clinicians.
    2. are prescribed by physicians.
    3. have been investigated by nurse researchers.
    4. are based on evidence of the efficacy of the intended treatment.

14. Nursing behaviors associated with the implementation phase of the nursing process are concerned with:
    1. self-analysis.
    2. participating in quality improvement activities.
    3. carrying out interventions and generating alternatives.
    4. comparing patient responses and expected outcomes.

15. The nurse clinician is attempting to explain the evaluation phase of the nursing process to a student. Which statement would help the student grasp the essentials?
    1. "It is a continuous, active process."
    2. "Patient and family participation is optional."
    3. "It takes place at the time of termination of services."
    4. "It is optional, based on patient readiness."

16. Which statement about the relationship of the Stuart Stress Adaptation Model and the patient assessment data is identified in Standard I?
    1. There is no relationship.
    2. The patient data to be identified is reflected by the components of the model.
    3. The patient data to be identified reflects several items not included in the model.
    4. The patient data to be identified is incomplete according to the components of the model.

17. Which action demonstrates nursing accountability?
    1. Volunteering to serve on a hospital committee
    2. Notifying the head nurse that a medication error was made
    3. Planning patient-care strategies for a newly admitted patient
    4. Coordinating a patient-centered conference for the health care team

18. A new male staff nurse has set a goal for himself of gaining greater autonomy over his practice. The two major components of autonomy that he will need to focus on are:
    1. valuing reciprocal interactions and taking responsibility for actions.
    2. exercising control over nursing tasks and participating in decision making.
    3. identifying ethical components of practice and exploring options.
    4. assuming responsibility for personal actions and the attitude of integrity and vigilance.

19. A new psychiatric staff nurse is asked to be a member of the Quality Improvement (QI) Committee. The nurse should be motivated to agree to do this because:
    1. QI is a requirement of one's job.
    2. evaluation of quality of care is a standard of professional performance.
    3. salary increments depend on performance variables such as committee work.
    4. QI is an activity mandated by the Joint Commission on Accreditation of Health Care Organizations.

20. A staff nurse is told in orientation that he will receive performance appraisals in two forms. He can expect that these will be:
    1. administrative and clinical.
    2. professional and interpersonal.
    3. nursing and collaborative practice.
    4. intradisciplinary and interdisciplinary.

21. A staff nurse is told at orientation that the department has a clinical advancement program in place. Upon what criteria is advancement usually based?
    1. Desire for professional growth
    2. Acceptance of peer feedback
    3. Attainment of an advanced degree in a nursing-related field
    4. Increased critical thinking ability and advanced application of nursing skills

22. As Ms. J., a mental health nurse, begins supervised clinical work with patients, she should keep in mind that which of the following is the major difference between supervision and therapy?
    1. Therapy is more intensive.
    2. Supervision extends to all aspects of life, whereas therapy is limited to problem areas.
    3. Supervision teaches psychotherapeutic skills, whereas therapy changes personal coping patterns.
    4. Therapy utilizes transferences, whereas supervision focuses on only personal limitations.

23. Nurse J. registers for a DSM-IV update workshop. This is an example of adherence to the standard of professional performance that refers to:
    1. education.
    2. ethical standards.
    3. resource utilization.
    4. performance appraisal.

24. According to the nursing standard related to research, Nurse V., a beginning psychiatric-mental health nurse with an associate's degree, can be expected to:
    1. engage with other staff in the research process.
    2. use research findings to improve clinical practice.
    3. plan small, independent, data-gathering research projects.
    4. collaborate in proposal development and data collection and analysis.

25. During a team conference, a nurse brings up the fact that the antidepressant being considered for a patient is very expensive and that the patient may have difficulty paying for the medication after discharge. This is an example of implementing:
    1. collaboration.
    2. participation.
    3. discharge.
    4. resource utilization.

26. Ms. M., a psychiatric nurse who has been a staff nurse for several years, seems to value other nursing roles less than she values her own. She is heard calling nurse educators "the ones who sit in ivory towers," and she refers to nurse administrators and researchers as "the irrelevant ones." This nurse can be assessed as having a problem with:
    1. ethics.
    2. education.
    3. collegiality.
    4. resource use.

CHAPTER 13: MENTAL HEALTH PROMOTION AND ILLNESS PREVENTION

1. A couple that has sought genetic counseling about bipolar disorder asks the nurse, "The geneticist mentioned that if we have a child we should next consider the avenue of primary prevention. What is primary prevention?" The nurse should begin by replying that primary prevention is considered to be the reduction of the:
    1. severity of mental disorders.
    2. duration of mental disorders.
    3. incidence of mental disorders.
    4. prevalence of mental disorders.

2. The psychiatric nurse has responsibility to assist in assessing the need for mental health services at the clinic. When trying to estimate the number of clients with bipolar disorder in the community, the nurse should place highest priority on using which of the following data-gathering techniques?
    1. Statistics from local public reports about race, marital status, population density, and substance abuse
    2. Epidemiological studies that indicate incidence and prevalence of disease
    3. Community forums that solicit data shared by patients and families
    4. Use of key informants, such as local social service personnel, nurses, and physicians

3. A nursing student asks the psychiatric nurse, "What is the essential difference between the nursing prevention model and the medical prevention model?" Which of the following responses by the nurse is most accurate?
   1. "The medical model targets universal populations; the nursing model targets a selective population."
   2. "The medical model assumes that all people are at equal risk; the nursing model attempts to identify those who are more vulnerable."
   3. "The medical model attempts to identify the most likely cause of the disease; the nursing model stresses that mental disorders are multicausal."
   4. "The medical model offers a continuum of nonspecific preventive measures; the nursing model offers one specific, tested, preventive measure."

4. A psychiatric nurse working in the community would foster which of the following traits or abilities in the health education of patients for primary prevention of mental health problems?
   1. Networking
   2. Resilience
   3. Trust
   4. Motivation

5. The nurse is working with the following patients diagnosed with depression. Which of them has the greatest likelihood of recovery based on self-efficacy?
   1. A 22-year-old who might begin taking a few courses at a local community college
   2. A 20-year-old living at home who believes her mother excessively tries to control her life
   3. A 23-year-old who works part time in a video game store for a living
   4. A 26-year-old who recently started his own business

6. A nurse who describes herself as working in tertiary prevention of mental disorders would achieve particular satisfaction in her work when:
   1. early case finding results in prompt treatment of an individual's mental disorder.
   2. health education and social support prevent the need for the hospitalization of an individual.
   3. rehabilitative activities reduce the disability associated with an individual's mental disorder.
   4. a preretirement counseling program is established by the psychiatric nurses interest group.

7. Ms. W. is a nurse who works in community mental health. During the course of her work, she identifies a Hispanic neighborhood group as having low self-efficacy and being particularly susceptible to a number of stressors. In which phase of the nursing process did this activity take place?
   1. Planning
   2. Evaluation
   3. Assessment
   4. Implementation

8. Of what concern is it when Nurse W., a community mental health nurse, identifies a Hispanic neighborhood group as having low self-efficacy? People with low self-efficacy:
   1. often engage in antisocial or criminal behavior.
   2. use more community health resources than their share.
   3. are motivated, handle stress well, and have low vulnerability to depression.
   4. give up in the face of difficulty, recover slowly from setbacks, and easily fall victim to depression.

9. When Nurse W., a community mental health nurse, elaborates on intervention strategies designed to increase self-efficacy among members of a Hispanic neighborhood group, a realistic primary prevention goal would be:
   1. elimination of mental illness in the community.
   2. resolving social problems in the community.
   3. reducing stress and suffering in the group.
   4. reducing the incidence of depression in the group.

10. The elaboration of intervention strategies designed to increase self-efficacy among members of a Hispanic neighborhood group is conducted in the phase of the nursing process identified as:
    1. planning.
    2. evaluation.
    3. assessment.
    4. implementation.

11. The nursing primary prevention model suggests there are many reasons why some people develop mental disorders. A nurse assessing a person who is deemed to be at high risk will find that, compared with others, the person has:
    1. fewer stressors.
    2. more protective factors.
    3. unusual developmental tasks.
    4. inadequate coping mechanisms.

12. In the event that a vaccine is developed to prevent schizophrenia, which population group would be selected to first receive it?
    1. The universal population
    2. The indicated population
    3. The developmental population
    4. The epidemiological population

13. Which person can be identified as vulnerable to the development of psychiatric illness based on sociocultural factors?
    1. Ann, 16, whose mother has bipolar disorder
    2. Juana, 67, who is poor and has no social support system
    3. Keith, 55, who has retired with full pay from his job as a high school teacher
    4. Jim, 24, who was raised by his grandfather after his parents died in a plane crash

14. To effectively use the nursing primary prevention model, it is most important for Nurse T. to have knowledge of:
    1. personality types.
    2. psychiatric medications.
    3. normal growth and development.
    4. the DSM-IV diagnostic categories.

15. A nurse working in a community health agency wishes to implement a primary preventive program in mental health for the elderly. To do so, the nurse will carry out each of the activities listed below. Which one should be the initial priority?
    1. Elaboration of specific preventive strategies
    2. Identification of a stressor that precipitates maladaptive responses
    3. Application of selected nursing interventions to enhance adaptation
    4. Determination of effectiveness of nursing activities and consideration of short-term and long-term outcomes

16. A psychiatric nurse is working with patients in a health education group on strategies to improve anger management. The nurse would best evaluate the effectiveness of this intervention by determining changes in the patient's:
    1. knowledge of people and events that trigger anger.
    2. coping skills.
    3. opinion about his or her self-worth.
    4. underlying mental health disorder that is exhibited by the symptom of anger.

17. Which nursing strategy of primary prevention in mental health is based on the assumption that many maladaptive responses result from a lack of competence derived from a perceived lack of control over one's own life, ineffective coping strategies, and subsequent loss of self-esteem?
    1. Social support
    2. Health education
    3. Group intervention
    4. Environmental change

18. The nurse working with adolescents would most likely refer them to which of the following types of groups that deals with issues of importance to that age group?
    1. Peer relationships
    2. Normal growth and development
    3. Childrearing
    4. Career selection

19. Nurse R. is working in primary prevention and focuses on increasing gang members' problem-solving and coping skills. This is an example of:
    1. crime reduction.
    2. community service.
    3. competency building.
    4. environmental manipulation.

20. Which intervention would be least helpful in achieving the goal of improving the social support system of an individual at risk for developing maladaptive coping responses?
    1. Hospitalization
    2. Encouraging participation in a self-help group
    3. Explaining to concerned others how they can help
    4. Providing services in a caring and supportive manner

21. An individual considering going to a self-help group mentions to the nurse, "I think I might go to the bereavement self-help group meeting at the community center, but I have some reservations. What if I don't like the group? What if I'm required to change in ways I don't want to?" The nurse can help most by replying:
    1. "Perhaps you're not quite ready to join a group. Give yourself a few more weeks."
    2. "These are natural concerns. Trying something new activates all our insecurities."
    3. "Most group members will feel just like you do. They will help you hold your own against aggressive group members."
    4. "Self-help groups are led by members like yourself, and each member has sole responsibility for making changes in his or her own life."

22. The patient asks the mental health nurse, "I've heard a lot about how self-help groups may be useful for people like me who have difficulty managing stress. Can you tell me more about what these groups are like?" Which of the following responses by the nurse is best?
    1. "Each of these groups is led by a therapist who specializes in the focus of the group."
    2. "These groups are supportive and educational in nature rather than therapeutic."
    3. "These groups provide a forum to which people can bring a variety of mental health issues and concerns."
    4. "These groups are for-profit and generally require small but mandatory membership fees."

CHAPTER 14: CRISIS INTERVENTION

1. The patient comes to the mental health clinic complaining of insomnia, irritability, increased tension, and headaches. His symptoms began a week ago after he lost his job. He states that he is concerned that he and his family may have to relocate. He is most likely experiencing:
    1. an anxiety reaction.
    2. a situational crisis.
    3. a maturational crisis.
    4. an adjustment disorder.

2. A jet plane carrying 140 passengers crashes in a nearby community. One can reliably predict that the survivors, families, and community will experience:
    1. a situational crisis.
    2. problem resolution.
    3. adjustment disorders.
    4. psychological equilibrium.

3. A patient comes to the mental health center and relates that he has been feeling very anxious since graduating from high school a week ago. He is having difficulty concentrating and feels shaky. This typifies:
    1. a situational crisis.
    2. a maturational crisis.
    3. psychological equilibrium.
    4. a pseudopsychological crisis.

4. A patient comes to the mental health center after being held hostage during a bank robbery 2 days ago. He relates a number of symptoms, including intrusive thoughts, nightmares, and feelings of helplessness. The nurse should consider the possibility that he is experiencing:
    1. a situational crisis.
    2. a maturational crisis.
    3. a developmental crisis.
    4. a pseudopsychological crisis.

5. The patient experiencing intrusive thoughts, nightmares, and feelings of helplessness after a hostage experience begins crisis intervention therapy. He asks, "How long before I will feel like myself again?" The reply that shows the best understanding of the parameters of crisis intervention therapy would patient:
    1. "My best guess would be 6 months."
    2. "This type of therapy usually lasts 6 weeks or less."
    3. "The experience may result in permanent changes in how you feel."
    4. "No one can really say. It may be as soon as a week, but it may take up to a year."

6. A patient, age 19, recently gave birth. Since bringing the baby home, she says she has felt apathetic, fatigued, and helpless. She cares adequately for the baby, but states, "I don't know what's expected of me." No cognitive impairment or thought disorder is noted. The nurse should consider the possibility that the patient may benefit from:
    1. crisis intervention.
    2. short hospitalization.
    3. neuroleptic medication.
    4. antidepressant medication.

7. The outcome of crisis intervention therapy that should be identified for a patient who has been apathetic, fatigued, and feeling helpless since the recent birth of her baby, is that she will:
    1. experience reduced anxiety.
    2. undergo personality change.
    3. identify the precipitating event.
    4. return to the precrisis level of functioning.

8. Ms. G. is being seen for crisis intervention. The precipitating event was receiving a poor job evaluation. The self-esteem need that nursing assessment will most likely reveal will be related to:
    1. dependency.
    2. role mastery.
    3. biological functioning.
    4. unmet financial responsibility.

9. When the crisis clinic nurse asks a patient, "Who takes care of you when you are sick?" the nurse is exploring the balancing factors of:
    1. situational support.
    2. problem resolution.
    3. coping mechanisms.
    4. perception of the event.

10. A crisis worker who is involved with helping a victim of spousal abuse move from home to a shelter for battered women is helping the patient meet a need related to:
    1. dependency.
    2. role mastery.
    3. biological function.
    4. financial responsibility.

11. To understand the effects of a precipitating event such as the loss of one's job, the nurse must assess the:
    1. patient's appraisal of the event.
    2. perception of the support group.
    3. patient's awareness or lack of awareness of options.
    4. patient's own feelings about his or her response to the situation.

12. Survivors of a hurricane are grieving the loss of loved ones and homes. Which level of crisis intervention would be most appropriate for the nurse to use?
    1. General support
    2. Generic approach
    3. Individual approach
    4. Environmental manipulation

13. A critically ill postsurgical patient tells the nurse about his emergency surgery and the long-term postoperative course he expects. As he speaks, the nurse notices that his speech lacks affect. Which technique of crisis intervention would be most therapeutic to use initially?
    1. Catharsis
    2. Manipulation
    3. Raising self-esteem
    4. Reinforcement of behavior

14. A nurse working with a mother in crisis suggests that the mother send two of her children to stay with their grandmother temporarily. This is an example of:
    1. reducing dependency.
    2. environmental manipulation.
    3. reducing the children's stressors.
    4. increasing contact with the extended family.

15. You have worked as a psychiatric nurse with a crisis team for many years. A patient with whom you are familiar because of past crises comes to the clinic stating that he has just lost his job and is at an age at which he is afraid he will no longer be able to find work in his career field. As the psychiatric nurse will probably use which level of approach for this patient?
    1. Environmental manipulation
    2. Generic approach
    3. Individual approach
    4. General support

16. A nurse working with a patient in individual crisis intervention would characterize the approaches used as:
    1. open-ended.
    2. passive and indirect.
    3. active, focused, and explorative.
    4. psychoanalytic-based techniques.

17. While working with a patient in crisis, Nurse G. attempts to help the patient identify the relationship between the event precipitating the crisis and the patient's subsequent feelings and behaviors. This is an example of:
    1. clarification.
    2. support of defenses.
    3. reinforcement of behavior.
    4. raising the patient's self-esteem.

18. Nurse G. notes that a client is using alcohol each evening as a means of coping with the loneliness associated with his recent divorce. Nurse G. points this out to the patient and encourages him to join an exercise club or try jogging in lieu of drinking. Nurse G.'s approach is called:
    1. clarification.
    2. support of defenses.
    3. raising self-esteem.
    4. reinforcement of behavior.

19. Nurse G., a crisis intervention clinic nurse, responds to a patient who has many concerns about his marriage by saying, "You seem to be very committed to the success of your marriage. I think you have the ability to work through these issues and end up with a stronger relationship." The technique used is:
    1. clarification.
    2. support of defenses.
    3. raising self-esteem.
    4. exploration of solutions.

20. The patient was a driver of a car that was car-jacked. She was released after 12 hours. In the crisis clinic, she repeatedly states, "I can't believe it happened to me!" She describes feeling anxious and afraid of strangers and she wonders whether she will ever be able to drive again. The nurse's interventions should target:
    1. basic needs and confusion.
    2. repression and sublimation.
    3. denial, anxiety, and self-efficacy.
    4. low self-esteem and suicide-potential.

21. The patient was the driver of a car that struck and killed a child who darted into the street. He tells the nurse, "I killed a child! I'm haunted by the sight of his body being thrown into the air. If I hadn't been drinking I might have been able to stop. I don't know how I can go on living with myself!" An avenue the crisis nurse should be sure to explore is:
    1 suicidal risk.
    2. hallucinations.
    3. recent drug use.
    4. the patient's physical condition.

22. When a patient in crisis intervention therapy alludes to the possibility of self-harm, the nurse should:
    1. arrange for constant 1:1 supervision for the patient.
    2. advise the patient that hospitalization will be necessary.
    3. tell the patient that he or she is too intelligent to consider only that solution.
    4. formalize a contract in which the patient agrees not to harm himself or herself.

23. When evaluating care of a crisis patient, a psychiatric nurse must remember that one of the primary goals of crisis intervention is to:
    1. support the patient through the process.
    2. help the patient return to the precrisis state.
    3. give the patient new coping mechanisms.
    4. attentively listen to the patient to help reduce the stress level of the patient.

24. Which statement made by a person in a crisis state indicates the presence of a balancing factor?
    1. "I've been drinking more than usual."
    2. "I've always been a loner. I don't need other people."
    3. "I pray when things get tough. It's always helped me survive trouble."
    4. "My husband went to the store. I don't believe it when they tell me he's dead."

25. A variety of crisis intervention methodologies are available in contemporary society depending on the needs of patients. Some of the methodologies are:
    1. available only during non-daytime hours.
    2. in PCP office settings.
    3. in mobile crisis programs.
    4. available only to certain age groups of patients depending on the setting.

CHAPTER 15: PSYCHIATRIC REHABILITATION AND RECOVERY

1. A psychiatric nurse whose area of practice is tertiary prevention of mental illness is asked to describe the focus of her practice. The nurse will say it is:
    1. the curing of mental illness.
    2. preventing mental illness from occurring.
    3. limiting disability related to an episode of mental illness.
    4. increasing community awareness of the symptoms of mental illness.

2. Which of the following professionals would be a multidisciplinary rehabilitative treatment team?
    1. Psychiatric nurse, nutritionist, psychologist, and psychiatrist
    2. Psychiatric nurse, nutritionist, pharmacist, and home health aide.
    3. Psychiatric nurse, social worker, rehabilitation counselor, and pharmacist.
    4. Psychiatric nurse, psychologist, social worker, and rehabilitation counselor.

3. The nurse asked to explain how psychiatric rehabilitation under the tertiary prevention model differs from the traditional medical model should explain that, in tertiary prevention, the focus is on:
    1. disease as opposed to the coping continuum.
    2. learning to receive treatment in institutional settings.
    3. health and wellness and not just symptoms of disease.
    4. proper diagnosis and appropriate medications to treat disorders.

4. Under the tertiary prevention model, Nurse G. is more likely to work with a patient with a psychiatric disorder:
    1. in a decision-making partnership.
    2. by authoritatively prescribing treatment.
    3. with the assumption that the patient knows best.
    4. from the position of requiring the patient to be compliant and dependent.

5. When an outpatient on Nurse W.'s caseload is hospitalized in the psychiatric inpatient unit, Nurse W. will implement the rehabilitation model by:
    1. assessing patient deficits.
    2. identifying and reinforcing patient strengths.
    3. reviewing the patient's former treatment plan for mistakes.
    4. considering lowering expectations when the patient is discharged.

6. Nurse W. notes that the attitude of a patient about his illness has become negative. The patient voices that he is ashamed because he has a mental illness and begins to isolate himself. Nurse W. will likely interpret this behavior as:
   1. unrelated to his serious mental illness.
   2. related to primary symptoms of serious mental illness.
   3. associated with secondary symptoms of serious mental illness.
   4. a coincidental response that has little relationship to his illness.
7. A new nurse asks, "What do psychiatric patients in the community perceive about their acceptance by others?" The best response would be:
   1. "Many feel stigmatized and alienated."
   2. "Most feel well-accepted and supported."
   3. "The majority are intensely angry and hostile."
   4. "Most are more concerned with their primary symptoms."
8. At a neighborhood meeting seeking to develop support for a supervised housing facility in a suburb, a homeowner states, "I don't want mentally ill people in the neighborhood. They're dangerous!" The community mental health nurse should respond:
   1. "Former patients need care and concern, not stigmatization."
   2. "I think your real concern is the fear that property values will decrease."
   3. "The way you act toward former patients will determine how they act toward you."
   4. "People who have come through mental illness are more apt to be withdrawn and timid than aggressive."
9. The psychiatric rehabilitation nurse is assessing the family and home of a patient who is being discharged to home within the next few days from an inpatient unit. One of the prioritized assessment components for which the nurse must assess is:
   1. how the family members will make changes to meet the needs of the patient.
   2. family members' attitudes about the mentally ill member.
   3. how the family members will divide up the responsibilities of caring for the patient.
   4. who will be the primary caretaker in the family for helping the patient with ADLs.
10. The nurse knows that daily "hassles" can be disruptive to rehabilitation outcomes for a patient in the community. Mr. O is a 24-year-old patient who is persistently and severely mentally ill. He lives with family in a rural setting and does not work. For which "hassles" should the nurse be particularly alert?
    1. Housing, school, and work problems
    2. Money problems, loneliness, and boredom
    3. Marriage concerns and medication problems
    4. Florid symptoms, odd dress, and bizarre behavior
11. A nurse is assessing Mr. T's community living skills. Mr. T. is 28 and the only child of working parents. The nurse ascertains that he has poor personal hygiene, has never worked, shopped, or cooked, and has never used a budget. He spends his social security check on cigarettes and beer. He has poor conversational skills and gets up and walks away from the nurse during conversation. The nurse can make the assessment that he:
    1. has low readiness to function in the community.
    2. will be too much of a burden to live with his family.
    3. is too psychotic to be considered for community placement.
    4. may be too old to profit from psychiatric rehabilitation to teach living skills.
12. Mr. D. is a severely and persistently mentally ill patient with schizophrenia who lives with his parents. Research suggests that some patient behaviors are more disturbing to the family than others. With this in mind, the nurse should explore the family's feelings about the patient's potential:
    1. wandering.
    2. suicide attempts.
    3. excessive arguing.
    4. poor grooming and personal care.
13. As a nurse assesses the family burden associated with having a mentally ill family member, he or she usually can expect to find:
    1. decreased family stress and conflict.
    2. family members blaming each other for the illness.
    3. increased understanding and acceptance of the illness.
    4. too little time, energy, and money given to the ill member.
14. To ensure that complete data about family social support needs are obtained, the nurse should consider seeking information relating to four categories designated as:
    1. anger quotient, resiliency, flexibility, and guilt.
    2. financial, dependency, worry, and involvement.
    3. emotional, feedback, cognitive, and instrumental.
    4. diagnosis, treatment, relapse prediction, and violence potential.
15. Which NANDA nursing diagnosis might the nurse working with families with a mentally ill member find almost universally applicable?
    1. Grief
    2. Anger
    3. Noncompliance
    4. Powerlessness

16. A patient in a psychiatric rehabilitation program mentions to the nurse, "I feel so guilty because my family gives me so much and I have so little to give in return." A helpful reply would be:
    1. "Your family feels good about giving to you."
    2. "Remember that and don't bite the hand that feeds you."
    3. "Following your treatment plan and helping with household tasks are ways you can give back."
    4. "You can help most by keeping your feelings to yourself and not burdening the family when you feel upset."

17. A highly effective way for a nurse working in psychiatric rehabilitation to gain firsthand knowledge about a community agency is to:
    1. read the description in a community social services directory.
    2. query patients who have used the services of the agency.
    3. go to the agency with someone who is requesting services.
    4. go to the agency pretending to be someone who needs services.

18. Ms. B, a 22-year-old diagnosed with major affective disorder, tells the nurse that she is worried about how she will spend her time after she is discharged. She states, "I don't want to vegetate, but I'm a little afraid of how others will respond to me." The nurse should suggest:
    1. "Just try to get out and meet people."
    2. "You should really take it easy when you get home."
    3. "Why not register to take a course or two in night school?"
    4. "Consider going to a consumer-run psychosocial program."

19. The rehabilitative treatment program Nurse T. heads is described as one in which staff are assigned to spend time with psychiatric patients who are in crisis in the community in lieu of hospitalizing the patient. The staff member assists the patient to learn to meet real-world demands. Such a program typifies:
    1. respite care.
    2. foster home care.
    3. halfway housing.
    4. training in community living.

20. To promote positive outcomes, nurses in psychiatric rehabilitation practice should be skilled in:
    1. confrontation, support, and negotiation.
    2. active listening, giving feedback, and medication teaching.
    3. helping develop strengths, teaching living skills, and accessing environmental support.
    4. helping to accept illness and disability, living with stigma, and accepting dependency.

21. Effective programs are essential for families of patients with severe mental illness. Which of the following components should be included to make a program effective?
    1. Education and empowerment
    2. Empowerment and the participation of political figures
    3. Political support and education
    4. Financial support and a large membership

22. As a psychiatric rehabilitation nurse, you are working with a patient with schizophrenia who repeatedly states, "I want to go get a job. I can work, I can do some things, I should be smarter." You know that this patient is very capable of completing more education to increase his chances for a better job. You also know that he lives at home with his parents and does not need to work full time right now so he could return to school if he was willing. He is also eligible for financial support to return to school. Which of the following would be your key points to help him look at all of his options to fulfill his need to feel more productive?
    1. "If you return to school and get a degree you can graduate from college and get a better job in 5 or 6 years."
    2. "You could return to school. You could start by taking one course at a school where classes have small enrollments; this would help you see yourself differently and help you find a career or future work skills that would make you more independent. You could also work part time while you are a student."
    3. "Why don't you just look at the want ads and find something you want to do for work?"
    4. "You don't need the money from a job right now, so let your parents support you. Go back to school while someone else is paying, and then in 10 years you'll get a good job."

23. The patient is a 27-year-old male living at home with his parents. You are the psychiatric rehabilitation nurse who is helping the family become more empowered to work with the family member, who has alcoholism and schizophrenia. What steps do you take?
    1. Help the family members with scheduling regular daily activities and suggest the family members allow the patient his privacy and personal space.
    2. Have the family members remind the patient often about appointments and the schedule of daily activities.
    3. Suggest to family members that they spend as much time as possible with the patient and continuously reassure the patient that they will never let him be alone or totally on his own.
    4. Suggest that a family member help the patient plan his activities of daily living and make sure that all family members understand the need for vigilance with the patient.

24. You are the psychiatric rehabilitation nurse who is conducting a workshop on family skill building. All participants have a family member living in their household with severe mental illness. Which of the following might be the most effective method to present coping skills to the participants?
    1. Have a rehabilitation counselor present coping skills that family members can learn.
    2. As a psychiatric rehabilitation nurse, present a skill and allow participants in the workshop to give you feedback on the usefulness of the skill for their family member.
    3. Arrange a workshop presenter who is a family member of a patient with alcoholism and bipolar disorder and who has lived in the same household with the patient for 9 years.
    4. Have someone who has worked in homecare for the mentally ill present a talk at the workshop.

25. All rehabilitation programs should be evaluated regularly to ensure:
    1. involvement with appropriate resources for grant funding and assure proper use of funds.
    2. appropriate grant funding documentation and competence.
    3. accountability for service providers, relevance, and cost effectiveness.
    4. cost effectiveness, geographic service area, and efficiency of administration.

CHAPTER 16: ANXIETY RESPONSES AND ANXIETY DISORDERS

1. Nurse G. is assessing a patient who gives the impression of being anxious. Nurse G. seeks to validate this impression because anxiety is:
    1. necessary for survival.
    2. communicated interpersonally.
    3. an emotion without a specific object.
    4. a subjective experience of the individual.

2. While completing the nursing admission of a patient admitted to the general hospital for surgery, the nurse observes that the patient is experiencing a narrowed perceptual field and seems to focus on immediate concerns. The patient is able to follow directions with assistance. The nurse determines that the patient is experiencing anxiety at the:
    1. mild level.
    2. panic level.
    3. severe level.
    4. moderate level.

3. A psychiatric patient has greatly increased seemingly non–goal-directed motor activity and seems terror-stricken. He does not respond to nursing staff efforts to calm him. He is noted to have distorted perceptions and disordered thoughts. The level of patient anxiety can be assessed as:
    1. mild.
    2. panic.
    3. severe.
    4. moderate.

4. A psychiatric patient has greatly increased seemingly non–goal-directed motor activity and seems terror-stricken. He does not respond to nursing staff efforts to calm him. He is noted to have distorted perceptions and disordered thoughts. The initial intervention of highest priority is:
    1. provide for the patient's safety.
    2. reduce environmental stimuli.
    3. respect the patient's personal space.
    4. encourage the patient to discuss his feelings.

5. A psychiatric patient has greatly increased seemingly non–goal-directed motor activity and seems terror-stricken. He does not respond to nursing staff efforts to calm him. He is noted to have distorted perceptions and disordered thoughts. Of the medications listed on the patient's medication administration sheet, which one, with the appropriate order, can be given as a prn anxiolytic?
    1. Buspirone (BuSpar)
    2. Lorazepam (Ativan)
    3. Phenytoin (Dilantin)
    4. Fluoxetine (Prozac)

6. A nurse explains a patient's behavior, "His anxiety stemmed from being unable to attain a desired goal." This nurse is basing care on:
   1. learning theory.
   2. behaviorist theory.
   3. interpersonal theory.
   4. psychoanalytic theory.

7. A patient tells the nurse he is feeling "edgy and can't concentrate." Earlier the nurse had noted the patient alternately smoking, pacing, and cursing. The nurse can assess the patient's level of anxiety as:
   1. mild.
   2. panic.
   3. severe.
   4. moderate.

8. During a staff conflict, one of your nursing peers defends her actions and asserts her own rights among the professional staff. Her behavior is best described as typifying the coping mechanism of:
   1. ego-oriented reaction.
   2. task-oriented reaction.
   3. physiological conversion.
   4. psychological conversion.

9. A nurse who works at an anxiety clinic states that she has discovered a truth about defense mechanisms that will help in nursing practice. Which is she most likely to relate? They:
   1. involve some degree of self-deception.
   2. are rarely used by mentally healthy people.
   3. seldom make the person feel more comfortable.
   4. are usually effective in resolving basic conflicts.

10. Ann tends to use the defense mechanism of displacement. When her husband, to whom she is devoted, bawls her out for being disorganized and flighty, she is most likely to react by:
    1. burning his dinner.
    2. scolding the paperboy for being late.
    3. telling her husband that she is furious with him.
    4. being an especially gracious hostess when they entertain his boss.

11. A 20-year-old woman was raped when she was 12 but can no longer remember the incident. The defense mechanism in use is:
    1. projection.
    2. repression.
    3. displacement.
    4. reaction formation.

12. If a miserly man rationalizes, the nurse expects that he is most likely to:
    1. call other people stingy.
    2. start spending money liberally.
    3. say that he exemplifies the virtue of thrift.
    4. give all his money to charity when he dies.

13. A school-age girl hits her playmate on his head. In response to the little boy's cries, the girl's mother comes over and asks what happened. The girl replies, "He hit me! He hit me!" The little girl is using:
    1. projection.
    2. sublimation.
    3. displacement.
    4. rationalization.

14. A policeman who is unconsciously afraid that he is a coward and who defends himself by the mechanism of reaction formation is most likely to:
    1. call others cowards.
    2. develop paralysis of his leg.
    3. volunteer for perilous SWAT duty.
    4. have daydreams in which he is wounded while on duty.

15. A woman calls the community mental health center and says that for the past 6 months she has been "terrified of leaving her home. My heart pounds, I shake and cry and feel dizzy when I even think about leaving the house." She adds, "I'm losing my friends. They've stopped calling because I always refuse to join them." These symptoms can be assessed as being most consistent with:
    1. panic disorder with agoraphobia.
    2. obsessive-compulsive disorder.
    3. posttraumatic stress disorder.
    4. generalized anxiety disorder.

16. Ms. H. is a 34-year-old woman who has obsessive-compulsive disorder (OCD). On her first clinic visit, she is pacing rapidly back and forth in the interview room counting her steps. The nurse practitioner most likely will consider prescribing which of the following?
    1. Clomipramine
    2. Chlorpromazine
    3. Chlordiazepoxide
    4. Buspirone

17. Mr. J., age 35, is admitted to the psychiatric unit and is so anxious that he can follow simple directions only with great difficulty. He tells the nurse that he is worried about how he can keep clean in such a public place and repeatedly dusts the furniture in his room. He folds and refolds his clothing and repeatedly brushes his teeth. The nurse should assess his level of anxiety as:
    1. mild.
    2. panic.
    3. severe.
    4. moderate.

18. Which nursing intervention would be most therapeutic for a newly admitted patient with obsessive-compulsive disorder (OCD) who is busily cleaning and straightening his room?
    1. "I've inspected the room and it's very clean."
    2. "Tell me why your clothes and room need to be cleaned."
    3. "You will not be allowed in your room if you cannot control your cleaning behaviors."
    4. "I can see how uncomfortable you are, but I would like you to take a short walk so I can show you the unit."

19. Mr. J., age 35, is admitted to the psychiatric unit with obsessive-compulsive disorder (OCD). He tells the nurse that he is worried about how he can keep clean in such a public place and repeatedly dusts the furniture in his room. He folds and refolds his clothing and repeatedly brushes his teeth. He sleeps only 1 hour the first night. The nurse planning his care establishes short-term goals and plans interventions. Within the next 48 hours, which outcome would indicate that nursing interventions to relieve anxiety had been successful?
    1. The patient sleeps 6 hours nightly.
    2. The patient engages in continual cleaning.
    3. The patient states that performing rituals is "silly."
    4. The patient states that he is acutely anxious and wants help.

20. To know the full range of symptoms to seek when assessing a patient who is experiencing anxiety, Nurse F. needs to know that the physiological responses associated with anxiety are modulated by the brain through the:
    1. autonomic nervous system.
    2. cardiovascular system.
    3. neuromuscular system.
    4. endocrine system.

21. Trent tells the psychiatric nurse that he was visiting New York when terrorists bombed a building. He was trapped in debris between two floors and waited many hours for rescue. At the time, he experienced the pain of his crush injuries and great thirst. He mentions that he wondered whether he would be left to die. Now, several months later, he states he feels "numb" and can't relate well with people. He sometimes re-experiences the terror and the sounds and sights associated with being trapped. The data collected about Trent are consistent with the symptoms of:
    1. agoraphobia.
    2. panic attacks.
    3. posttraumatic stress disorder.
    4. obsessive-compulsive disorder.

22. The nurse who has spent an hour with a highly anxious patient mentions to a peer, "I'm really feeling uptight! I need a quiet place." This can be attributed to:
    1. hypersensitivity on the nurse's part.
    2. communication of anxiety interpersonally.
    3. fatigue from the effort of establishing a relationship.
    4. a threat to the nurse's self-esteem created by this difficult patient.

23. Ms. O. is assessed by the physician as experiencing double approach-avoidance conflicts associated with the need to replace maladaptive behaviors with more adaptive behaviors. How will this be made apparent to the nurse? The patient will:
    1. wish to both pursue and avoid the same goal.
    2. have to choose between two undesirable goals.
    3. seek to pursue two equally desirable but incompatible goals.
    4. see both desirable and undesirable aspects of two alternatives.

24. Ms. J., age 44, is admitted with the diagnosis of generalized anxiety disorder r/o (rule out) depression. The nurse providing her care knows that careful assessment is important. In the cognitive realm, which assessment points to depression?
    1. Selective and specific negative appraisals
    2. Uncertainty in negative evaluations
    3. Global view that nothing will turn out right
    4. Tentatively regards defects or mistakes as revocable

25. If a patient with obsessive-compulsive disorder (OCD) or a phobia makes a derogatory comment about his or her symptom, such as "I'm such a stupid person for behaving this way," the best response for the nurse would be to:
    1. change the subject.
    2. join in the ridicule of the symptom.
    3. ask about the feelings experienced before using the behavior.
    4. support the insight by asking for immediate behavioral change.

26. Quentin, a police officer, did not write a report about a family dispute in which he intervened, thinking the problem was resolved. Later, the husband shot the wife. Quentin became severely anxious and sought help. At the interview he repeated over and over "I'm going to be fired." The nurse decides to use cognitive techniques. Which approach would be most useful?
    1. "Let's look at the evidence that you'll lose your job."
    2. "I'm going to teach you how to make your body relax."
    3. "Before we talk about this problem, you are going to the gym to work out."
    4. "I'm going to use role playing to help you work out a strategy for explaining your action to your superior officers."

CHAPTER 17: PSYCHOPHYSIOLOGICAL RESPONSES AND SOMATOFORM AND SLEEP DISORDERS

1. Which of the following patients is most likely exhibiting a somatization disorder?
    1. A woman with chronic pain in the right ankle after a skiing injury
    2. A college graduate who cannot maintain steady employment because of multiple vague complaints that result in absenteeism
    3. A man who experiences occasional chest pain after a myocardial infarction (heart attack)
    4. A teenager who dislikes going out to social events with large groups because of embarrassment about facial acne

2. Of the following patients, which is most likely exhibiting a conversion disorder?
    1. A 2-year-old with frequent ear infections
    2. An 18-year-old athlete with exercise-induced asthma
    3. A 53-year-old night watchman who suddenly goes blind
    4. A 63-year-old woman whose broken foot is not healing well

3. Ms. A. has conversion disorder that is evidenced by paralysis of her right hand. Which nursing intervention should be implemented?
    1. Focus discussions on the patient's inability to fulfill usual roles.
    2. Focus discussions on the patient's unusual and unexplainable physical symptom.
    3. Spend time with the patient to give recognition for positive qualities and strengths.
    4. Spend time with the patient during situations when the paralysis renders her helpless to perform self-care activities.

4. Which intervention should the nurse select to help a patient with chronic pain disorder cope more effectively?
    1. Mild opioids
    2. Benzodiazepines
    3. Relaxation techniques
    4. Response prevention

5. Which patient would be at the greatest risk of encountering the exhaustion phase of the general adaptation syndrome?
    1. Ms. F., 67, who is scheduled for knee joint replacement surgery
    2. Mr. B., 46, who has high self-efficacy and has recently accepted a job promotion
    3. Ms. D., 24, who has had elective rhinoplasty to correct a prominent hump in the bridge of her nose
    4. Ms. C., 74, who has severe osteoarthritis and was admitted to a nursing home after the death of her caretaker husband 2 months ago

6. The nurse assesses Ms. G. as being at risk for the development of a psychophysiological disorder associated with multiple stressors. In the assessment of Ms. G.'s coping resources, which factor would the nurse consider?
    1. The social support available to Ms. G.
    2. Whether Ms. G. has sustained recent loss
    3. Whether Ms. G. is overworked and has too many commitments
    4. The existence of strain associated with Ms. G.'s marriage and parenting duties

7. Ms. H. has essential hypertension. She has reported that she feels pressured by the demands made on her by family, friends, and employer. Which role play, as part of a patient education plan for coping with stress, would most likely help the patient develop effective stress-reduction skills?
    1. Patient offering to help a friend organize a church group activity
    2. Patient saying "no" to a request made by the employer to work overtime
    3. Patient accepting a verbal demonstration of caring and concern from husband
    4. Patient asking a work subordinate to change his behavior and come to work on time

8. Mr. I. has been told he has a peptic ulcer. He is being treated with medication and a free-choice diet. He has been advised to get more rest, to stop smoking and drinking, and to reduce the amount of stress in his life. A week after the ulcer has been diagnosed, Mr. I.'s wife reports to the nurse that he is more active than previously, has taken on more responsibility at work, behaves more competitively, spends more time in meetings, misses meals, and continues to smoke and drink. The nurse can assess this behavior as evidence the patient is employing:
   1. projection.
   2. regression.
   3. rationalization.
   4. compensation.

9. Ms. M., age 30, is dissatisfied with the appearance of her nose and believes that it is too long. She has had two surgeries to reshape the nose and has recently visited several plastic surgeons and asked for further surgery. Each has told her that further surgery is not indicated. She tells the nurse that her life will be ruined unless her appearance can be improved. She suggests that she will be unable to marry and will be passed over for a promotion at work. Ms. M.'s thinking suggests:
   1. hypochondriasis.
   2. conversion disorder.
   3. somatization disorder.
   4. body dysmorphic disorder.

10. Ms. M., age 30, is dissatisfied with the appearance of her nose. The nurse, however, thinks Ms. M. is attractive. Ms. M. tells the nurse that her nose is ruining her life. She adds that she is so homely she is sure no one will ever marry her and that she will be passed over for a promotion at work. A possible nursing diagnosis to consider for this patient is:
    1. activity intolerance.
    2. disturbed body image.
    3. ineffective role performance.
    4. ineffective sexuality pattern.

11. Which type of treatment is likely to be effective for Ms. M., a 30-year-old woman who is preoccupied with the appearance of her nose?
    1. Short-term benzodiazepine use to reduce anxiety
    2. Biofeedback to control physical responses to anxiety
    3. Antidepressant therapy to improve her lowered self-esteem, increase her self-confidence, and improve her outlook
    4. Cognitive-behavioral therapy to challenge distorted thinking and interrupt self-critical thoughts

12. What nursing action would deter the development of a relationship with a patient with a psychophysiological disorder?
    1. Convey to the patient that the problem is mostly in his or her mind.
    2. Approach the patient with understanding that his or her symptoms are real.
    3. Encourage the patient to identify things that make his or her symptoms worse.
    4. Encourage the patient to identify things that make his or her symptoms better.

13. Mr. X. believes he has a brain tumor. He has seen several doctors and has had many diagnostic tests over the past year that have shown no evidence of organic disease. He presents as anxious and distraught. The nurse who interviews him should suspect the presence of:
    1. hypochondriasis.
    2. chronic pain disorder.
    3. conversion disorder.
    4. body dysmorphic disorder.

14. Mr. X. believes he has a brain tumor. He has seen several doctors and has had many diagnostic tests that have shown no evidence of organic disease. He tells the nurse, "No one believes me! I have the symptoms: terrible headaches and episodes of blurred vision. Last week I felt weak and even vomited. I'm going to die." The physician has suggested that cognitive behavioral therapeutic approaches may be useful. Which nursing approach fosters cognitive restructuring?
    1. "Tell me about your relationships with the significant women in your life."
    2. "You must be very worried about your condition. Let's discuss these feelings."
    3. "Let's look at the evidence that you have that suggests a brain tumor and consider the possible explanations for the symptoms."
    4. "Your concern is unfounded. The more you talk about it, the more your false idea is perpetuated. Let's talk about something else."

15. "Doctor shopping," which is common among patients with somatoform disorders, suggests to the nurse that the patient:
    1. is denying the psychological component of the illness.
    2. cannot be successfully treated on an outpatient basis.
    3. uses rationalization to cope with anxiety aroused by the physical symptoms.
    4. has consciously chosen to display symptoms of a physical illness to avoid certain responsibilities.

16. Ms. O. is a staff nurse who has received an unfavorable evaluation of her work from the head nurse. Although she disagrees with the evaluation, she decides not to protest it. She complains that now she gets little satisfaction from her work, feels tired all the time, and can't wait for her shift to end. Her behavior is characteristic of the stage of Selye's general adaptation syndrome called:
    1. alarm reaction.
    2. the stage of resistance.
    3. the stage of resolution.
    4. the stage of exhaustion.

17. The nurse is working with a patient who is exhibiting psychophysiological symptoms. It is important to care planning that the nurse understands that the patient's symptoms are:
    1. feigned.
    2. psychosomatic.
    3. serious and possibly fatal if untreated.
    4. only serious if associated with actual pathology.

18. The nurse is working with a patient who has been diagnosed as having somatization disorder. The patient asks, "My last tests didn't show anything. When will they be doing more diagnostic testing?" Which would be the best response by the nurse?
    1. "You are resisting the idea that you do not have a physical illness."
    2. "No more tests will be ordered. Your HMO won't pay for repeating any tests."
    3. "We think you need a rest from all the testing. We'll consider more tests at a later time."
    4. "No other diagnostic testing is scheduled. We will focus next on evaluating the role of stress in your life."

19. The nurse planning care for a patient who has somatization disorder needs to be aware that these patients often have relationship problems associated with:
    1. anger.
    2. dependency.
    3. detachment.
    4. misplaced objectivity.

20. Mr. T., an executive in an advertising firm, is a patient in the CCU after a myocardial infarction. He tells the nurse that he must have a telephone in his room. When the nurse tells him that this is not possible, he angrily berates the nurse and demands to see his physician. Which would be the most helpful nursing intervention?
    1. "I'll call your physician."
    2. "I'll arrange for you to have a telephone."
    3. "I can see that being ill is difficult for you."
    4. "You are just too ill to make business calls."

21. Which expected outcome would be appropriate for a patient with a somatoform disorder?
    1. Patient's anxiety level will decrease from severe to moderate.
    2. Patient will demonstrate compliance with anti-anxiety medication regimen.
    3. Patient will be able to cope with stress without being preoccupied with physical symptoms.
    4. Patient will express feelings verbally rather than through the development of physical symptoms.

22. Which strategy would be most useful to help a patient with a psychophysiological disorder develop insight?
    1. Spend time with the patient to identify strengths
    2. Identify dysfunctional coping mechanisms for the patient
    3. Suggest that the patient's use of denial is interfering with developing insight
    4. Help the patient become aware of feelings when physical symptoms are present

23. A patient with a history of insomnia has been taking chlordiazepoxide (Librium) 15 mg po hs for the past year. She says she currently has difficulty getting to sleep and wakes up frequently during the night. The most appropriate nursing diagnosis to consider is:
    1. disturbed sleep pattern related to anxiety.
    2. moderate anxiety related to disturbed sleep pattern.
    3. disturbed sleep pattern related to tolerance to chlordiazepoxide (Librium).
    4. thought disorder related to a disturbed sleep pattern and chlordiazepoxide (Librium).

24. Ms. T., a patient admitted with conversion disorder, was prematurely forced to acknowledge the psychological nature of her paralysis. The morning after this happened, Ms. T. called the nurse to say that she could not see. This set of circumstances is evidence of the:
    1. unpredictability of the disorder.
    2. defensive nature of the disorder.
    3. intentional nature of the disorder.
    4. manipulative tendencies of patients with conversion disorder.

25. The nurse who is working with a patient who is currently suffering from extreme stress wishes to focus interventions on promoting adaptive psychophysiological patient responses. Which intervention has this focus?
    1. Monitoring the patient's medication
    2. Monitoring the patient's physical health
    3. Shifting the patient's attention away from the symptoms
    4. Providing education to promote change in patient health habits

CHAPTER 18: SELF-CONCEPT RESPONSES AND DISSOCIATIVE DISORDERS

1. Which individual would be at greatest risk for self-esteem disturbance?
   1. Tony, 5, who is starting school
   2. Kim, 16, a high school junior
   3. Janet, 26, an LPN who is entering a college nursing program
   4. Jim, 45, who is working toward a master's degree in business administration

2. A patient tells the nurse that he is a "weak person." He sees himself as inadequate and vulnerable and states that he often feels helpless and frightened. The nursing diagnosis most likely to fit this situation is:
   1. personal identity disturbance.
   2. self-esteem disturbance.
   3. personality fusion.
   4. depersonalization.

3. The psychiatrist states that Ms. W. has classic symptoms of identity diffusion. The nurse can expect to see a patient who demonstrates behaviors that are:
   1. empathetic, warm, and friendly.
   2. depressed, apathetic, and helpless.
   3. out of contact with reality and confused.
   4. exploitative, amoral, and nonempathetic.

4. A patient reports feeling detached and says, "It feels as though I'm watching a movie as life unfolds. I'm isolated, on the outside, a pawn and not a player, untouched. I really don't feel anything. I don't know if I'm alive or dead, awake or sleeping." The nurse can determine that the patient is describing:
   1. akathisia.
   2. conduct disorder.
   3. depersonalization.
   4. boundary violation.

5. Which of the following individuals is most in need of measures to reduce the risk potential for self-concept disturbance associated with health-illness transition?
   1. Ed, 30, blind due to glaucoma, who states, "My wife will help me learn Braille"
   2. Ann, 52, who has breast cancer and states, "My life is more valuable than any body part"
   3. Gloria, 15, who has Crohn's disease, who states, "An ileostomy will mean I won't be able to do stuff with my friends"
   4. Jim, 18, an above-the-knee double amputee, who states, "I guess I'll be a wheelchair athlete instead of a marathon runner"

6. Mr. K. is an acutely psychotic, withdrawn patient who states that he is a robot, adding, "I can't relate to others. I have no feelings. I can't talk because I have no ideas in my head." The nurse plans to help Mr. K. by adopting an accepting attitude. Acceptance is shown when the nurse remarks to this patient:
   1. "I'd like to sit here with you for a while."
   2. "You need to loosen up and be less rigid."
   3. "I'll help you get in touch with the feelings you're trying to deny."
   4. "I'll make decisions for you and care for your needs until you get yourself back under control."

7. Mr. K., an acutely psychotic, withdrawn patient, states that he is a robot. An early intervention designed to help this patient expand self-awareness would be to:
   1. confirm the patient's identity.
   2. set up a schedule for him.
   3. introduce him to two other withdrawn patients.
   4. explain to him the need to express his feelings more openly.

8. When Mr. K., an acutely psychotic, withdrawn patient, states that he is a robot and cannot think of how to take a shower, which response by the nurse is best?
   1. "You must shower independently, or the staff will give you a bed bath."
   2. "I will turn on the water for you and give you step-by-step directions."
   3. "Don't jest. You must shower, or you'll risk having people avoid being around you."
   4. "We can put off the shower for another day, because you don't have a body odor."

9. Ms. R. was abused by her mother during her childhood. She tells the nurse of the abuse in a stilted, unemotional way. Which intervention would promote attainment of the goal that the patient will examine feelings associated with childhood abuse?
   1. "You poor thing! I feel deeply sorry for what you endured."
   2. "When you described this relationship, you didn't tell me how you felt."
   3. "You must be feeling so angry with your parents that you'd like to harm them."
   4. "I think, as a child, I would have felt betrayed, confused, and frightened."

10. During the process of self-exploration, it is important for the nurse to convey the message that the patient:
    1. may be the victim of circumstances beyond his or her control.
    2. is responsible for his or her own behavior, including maladaptive coping responses.
    3. cannot hope to make significant changes without therapeutic guidance.
    4. may need to focus on changing the attitudes and behaviors of significant others.

11. During the process of working with a patient with self-concept disturbance, which type of communication would initially be most useful?
    1. Probing
    2. Empathic
    3. Confrontive
    4. Sympathetic

12. Which patient could be evaluated as having achieved the desired outcome of therapy to improve self-concept?
    1. Ken: "My abilities are still a long way from comparing favorably with my self-ideal."
    2. Meg: "I felt pushed to do what the nurse wanted. I wasn't always ready to move forward when she was."
    3. Tom: "I understand myself better, but I haven't worked out what alternative behaviors will serve me best."
    4. Abby: "I understand that no one else can make me happy. I'm using my strengths and making my wishes become realities."

13. Mr. B. states, "Ever since I was a kid, I knew I should study, get good grades, and go to medical school. I wanted to be helpful and do good for others." From this statement, the nurse obtains information to assess this patient's:
    1. self-ideal.
    2. self-esteem.
    3. self-concept.
    4. self-actualization.

14. K. is age 3 and lives with her parents and her two siblings. She has a number of aunts, uncles, and cousins, all of whom she sees frequently, and she goes to nursery school 3 days a week. In a parenting class, K.'s mother asks, "Which relationships most significantly affect my child's development of self-concept?" The nurse should respond:
    1. "Relationships with her peers."
    2. "Relationships with her parents."
    3. "Relationships with her extended family."
    4. "Relationships with the teachers in nursery school."

15. Ms. L., a patient who is seeking help at the mental health clinic, states, "I know my work has gone downhill. I'm a poor wife, mother, and teacher. I should be able to do better." The best response by the nurse to Ms. L. would be:
    1. "You have very high expectations for yourself."
    2. "Why do you feel you should be all things to all people?"
    3. "Have you talked this problem over with your husband?"
    4. "Perhaps it would be better if you quit work and concentrated on your other responsibilities."

16. A nurse is working with a patient to alter the patient's self-concept. Place the following nursing interventions in the correct sequence as to when they should be implemented.
    A. Assist the patient's self-evaluation.
    B. Encourage the patient's self-exploration.
    C. Expand the patient's self-awareness.
    D. Help the patient formulate a plan of action.
    E. Support the patient in the achievement of goals.
    1. A, B, C, D, E
    2. B, C, D, E, A
    3. C, B, A, D, E
    4. E, B, D, C, A

17. Which of the following best describes the final expected outcome when working with a patient who has an alteration in self-concept?
    1. The patient will develop insight into her problems and life situation.
    2. The patient will clarify his or her concept of self in relation to relationships with others.
    3. The patient will attain the maximum level of self-actualization to realize his or her potential.
    4. The patient will evaluate coping choices made in the past and their consequences.

18. When working with a patient with an alteration in self-concept evidenced by dissociative amnesia, the nurse should begin by:
    1. identifying and supporting patient ego strength.
    2. taking measures to prevent identity diffusion.
    3. helping the patient develop a realistic self-ideal.
    4. setting mutual goals for attitudinal and behavioral change.

19. How does the nurse's use of sympathetic communication hinder a patient's work in developing a more realistic self-concept?
    1. Sympathy can reinforce self-pity.
    2. Sympathy reduces patient ego strength.
    3. Sympathy encourages premature self-revelation.
    4. Sympathy limits potential positive effects of transference.

20. The nurse is completing an assessment of an adolescent patient's self-esteem. The nurse concludes that which of the following patient statements represents an indirect expression of low self-esteem?
    1. "It seems as if I have been a loser almost since I was born."
    2. "Drinking beer helps me to forget my problems."
    3. I don't have many friends, and these days I tend to stay away from the ones I do have."
    4. "If I had only gotten that after-school job, then I could have finally been happy in life."

21. The nurse is working with a patient to improve self-concept. To assist the patient using an intervention at level 1 expanded self-awareness, the nurse should do which of the following?
    1. Encourage the patient to examine feelings and behavior related to a stressor
    2. Create a climate of acceptance toward the patient
    3. Discuss all possible alternatives and solutions
    4. Challenge the patient's faulty beliefs

22. The nurse is working with a patient to improve self-concept. To assist the patient using an intervention at level 2 self-exploration, the nurse should do which of the following?
    1. Discuss all possible alternatives and solutions
    2. Challenge the patient's faulty beliefs
    3. Encourage the patient to examine feelings and behavior related to a stressor
    4. Create a climate of acceptance toward the patient

23. The nurse is working with a female patient to improve self-concept. To assist the patient in using an intervention at level 3 self-evaluation, the nurse should do which of the following?
    1. Provide support measures to reduce the patient's anxiety
    2. Clarify that the patient's beliefs affect her feelings and behaviors
    3. Note her use of logical and illogical thinking
    4. Help the patient to understand that she can only change herself, not others

24. The nurse is working with a female patient to improve self-concept. To assist the patient in using an intervention at level 4 realistic planning, the nurse should do which of the following?
    1. Note the patient's use of logical and illogical thinking
    2. Help the patient to understand that she can change only herself, not others
    3. Provide support measures to reduce the patient's anxiety
    4. Clarify that the patient's beliefs affect her feelings and behaviors

25. A male patient in counseling who has low self-esteem has begun making behavior changes, such as taking on home repair projects and taking an interest in his children's activities. The nurse positively reinforces these changes during a therapy session. The patient and nurse are actively engaged in which level of intervention?
    1. Commitment to action
    2. Self-evaluation
    3. Realistic planning
    4. Expanded self-awareness

CHAPTER 19: EMOTIONAL RESPONSES AND MOOD DISORDERS

1. According to the Stuart Stress Adaptation Model, which person can be assessed as being the farthest from the adaptive responses end of the continuum of emotional response?
    1. Mr. T., whose wife died 6 months ago, who states, "I hate the fact that she died and left me alone after all the years we shared."
    2. Ms. B., whose daughter died 2 weeks ago of SIDS, who states, "I can't believe I'll never hold her in my arms again."
    3. Ms. S., whose fiancée died 6 weeks ago, who tells the nurse, "My life will never be the same. I find myself crying every day when I think of him."
    4. Mr. C., whose wife died 2 years ago, who states, "Men don't mourn. I've kept busy and focused on supporting the kids."

2. Mr. J. is a 35-year-old steelworker who has been told that he no longer has a job because the company plans to use robots in his department. His initial response was disbelief, and then he shouted, "How am I supposed to support a family?" He left the premises muttering that he would sue the company. At home he told his wife that he had lost his job, but retreated to the bedroom saying, "I'm too choked up to talk about it right now." Mr. J. is exhibiting behaviors characteristic of:
    1. mania.
    2. depression.
    3. normal grief reaction.
    4. delayed grief reaction.

3. Which coping mechanism should the nurse expect to see Ms. T use as she begins to mourn the death of her husband?
    1. Denial
    2. Introjection
    3. Suppression
    4. Dissociation

4. Ms. R., 67 years old, was widowed 8 months ago. Her family was amazed at the fortitude during and immediately after the funeral. She did not cry and always spoke of her husband as if he were still sharing her life. Now her son has brought her to the emergency room after she called him on the telephone to say she was going to take an overdose of sleeping pills because she "was too weak to go on alone." The prominent defense mechanism used by Ms. R. has been:
   1. denial.
   2. projection.
   3. introjection.
   4. sublimation.

5. Mr. C. is distraught over his wife's behavior. Their 17-year-old son died in a car accident 1 month ago, he explains, and his wife still cries herself to sleep each night. He asks the clinic nurse to "help my wife control herself." The nurse's best response to him would be:
   1. "I wonder why it is that you are so bothered by her crying."
   2. "I'll spend some time with her to help her see that crying is counterproductive."
   3. "It's hard to see her so upset, but crying is one way of expressing her feelings."
   4. "Her response is entirely normal, but I'm concerned that you don't seem to be grieving."

6. While talking with a patient about her mother, the patient remarks, "My father's been dead for months. I think Mom needs to get on with her life." The most appropriate response by the nurse is:
   1. "Giving her support will be more helpful than being critical."
   2. "Have you thought of ways you might help her find more pleasure in her life?"
   3. "It's possible that she still needs more time. Grieving often takes a year or more."
   4. "A death is usually a crisis for the whole family as well as the spouse. How has it affected you?"

7. A patient who goes to the mood disorders clinic in January tells the nurse, "My mood is really low. I'm tired all the time even though I sleep for 10 or 12 hours a day. I've gained weight because I want to eat sweets all the time. It seems like it happens every fall and winter." This patient is most likely experiencing:
   1. bipolar disorder.
   2. delayed grief reaction.
   3. postpartum depression.
   4. seasonal affective disorder.

8. The critical element a nurse must consider when completing a behavioral assessment of a patient with a mood disturbance is:
   1. the level of anxiety present.
   2. the degree of agitation noted.
   3. the depth of depression reported.
   4. a change in usual patterns and responses.

9. Ms. R. was admitted with major depressive disorder 3 weeks ago. Suicidal ideation was present, but Ms. R. had no plan. She has received sertraline (Zoloft) and according to her self-report is feeling somewhat less depressed. A factor of importance for the nurse to consider when planning care for Ms. R. is that:
   1. the patient is no longer considered a suicide risk after 3 weeks on medication.
   2. the patient may be at increased risk for suicide as the depression lifts.
   3. the patient will be at decreased risk for suicide as the depression lifts.
   4. no relationship between the depth of depression and suicidality exists.

10. Ms. V., a 30-year-old accountant, paces the unit continuously. She wrings her hands and repeats, "I'm worthless. It's all hopeless." Which measure would be most helpful in establishing a relationship with Ms. V?
    1. Greet her with a cheerful smile.
    2. Insist that she go to her room to talk with you.
    3. Walk with her and make occasional empathic observations.
    4. Tell her that you do not agree with her assessment of worthlessness.

11. Mr. C. is being treated for severe depression. He evidences resistance to involvement in the nurse-patient relationship by being withdrawn and unresponsive. He is preoccupied with guilt and hopelessness. When a nurse interacts with him, a highly therapeutic approach could be summarized as:
    1. "Everything will work out."
    2. "Let's explore the origins of your pessimism."
    3. "You will feel better as your treatment continues."
    4. "You have to help yourself by getting rid of your negative thoughts."

12. A depressed patient eats very little and has recently lost 8 pounds. At meal times the nurse sits with him and encourages him to eat, but after a few bites, he refuses to eat more, saying, "I'm full. All that food makes me sick just to look at it." The most effective way to increase his dietary intake would be to:
    1. provide a high-calorie liquid diet.
    2. serve six small, calorie-dense meals daily.
    3. take him to the hospital cafeteria for meals.
    4. have his family bring his favorite foods from home.

13. Mr. T. is hospitalized for depression. He demonstrates dysfunctional thinking as evidenced by persistent pessimism and predictions of disastrous outcomes. The nurse using cognitive therapy will focus on:
    1. uncovering unconscious conflicts that affect the "here and now" behavior.
    2. finding an area of mutual understanding to serve as a basis for therapy.
    3. patient recognition and replacement of automatic negative evaluations.
    4. analyzing and enhancing relationships with significant others.

14. In deriving nursing outcomes for a patient with depression, Nurse T. should focus on the patient:
    1. never being depressed again.
    2. being physically recovered and able to take on new responsibilities.
    3. being emotionally responsive and functioning at the pre-illness level.
    4. being able to tolerate high levels of stress and exceeding pre-illness hardiness.

15. Ms. G. is severely depressed. Her psychomotor retardation and sense of worthlessness have resulted in poor personal hygiene with noticeable body odor and halitosis present at admission. After the admission interview, when the nurse suggests showering, the patient flatly states, "I can't." The nurse should:
    1. not force the issue before a nurse-patient relationship has been established.
    2. matter-of-factly help the patient to shower and dress in clean clothes.
    3. tell the patient that she will be required to shower the following morning.
    4. explain that other patients will respond negatively to someone with poor hygiene.

16. When Ms. P. is begun on the SSRI medication fluoxetine (Prozac), which of the following should be included in the plan for patient education?
    1. The onset of action is 2 to 6 weeks.
    2. Foods containing tyramine should be restricted.
    3. The patient should be alert for symptoms of hypomania.
    4. Intake of salt and salty foods should be restricted.

17. A nursing student mentions to her preceptor, "Although manic patients tire me out, at least I don't have to worry about loss of life as a complication like I do when I'm caring for a depressed patient." The best reply for the preceptor would be:
    1. "That's quite an astute observation."
    2. "Let's consider the ways that acute manic states can also be life threatening."
    3. "You're right in assessing that suicide potential always exists with depression."
    4. "Don't focus only on depression. The potential for suicide is high for all patients with psychiatric disorders."

18. Ms. W. goes to the mood disorders clinic at the urging of her mother. The physician who examines her tells the nurse, "She's hypomanic." The nurse can expect to assess:
    1. clinical symptoms more severe than mania.
    2. some motor hyperactivity but depressive affect.
    3. symptoms less severe than those of a manic state.
    4. grandiosity, distractibility, flight of ideas, and excessive psychomotor activity.

19. Ms. R. was referred to the hospital by the court. An unemployed secretary, she was arrested after writing several large personal checks on her account that had a balance of $10. Her purchases included a large-screen television, exercise equipment, a South Seas cruise, and a new wardrobe. She danced a hula, planted kisses on all the men in the courtroom, and explained in rapid-fire speech to the judge, "I've been watching life go by on a small screen TV. Now, I'm going to expand my outlook, shape-up, sail away, and be a bird in paradise." She reports that she's been too busy shopping and packing to eat or sleep for the past several days. These behaviors are consistent with a DSM-IV diagnosis of:
    1. mania.
    2. dysthymia.
    3. depression.
    4. delayed grief reaction.

20. The emergency department calls to say Mr. A., a patient experiencing symptoms of mania, is being admitted. Which of the following available room placements should the nurse choose for him?
    1. A single room near the unit entrance
    2. A single room near the nurse's station
    3. A double room shared with a patient with depression
    4. A double room shared with a patient with schizophrenia

21. Mr. A., a patient displaying symptoms of mania, has been in constant motion for 1 hour. Despite attempted verbal intervention, he has run in the halls, exercised vigorously, and pushed furniture around the solarium. Now, he approaches an elderly man and tells him he must do push-ups or be pushed down. The elderly patient looks fearful, but gets down on the floor. The nurse should:
    1. obtain an order for seclusion for Mr. A.
    2. forbid Mr. A. to coerce or threaten other patients.
    3. gather several staff to provide an escort to take Mr. A. to his room.
    4. allow the elderly patient to do a few pushups knowing Mr. A. will soon be distracted.

22. During discharge planning for Miss Y., a patient whose symptoms of manic disorder are remitting, the patient asks, "Do I have to take lithium even though I'm not high any longer?" The most appropriate response is:
    1. "You can stop the medication 1 week after discharge."
    2. "You will need to take medication for about 12 weeks."
    3. "Usually patients take medication for 6 months after discharge."
    4. "Taking the medication daily will help you avoid relapses and recurrences."

23. The care plan for Mr. K., a manic patient who is displaying elation, hyperactivity, grandiosity, verbosity, disturbed sleep pattern, and poor judgment, should take into consideration the need to:
    1. maintain physiological equilibrium.
    2. show good humor when interacting with him.
    3. provide a permissive, unstructured environment.
    4. provide large amounts of sensory stimulation and social interaction.

24. Ms. J. is extremely hyperactive and distractible. She sleeps little and leaves the dining room before she eats more than a few mouthfuls from her plate. She has lost 6 pounds since admission 3 days ago. Which of the following measures is least important to include in her plan for care?
    1. Set limits that she must remain in the dining room for at least 15 minutes per meal.
    2. Offer high-calorie "portable" finger foods and nutritionally fortified fluids hourly.
    3. Record all food and fluid intake.
    4. Weigh the patient daily.

25. Which data set would indicate that the goal of returning to appropriate emotional responsiveness has been attained by Mr. F., a manic patient?
    1. The patient interacts superficially with staff but refuses involvement in a therapeutic alliance.
    2. The patient manipulates another patient to create a disturbance on the unit and laughs at the outcome.
    3. The patient identifies two attainable goals for himself and offers a realistic (nongrandiose) self-appraisal.
    4. The patient maintains aloof relationships with other patients and advises others based on his own preferences.

26. Mr. P., a patient with severe depression, somatic delusions, and suicidal ideation, has not improved after trials with SSRI medications and tricyclic antidepressants. Which treatment option can the nurse assume the psychiatrist now will consider?
    1. ECT
    2. Neuroleptics
    3. Light therapy
    4. Benzodiazepines

CHAPTER 20: SELF-PROTECTIVE RESPONSES AND SUICIDAL BEHAVIOR

1. Which patient should be assessed as using indirect self-destructive behavior?
    1. Cathy, 28, who scratches her wrists with safety pins
    2. Betty, 62, who drinks nearly a quart of whiskey a day
    3. Ann, 47, who took an overdose of sedative-hypnotic drugs
    4. Amy, 19, who calls a friend when she is contemplating suicide

2. What nursing diagnosis should be considered when caring for a patient who has engaged in direct or indirect self-destructive behavior?
    1. Death anxiety
    2. Chronic or situational low self-esteem
    3. Disturbed body image
    4. Disturbed personal identity

3. The nurse assessing Ms. D., a patient who has been noncompliant with the prescribed diabetic diet and exercise regime, should consider planning strategies to overcome patient use of:
    1. denial.
    2. projection.
    3. dissociation.
    4. displacement.

4. The nurse caring for a patient who has been noncompliant with the prescribed diabetic diet and exercise regime will be most successful in promoting compliance if the nurse can enhance the patient's sense of:
   1. control.
   2. well-being.
   3. fear of the sequelae of illness.
   4. dependence on health care workers.

5. When planning care for patients who have attempted self-injury and for patients who have attempted suicide, the nurse must understand that the major difference in self-injury versus suicide lies in whether the patient has:
   1. intoxication or psychosis.
   2. the wish to relieve tension or the wish to die.
   3. a need to control or a need to be controlled.
   4. an indirect or direct expression of self-destructive urges.

6. A novice nurse asks the mentor, "Not all patients present with blatant suicidal ideation. How will I know when to assess for suicide risk?" The best reply would be, "Nurses working with psychiatric patients should pursue assessment of suicide risk for individuals who display tendencies to be:
   1. blaming, abusive, or confused."
   2. hostile, impulsive, or depressed."
   3. compulsive, obsessive, or weak."
   4. risk-taking, aggressive, or controlling."

7. Based on research findings, which patient on the psychiatric unit probably would be assessed as having the lowest risk for suicide?
   1. Mr. Jones, age 72, admitted for treatment of depression
   2. Mr. Kilmer, age 28, admitted for treatment of paranoid schizophrenia
   3. Mr. I., age 32, admitted for treatment of rapid cycling bipolar disorder
   4. Mr. Tracey, age 18, admitted for treatment of body dysmorphic disorder

8. A depressed patient tells the nurse, "I hope someone will make sure my family gets my jewelry when I'm gone." This statement can be assessed as a:
   1. suicide threat.
   2. suicide gesture.
   3. suicide attempt.
   4. completed suicide.

9. The nursing diagnosis for Ms. Z, who is depressed and suicidal at admission, is "Risk for suicide." An appropriate outcome for this diagnosis at discharge from the hospital is, "The patient will:
   1. increase feelings of self-worth."
   2. not harm self while hospitalized."
   3. be able to problem-solve effectively."
   4. develop a trusting relationship with one staff member."

10. Mr. M. calls the crisis hotline and tells the nurse who answers, "Nobody can help me now. I just want to say goodbye to somebody before I do it." The best response to this statement would be:
    1. "I can help you, if you'll let me try."
    2. "You're still alive, so you can still get help."
    3. "You sound very discouraged. What do you plan to do?"
    4. "I'll arrange transportation so you can come here and tell me about the problem."

11. Mr. J. is a 55-year-old married man who has lost his job. He telephones the mental health clinic and tells the nurse, "I feel so overwhelmed that I've decided to take an overdose of sleeping medicine I bought over-the-counter at the drugstore. I wish I didn't have to do it, but there's no other way." The nurse asks several questions and learns that his wife is in the next room. Which approach should the nurse take?
    1. Convince him to drive himself to the hospital.
    2. Get his address and go to his home and take him to the hospital.
    3. Keep him on the telephone and send the police to bring him to the hospital.
    4. Persuade him to call his wife to the telephone and ask her to bring him to the hospital.

12. The patient states, "I don't want to try anymore, it's too hard. I'm tired. I just want to end it all. Please leave me alone." You are the psychiatric nurse on the telephone with this patient. You are trying to keep the patient talking until you can get help for him because you know that most individuals in this country who carry out successful suicides are:
    1. female age 65 or older
    2. male age 50 or older
    3. male age 19-27
    4. female age 13-19

13. A suicidal patient is found by a nurse as he tries to hang himself from the shower in the bathroom. What nursing intervention would address the patient's need for safety while maintaining his self-esteem?
    1. Assign a staff member to remain with him at all times.
    2. Place him the seclusion room with 15-minute checks.
    3. Request that he remain with the patient group at all times.
    4. Tell him he may use the bathroom only with staff supervision.

14. In evaluating the effectiveness of the care provided for a self-destructive patient, the best approach is to:
    1. identify maladaptive coping behaviors.
    2. involve the patient in the process of evaluation.
    3. make sure the staff has followed the original care plan.
    4. modify the plan as little as possible to avoid confusing the patient.

15. You arrive on the locked inpatient unit today where you are one of the psychiatric nurses who make up the unit's interdisciplinary team. You learn that Mr. T., whom you discharged 2 weeks ago from the unit, successfully committed suicide yesterday afternoon. You are very saddened by the news and decide to participate in the multidisciplinary debriefing today and for the next few days because you know that the primary effect of a patient's successful suicide can:
    1. produce blaming among the nurses.
    2. be devastating to the nurses on the team because nurses are with patients 24 hours a day while they are hospitalized.
    3. split the interdisciplinary treatment team.
    4. reduce the quality of the treatment team's effectiveness because they have failed the patient.

16. At a staff meeting a psychiatric technician states, "Ms. T. is really difficult. She makes suicidal gestures but never really hurts herself. They should send her home instead of admitting her." The best response on the part of the nurse would be:
    1. "She has no family to provide social support."
    2. "Any suicide attempt deserves serious attention and concern for safety."
    3. "You seem to have a real problem when patients lose emotional control."
    4. "Nursing staff have no part in the decision to admit. Tell your concerns to the physician."

17. Nurse O. performs the admission interview for Mr. P. and identifies a need for one-to-one supervision. This determination is based on Mr. P.'s constant thoughts of suicide on admission and his plan to escape from the hospital at the first opportunity so that he may kill himself. The best way to inform him of the nursing plan is to say:
    1. "We cannot trust you to remain safe, so someone will always be with you."
    2. "It is our policy to assign a staff member to stay with all new admissions to the unit."
    3. "The hospital can't let you hurt yourself. Someone will stay with you at all times to keep you from self-harm."
    4. "I understand your impulse to harm yourself. A staff member will stay with you to help you control that impulse."

18. Nurse W. is admitting a patient that she suspects is having suicidal ideation. The best course of action for Nurse W. to take is to:
    1. ask the patient if he's having thoughts of suicide.
    2. ask the patient's significant other if the patient is suicidal.
    3. arrange for commitment to avoid harm to self or others.
    4. avoid the subject to avoid pushing him into further thoughts of self-harm.

19. Nurse H. is working with a depressed patient who had an identical twin who committed suicide. In assessing this patient for suicidal risk, Nurse H. should consider that this patient:
    1. is at increased risk for suicide.
    2. has the same risk as the general population.
    3. is at low risk because he has experienced the trauma of suicide.
    4. cannot be assigned a level of risk on such limited data.

20. You are discussing a psychoeducational group concentrated on increasing self-esteem and positive coping skills with a 27-year-old female patient who was admitted to the inpatient unit after a serious suicide attempt. The patient is scheduled to be discharged to home tomorrow. You would like to have the patient attend an outpatient weekly psychoeducational group in the clinic to help her increase her self-esteem and coping mechanisms. You know that while she has been in the unit she has been responding to the daily group therapy. She has participated in group activities and continues to respond positively because:
    1. she discusses her positive attributes in the group, thanks you and other members of the group who give her genuine praise, and is beginning to demonstrate positive behavioral changes.
    2. she continuously seeks praise from multidisciplinary team members.
    3. she continuously says, "I'm trying to change, I can't do it all at once but I want to continue to try."
    4. she says that she will go to every meeting that you schedule for her after she is discharged.

21. The assessment has been made that Mr. T. is highly suicidal. One-to-one constant supervision with unit restriction has been ordered. How will this order be implemented?
    1. Observe Mr. T. while he is awake, on or off the unit.
    2. Obtain a no-suicide contract, remove harmful objects from the environment, and keep him on the unit.
    3. Observe Mr. T. every 15 minutes around the clock. Document his whereabouts and activity level.
    4. Remove harmful objects from his possession; stay with him at all times, awake or asleep, even in the bathroom; keep him on the unit.

22. The nurse caring for a hospitalized suicidal patient on one-to-one supervision should initially focus on:
    1. mobilizing social support for the patient and family.
    2. facilitating awareness, expression, and labeling of feelings.
    3. helping the patient test new mechanisms for coping with stress.
    4. talking to the patient about the effect his or her suicide would have on his or her family.

23. Which remark by the nurse represents an attempt to assess the patient's current ability to organize and enact a suicide wish?
    1. "What is your educational background?"
    2. "What plan do you have for committing suicide?"
    3. "Have you ever thought about or tried to hurt yourself?"
    4. "Are your self-destructive thoughts constant or intermittent?"

24. An individual anonymously calls the crisis line. The nurse obtains the following information: The caller is a widow with no children and no close friends. She has frequent suicidal thoughts. She plans to drive her car to a high bridge over a rapidly flowing river at 4 AM when there is minimal traffic and jump from the bridge. She cannot swim. What level of lethality would the nurse assess for this plan?
    1. Low level of lethality
    2. Moderate level of lethality
    3. High lethality
    4. Lethality cannot be determined from this data.

25. Ms. G., age 40, was admitted after taking sedatives and deeply slashing her wrists. Her husband had gone to work, and she had called her employer to say that she was ill and would not be at work. She had expected that she would not be found until her husband returned from work. A maintenance worker unexpectedly entered the apartment to fix a faucet and found her unconscious and bleeding in the bathtub. Now, she mentions that it was her typical bad luck to be found, and that another time she will make sure no one will find her. She refuses to sign a no-suicide contract. What, if any, level of suicide precautions should be ordered?
    1. None
    2. Routine checks
    3. Every-15-minute check
    4. One-to-one supervision

CHAPTER 21: NEUROBIOLOGICAL RESPONSES AND SCHIZOPHRENIA AND PSYCHOTIC DISORDERS

1. T., 22, has schizophrenia. The nurse notes that he is often forgetful and seems uninterested in activities. Furthermore, he has difficulty completing tasks. The nurse planning care for T. will select successful strategies by understanding that these behaviors are due to:
    1. a lack of self-esteem.
    2. manipulative tendencies.
    3. shyness and embarrassment.
    4. problems in cognitive functioning.

2. K., a young woman with schizophrenia, is standing naked after showering. She seems dazed and indecisive. The nursing intervention that will be most helpful to promote dressing would be to:
    1. say, "These are your clothes. Please get dressed."
    2. say, "These are your underpants. I'll help you put them on."
    3. show her two outfits and ask, "Which outfit would you like to wear?"
    4. ask, "Is something the matter with your clothes that you are not dressing?"

3. Patients in occupational therapy are engaged in making collages. M., a young patient with schizophrenia, sits staring at a piece of paper in her hand. What intervention should a staff member employ?
    1. None. If the patient prefers to sit and stare for a time, it is acceptable.
    2. "You seem immobilized by anxiety. What can I do to help you?"
    3. "Are you having trouble deciding where you want to glue that piece?"
    4. "Rub the glue stick on the back of the paper."

4. P., a person with schizophrenia, reveals to the nurse that voices have told him he is in danger. He is safe only if he stays in the room and wears the same clothes. He goes on, "They're so loud they frighten me. Do you hear them?" The nurse's best initial response would be:
   1. "I know these voices are very real to you, but I don't hear them."
   2. "Don't worry. You're safe in the hospital. I won't let anything happen to you."
   3. "Tell me more about the voices. Are they men or women? How many are there?"
   4. "You need to get out of your room and get your mind occupied so you don't hear the voices."

5. The nurse is explaining to the family of a patient with schizophrenia that the disorder is considered to have neurobiological origins. The patient's mother is a first-year nursing student who asks, "Just what part of the brain is dysfunctional?" The nurse should reply, "Research has implicated the:
   1. medulla and cortex."
   2. cerebellum and cerebrum."
   3. hypothalamus and medulla."
   4. prefrontal and limbic cortices."

6. Ms. A., a severely withdrawn patient with schizophrenia, allows herself to be escorted to the dayroom. However, she does not speak. The most therapeutic nursing intervention in response to this behavior would be to:
   1. have her sit with a group of patients who will encourage her to talk.
   2. ignore her silence and talk about superficial topics such as the weather.
   3. point out that by not speaking she makes those about her feel uncomfortable.
   4. plan time with her even though she does not verbally communicate with the nurse.

7. The new nurse tells the assigned mentor, "I admitted a patient today who has several bizarre delusions. I wanted to tell him that his ideas and conclusions simply are not logical. What do you think will happen if I do?" Which of the following is the best reply by the mentor?
   1. "I think you'll give him something to think about."
   2. "He'll probably incorporate you into the delusions as a persecutor."
   3. "Don't point out discrepancies just yet. Develop trust using empathy and calmness."
   4. "It would be better to go along with his thinking to gain his cooperation."

8. Ms. K., who has been hospitalized for 2 days, remains delusional and anxious. The nurse perceives that the patient is not yet ready to give up her delusions. What intervention can the nurse use to help the patient focus less on the delusion?
   1. Schedule time for the patient to read and listen to music.
   2. Plan activities that require physical skills and constructive use of time.
   3. Begin planning for discharge by engaging the patient in psychoeducation.
   4. Discuss personal goals related to improved socialization with the patient.

9. A useful strategy for helping a patient with schizophrenia to manage relapse is to:
   1. have the patient attend group therapy.
   2. advise the patient to continue taking medication daily.
   3. teach the patient and family about behaviors that indicate impending relapse.
   4. schedule appointments for periodic blood tests to determine serum medication levels.

10. Which point should be included in teaching patients and families about relapse?
    1. Patients who relapse are those who have failed to take their medications.
    2. Caffeine and nicotine can reduce the effectiveness of antipsychotic drugs.
    3. With support, education, and adherence to treatment, patients won't relapse.
    4. Posthospitalization education about medication actions and side effects is ineffective.

11. A short-term goal for R., a withdrawn, isolated patient with schizophrenia, is, "The patient will:
    1. participate in all therapeutic activities."
    2. define major barriers to communication."
    3. talk about feelings of withdrawal in group."
    4. consistently interact with an assigned nurse."

12. The nursing diagnosis most likely to be used for a person who has a diagnosis of schizophrenia, paranoid type, is:
    1. social isolation related to impaired ability to trust.
    2. impaired mobility related to fear of losing control of hostile impulses.
    3. fear of being alone related to lack of confidence in significant others.
    4. impaired memory related to poor information processing associated with brain deficits.

13. Mr. L. has schizophrenia. His medical record states the patient has cognitive dysfunction. From this statement, the nurse can expect to see evidence of:
    1. anxiety, fear, and agitation.
    2. aggression, anger, hostility, or violence.
    3. blunted or flat affect or inappropriate affective responses.
    4. impaired memory and attention as well as formal thought disorder.

14. Mr. L., a patient with schizophrenia, repeatedly asks for directions or asks for the time. The nurse should:
    1. repeat the information in a kind, matter-of-fact manner.
    2. write out the information so the patient can easily refer to it.
    3. tell the patient that his habit of frequent questioning is annoying.
    4. provide the information once, then remind him that he asked the same question.

15. Which neurological deficit(s) would the nurse be most likely to encounter when assessing Ms. T., a patient with schizophrenia?
    1. Deafness
    2. Weakness and loss of function
    3. Paralysis and diminished reflexes
    4. Increased blinking and impaired fine motor skills

16. The nurse observes a patient, who is sitting alone in her room, put her hands over her ears and vigorously shakes her head as though saying, "No." Later the patient cries and mutters, "You don't know what you're talking about! Leave me alone." What assessment should the nurse attempt to validate? The patient is:
    1. seeking the attention of staff.
    2. inappropriately expressing emotion.
    3. experiencing auditory hallucinations.
    4. displaying negative symptoms of schizophrenia.

17. The emergency department note states, "This patient displays positive symptoms of schizophrenia as evidenced by psychotic disorders of thinking." The nurse can expect the patient to evidence:
    1. delusions and hallucinations.
    2. grimacing and mannerisms.
    3. echopraxia and echolalia.
    4. avolition and anhedonia.

18. Ms. H. has delusions that her "brain is tapped." She says that the government has implanted a device in her head that tells agents where she is at all times and transmits her thoughts to a special receiver. What outcome would the nurse identify for Ms. H.? The patient will, within 1 week of admission:
    1. take antipsychotic medication as prescribed without objection.
    2. give coherent data to support her beliefs that her brain is "tapped."
    3. interpret reality correctly by stating no "brain tap" has been implanted.
    4. report feeling less anxious about having the government listening to her thoughts.

19. Ms. H. has delusions that her "brain is tapped" by government agents who can trace her whereabouts and listen to her thoughts. When she tells the nurse of her delusional beliefs, an appropriate response for the nurse would be:
    1. "Your story is too strange for me to believe."
    2. "Tell me more about what you are experiencing and why you think your brain is tapped."
    3. "What was happening in your life just before you began to think your brain was tapped?"
    4. "It's not clear to me whether you're feeling frightened or angry about the violation of your body."

20. The nurse has been working for several days with Ms. P., a patient with schizophrenia who experiences auditory hallucinations. The patient relates, "When I first heard the voices they said nice things about me. Lately, they've changed and they say bad things." What information is least important to obtain?
    1. "Do you trust me to help you with the voices?"
    2. "Are the voices commanding you to do something?"
    3. "How often during 24 hours do you hear the voices?"
    4. "Do the voices trouble you more if you are in a quiet place or if it's busy and noisy around you?"

21. Which data gathered from the assessment of a family with a schizophrenic member would be of greatest importance in discharge planning for the patient?
    1. The patient is the middle sibling.
    2. The patient's mother is a talented artist.
    3. The patient's paternal grandfather was considered "eccentric."
    4. The patient becomes anxious when family members are hostile and critical of one another.

22. Ms. J. is a psychotic patient who is delusional and has auditory hallucinations. The best approach when the nurse needs to take an oral temperature with an electronic thermometer would be to say:
    1. "I need your vital signs. Put this in your mouth."
    2. "I hope I can count on you to hold still while I take your temperature."
    3. "Please sit here. I must take your temperature. I'll put the thermometer under your tongue and hold it there for a few seconds."
    4. "Don't be afraid. This probe is only a thermometer that will tell us whether you have a fever. It will be all over in just a few seconds."

23. Ms. C. was admitted in a semistuporous catatonic state. Her family states that she has not left her apartment for several weeks and has not attended to personal hygiene. She had spent the last 48 hours at home in her bed, mute and motionless without eating or going to the bathroom. Her bladder is distended. A nursing diagnosis that should be considered a priority is:
    1. self-care deficit.
    2. situational low self-esteem.
    3. disturbed thought processes.
    4. impaired verbal communication.

24. Mr. M. tells the nurse, "I can't go to community meeting. When I get in that room with all those people, they can hear my thoughts." The nurse can correctly assess this symptom as:
    1. concrete thinking.
    2. auditory hallucinations.
    3. thought broadcasting.
    4. loose associations.

25. A patient with schizophrenia approaches the nurse and says, "Cats eat birds… east now… job is new… you father." This speech pattern can be assessed as:
    1. hyperverbosity.
    2. circumstantiality.
    3. loose associations.
    4. expressing delusions.

26. Mr. K. has been rehospitalized for a short stay after a relapse of his schizophrenia. A priority intervention in designing a discharge plan to prevent relapses will be:
    1. helping his family develop tolerance for his cognitive symptoms.
    2. mobilizing the family to provide structure to reduce social dysfunction.
    3. working on self-concept to reduce avolition, anhedonia, and dysphoria.
    4. early identification of signs of impending relapse and coping strategies for prevention.

27. Mr. S. was hospitalized for a short stay after a first relapse resulting in part because he stopped taking the haloperidol that was prescribed. He mentioned that he obtained only partial relief from his hallucinations and the medication made his muscles feel tight, caused a hand tremor, and made him take little steps when he walked. Discussion by the treatment team will probably result in a medication change to:
    1. clozapine.
    2. olanzapine.
    3. risperidone.
    4. chlorpromazine.

CHAPTER 22: SOCIAL RESPONSES AND PERSONALITY DISORDERS

1. Ms. K. tells the nurse that she has been involved in a relationship with her boyfriend for more than a year. She states, "I can rely on him when I need support, but he's okay with my being an independent person, too. We're close but neither of us tries to control the other." The nurse can correctly assess this relationship as:
    1. narcissistic.
    2. enmeshed.
    3. disconnected.
    4. interdependent.

2. When the nurse plans education for the family of a patient with personality disorder who uses maladaptive social responses, which information can be included?
    1. The patient has considerable resilience when faced with stressful life situations.
    2. The patient's maladaptive behaviors involve only a single aspect of personality.
    3. The patient has enduring ways of relating that provoke others' negative reactions.
    4. Treatment can be expected to provide personality change and effect complete cure.

3. Which thinking about relationships would be most characteristic of a patient with antisocial personality disorder?
    1. "The only reason for relating is to take advantage of others."
    2. "'Live and let live' is as good a philosophy as any to live by."
    3. "I've always found that 'help one another' is a good policy."
    4. "I'll be your doormat. Feel free to take advantage of me."

4. A nursing diagnosis that is appropriate to consider for a patient with antisocial personality disorder is:
   1. anxiety.
   2. impaired social interaction.
   3. disturbed personal identity.
   4. disturbed sensory perception.

5. Which behavior would be most characteristic of an individual with narcissistic personality disorder?
   1. A lifelong pattern of social withdrawal
   2. Refusal to enter into relationships for fear of rejection
   3. Belief that he is entitled to special privileges that others may not have
   4. Belief that he has a sixth sense and knows what others are thinking

6. Ms. A. uses the maladaptive social behavior of manipulation. Staff working to reduce this behavior should convey the message that:
   1. she is accepted, but her behavior may be rejected as inappropriate.
   2. if she cannot control her own behavior, staff will establish external controls.
   3. manipulative behavior results in frustration and anger among staff and patients.
   4. manipulation of patients and family is more acceptable that manipulation of staff.

7. Before the community meeting, Mr. K., a patient with antisocial personality disorder was overheard coaching several other patients to bring up the topic and to strongly object to the "no smoking" policy of the unit. When the group leader confronts Mr. K. with this behavior, what remark would be most characteristic of this patient?
   1. "Never send boys to do a man's job. I'll be my own spokesman in the future."
   2. "Hey, it's not my fault. These guys object to you people running this place like a jail."
   3. "I think the patients and staff should talk about the rules and negotiate some changes."
   4. "I've learned something valuable from this. Can we talk about this in my therapy session?"

8. Mr. K., a patient with antisocial personality disorder, tells the nurse that he doesn't deserve unit restriction for smoking because, "A janitor gave me the matches. I assumed you folks knew what you were doing. Give him hell, not me!" Mr. K. is using which of the following coping mechanisms?
   1. Denial
   2. Projection
   3. Sublimation
   4. Reaction formation

9. In a staff meeting, two nurses point out that the treatment plan for Mr. K., a patient with antisocial personality disorder, seems too rigid, saying, "The poor guy doesn't have any freedom. He's really a pleasant guy. Why is everybody so uptight with him?" The rest of the treatment team maintains that Mr. K. needs external limits and careful observation by staff. What patient coping mechanisms are most likely responsible for the difference in staff opinions?
   1. Idealization and devaluation
   2. Projection and rationalization
   3. Splitting and projective identification
   4. Reaction formation and identification

10. Ms. M., a patient with borderline personality disorder, tells the nurse about her relationship with her ex-boyfriend. "When I met him he was simply perfect. He showed he loved me. He granted my every wish. But then he turned into the worst person in the world. I wanted to go to a movie and he told me to go by myself, because he was going to go to a baseball game with the guys. I screamed and shouted at him, but he left me and went to the game. I felt so empty and awful that I had to cut myself." Ms. M's description of her boyfriend shows that she:
    1. is using splitting.
    2. is attention-seeking.
    3. has antisocial tendencies.
    4. has formal thought disorder.

11. Ms. M., a patient with borderline personality disorder, tells the nurse about her relationship with her ex-boyfriend. "When I met him he was simply perfect. He showed he loved me. He granted my every wish. But then he turned into the worst person in the world. I wanted to go to a movie and he told me to go by myself, because he was going to go to a baseball game with the guys. I screamed and shouted at him, but he left me and went to the game. I felt so empty and awful that I had to cut myself." Ms. M's inference that she was entitled to all her boyfriend's time and attention is consistent with:
    1. impulsivity.
    2. narcissism.
    3. magical thinking.
    4. passive-aggression.

12. Which behavior would be most characteristic of a young man diagnosed as having an antisocial personality disorder?
    1. Having been convicted of a felony, to serve a jail sentence and then "go straight"
    2. When apprehended for committing a crime, to withdraw from contacts and remain mute and unresponsive
    3. Having committed a crime, to persuade the judge to suspend the sentence and later violate probation
    4. To plead guilty to his crime, show remorse, and develop symptoms of severe depression when he realizes the impact of his crime on his family

13. The nurse is assigned to work with Ms. A., a patient with borderline personality disorder. The nurse will need to consider in advance strategies for dealing with:
    1. grief, appropriate anger, and social isolation.
    2. a strong sense of self and interdependence.
    3. clinging, acting out, mood shifts, and impulsivity.
    4. altered sensory perceptions and formal thought disorder.

14. The nurse has been working with Ms. A., a patient with borderline personality disorder for several days. Ms. A. tells other staff, "My nurse is wonderful! She's the only person who has ever really understood me." The nurse will need to monitor his or her responses to Ms. A. to make sure to avoid the tendency fostered by projective identification to be:
    1. aloof, unconcerned, and blasé.
    2. overly stringent, or persecutory.
    3. involved, indulgent, and overly protective.
    4. prejudicial, blaming, and overly impersonal.

15. Milieu work with patients with personality disorders is most effective when it:
    1. focuses on interactional behaviors in the here and now.
    2. facilitates a process of delving into the patient's early childhood.
    3. provides strict structure to compensate for a lack of personal boundaries.
    4. promotes regression to help the patient work through earlier conflicts.

16. The admitting officer describes Ms. R. as lively, excessively emotional, attention-seeking, and superficial. The patient's history reveals stormy relationships with friends and lovers. The nurse notes that she seems comfortable on the unit while she is the focus of attention, but seems to become anxious when not the center of attention. The nurse anticipates that the DSM-IV diagnosis that is being considered is:
    1. paranoid personality disorder.
    2. antisocial personality disorder.
    3. histrionic personality disorder.
    4. obsessive-compulsive personality disorder.

17. The relationships of patients with borderline and narcissistic personality disorders are said to move through predictable stages. Initially there is idealization and overvaluation of the object; then disappointment when unrealistic needs are not met. The nurse can predict that the final stages will be:
    1. devaluation and rejection of the object.
    2. forgiveness and reinvestment in the object.
    3. reaction formation to the object and distancing.
    4. projection and incorporation of the object into a delusion.

18. A patient with a personality disorder has revealed to staff that her family treats her cruelly. At the same time she has told the family that she is receiving indifferent care from staff that ignores her. The patient's goal is to:
    1. learn how much acing out will be tolerated.
    2. align family and staff to maximize efforts for patient behavioral change.
    3. seek a structured environment while internal controls are being developed.
    4. create family-staff conflict that diverts the focus from the patient's need for self-examination.

19. The nurse caring for a patient with a personality disorder states, "When I started working with her I was sure I could be of help. She seemed like such a sweet, helpless little waif. Now after 3 weeks of her antics, I realize no one can help her. She's incorrigible! Working with her is like working with the devil." The two different views held by the nurse are most likely the result of:
    1 countertransference.
    2. lack of emotional self-control.
    3. objective assessment of the patient.
    4. inability of the patient to profit from therapy.

20. The patient with a personality disorder tells the nurse, "Let's skip the therapy stuff today and do something pleasant, like watch a good movie on the VCR. What do you say?" Which of the following is the best reply by the nurse?
    1. "Don't be manipulative."
    2. "This isn't a social occasion."
    3. "You'd rather not work on your problems today?"
    4. "You know our time together has to be spent problem solving."

21. To assess a patient as being impulsive, the nurse would have to see behavior that:
    1. postpones gratification.
    2. adheres to a strict moral code.
    3. uses manipulative, controlling strategies.
    4. shows inability to plan, unreliability, and unpredictability.

22. Which characteristic in an individual with a personality disorder makes it advisable for staff to have frequent meetings? The patient's ability to:
    1. manipulate to circumvent limits.
    2. rapidly and successfully adapt to stress.
    3. achieve interdependent relationships.
    4. behave responsibly in a group of peers.

23. A goal for Mr. R., a patient who displays impulsive behavior, is, "The patient will explore the causes and consequences of impulsive behavior." A strategy that will assist the patient to do this is:
    1. using rewards for appropriate behavior.
    2. using relaxation exercises to reduce interpersonal anxiety.
    3. keeping a diary to describe events before and after the behavior.
    4. frequent clinical supervision for the nurse providing therapy for the patient.

24. The frustration of caring for a patient who displays maladaptive social responses such as manipulation, impulsivity, and self-mutilation can be most effectively mitigated when staff:
    1. focus on patient strengths.
    2. are vigilant about patient limits.
    3. rely on the milieu to cue responsible behavior.
    4. are experienced enough to no longer require clinical supervision.

25. The nurse is caring for Ms. U., a patient with borderline personality disorder, who cut her forearms with scissors from the activities therapy department shortly after learning that her psychiatrist was going on vacation. While changing the dressing daily, it would be advisable for the nurse to:
    1. express sympathy and concern.
    2. maintain a matter-of-fact attitude.
    3. encourage discussion of the self-mutilation.
    4. reassure the patient that she will not abandon her.

26. The care plan for a patient with a personality disorder contains the following interventions: demonstrate accessibility, maintain confidentiality, and maintain consistent behavior by all nursing staff. The goal of these interventions is:
    1. the patient's serotonin levels will stabilize.
    2. the patient will not engage in self-mutilation.
    3. the patient will participate in a therapeutic nurse-patient relationship.
    4. the patient will not use manipulation as a way of relating to staff and family.

27. A nursing diagnosis that would be appropriate to consider for any patient with a personality disorder is:
    1. anxiety.
    2. risk for self-mutilation.
    3. disturbed thought processes.
    4. impaired social interaction.

CHAPTER 23: COGNITIVE RESPONSES AND ORGANIC MENTAL DISORDERS

1. Mr. B. is a 25-year-old man who is brought by ambulance to the emergency room. He is strapped to the gurney but fights against the restraints and shouts incoherently. He is accompanied by his girlfriend, with whom he lives. She reports that he was fine the previous night but was weak and confused when he awoke in the morning. She states that somewhat later he began "rambling and talking crazy." The nurse notes that his skin is flushed and dry. The priority nursing action is to:
    1. take his vital signs.
    2. start intravenous fluids.
    3. administer a sedative.
    4. perform a mini-mental status examination.

2. Mr. B. is a 25-year-old man who is brought by ambulance to the emergency room. He is strapped to the gurney but fights against the restraints and shouts incoherently. His girlfriend reports that he was fine the night before but was weak and confused when he awoke in the morning. She states that somewhat later he began "rambling and talking crazy." The nurse notes that his skin is flushed and dry. When he is transferred to a bed, he strikes out at the staff, tries to get out of bed, and shouts, "You're not going to kill me!" The most likely analysis of this behavior is:
    1. disturbed self-esteem related to catastrophic reaction.
    2. disturbed sensory-perception related to altered brain function.
    3. other-directed violence related to fear associated with hospitalization.
    4. impaired environmental interpretational syndrome related to metabolic disturbance.

3. Mr. B. is a 25-year-old man who was brought by ambulance to the emergency room. He was strapped to the gurney but was fighting against the restraints and shouting incoherently. He is accompanied by his girlfriend, with whom he lives. She reports that he was fine the night before but was weak and confused when he awoke in the morning. She states that somewhat later he began "rambling and talking crazy." The nurse notes that his skin is flushed and dry. His aggressive behavior and attempts to get out of bed present a safety issue. The nurse should first consider:
   1. applying four-point restraints.
   2. using a calm tone to orient the patient.
   3. leaving him alone with his girlfriend.
   4. calling for security guards to hold him down.

4. Mr. B. is a 25-year-old man who was brought by ambulance to the emergency room. He was strapped to the gurney and was fighting against the restraints and shouting incoherently. His girlfriend reports that he was fine the night before but was weak and confused when he awoke in the morning. She states that somewhat later he began "rambling and talking crazy." The nurse notes that his skin is flushed and dry. Further assessment reveals he has not voided or ingested food or fluid in 18 hours. His temperature, pulse, blood pressure, and respirations are elevated, and his sensorium is alternately clouded and then clears. The physician diagnoses fever of unknown origin and orders several diagnostic tests. Because the patient is restless and agitated, the plan is to attempt oral hydration before attempting to start an IV. The intervention most likely to be effective will be:
   1. placing a pitcher of water at his bedside.
   2. placing a "Force Fluids" sign at the head of his bed.
   3. asking his girlfriend to give him a drink whenever he is alert.
   4. staying with him while he drinks a glass of juice, water, or soft drink every hour.

5. Mr. B. is a 25-year-old man who is brought by ambulance to the emergency room. He is strapped to the gurney but fights against the restraints and shouts incoherently. His girlfriend reports that he was fine the night before but was weak and confused when he awoke in the morning. She states that somewhat later he began "rambling and talking crazy." The nurse notes that his skin is flushed and dry. Further assessment reveals that he has not voided or ingested food or fluid in 18 hours. His temperature, pulse, blood pressure, and respirations are elevated, and his sensorium is alternately clouded and then clears. Mr. B.'s cognitive impairment is most consistent with:
   1. delirium.
   2. dementia.
   3. sundown syndrome.
   4. early-onset Alzheimer's disease.

6. A 78-year-old woman tells the nurse preparing her for bed that the nurse should leave the door unlocked because her husband will be coming home soon. The nurse knows that the patient's husband has been dead for 10 years. The best response would be:
   1. "You've forgotten that your husband's dead, haven't you?"
   2. "Just try to sleep. He won't be home for a long time yet."
   3. "You must miss him a lot. It almost seems he's here with you."
   4. "Your husband died 10 years ago. He won't be coming here."

7. The physician's admission note mentions that Ms. Y., age 67, has sundown syndrome. The nurse can expect that the patient will:
   1. exhibit chronic fatigue.
   2. evidence extreme lethargy at night.
   3. manifest confusion and agitation at night.
   4. be more alert between 6 PM and 11 PM.

8. The most useful intervention to prevent or lessen the symptoms associated with sundown syndrome is to:
   1. place the patient in a quiet, dimly lit room.
   2. interact frequently with the patient during evening hours.
   3. offer a bedtime snack and take the patient to the bathroom at bedtime.
   4. give the patient a soft stuffed animal to keep with him or her.

9. A nursing diagnosis that would be appropriate for a patient with Alzheimer's disease is:
   1. disorientation related to hyperthermia.
   2. anxiety (moderate) related to dementia.
   3. disturbed thought processes related to irreversible brain disorder.
   4. disturbed sensory perception (visual) related to alcohol abuse.

10. Ms. S., age 45, shows marked cognitive impairment that has developed progressively over several months. The history reveals that his father also had early-onset dementia. Ms. S.'s young adult children are concerned that they also may develop early-onset dementia. What information, made available by research, can be given to this family?
    1. There is no substantial added risk for family members of a person with Alzheimer's disease.
    2. The risk for relatives of people who develop Alzheimer's disease before age 55 is greater than for those with no family history.
    3. Added risk is present only for people with Down syndrome, so "normal" relatives are essentially "safe."
    4. Alzheimer's disease is transmitted as an autosomal dominant trait, meaning that offspring have a 1 in 2 chance of developing the disorder.

11. Ms. S., age 72, has the medical diagnosis of delirium secondary to anticholinergic medication toxicity. Her family members are very concerned and express their concerns about placing her in a nursing home. The information that should serve as a basis for the nurse's reply is:
    1. delirium is reversible, and Ms. S. will recover.
    2. her symptoms are related to depression, which can be treated.
    3. delirium usually progresses to dementia, and Ms. S. will be permanently impaired.
    4. home care should be attempted; a nursing home should be the last resort.

12. Ms. S., age 72, has the medical diagnosis of delirium secondary to anticholinergic medication toxicity. The nurse planning discharge care must consider the need to teach the family to be alert for maladaptive cognitive symptoms because:
    1. delirium is a hypersensitivity reaction.
    2. the elderly often deny changes in cognition.
    3. elderly females are more prone to delirium than elderly males.
    4. slower metabolism in the elderly predisposes to medication toxicity.

13. The nurse is caring for a patient who is confused, disoriented in all three spheres, and experiencing visual hallucinations. In preparation to providing personal care, the nurse should:
    1. ask the patient, "Do you remember who I am?"
    2. speak minimally so as not to disturb the patient.
    3. pat the patient on the forearm and say, "Let's get started."
    4. tell the patient his or her name and position and what he or she is going to do.

14. Ms. V., age 25, is experiencing delirium secondary to corticosteroid toxicity. She is manifesting paranoid thinking and noisy, assaultive behavior. She has pulled out her IV and swung the pole at staff members. A CNA was assigned to stay with her to calm her, but she punched the CNA, breaking her nose. She is currently pacing the hall and shouting. The nurse has called the physician to come to the unit. The nurse can anticipate that the physician may order:
    1. the use of restraints and 1:1 supervision.
    2. a loading dose of phenytoin.
    3. a small dose of prednisone.
    4. an IV dose of thiamine.

15. Ms. N. has dementia associated with excessive alcohol use. At admission the nurse showed her a pencil, a nickel, and safety pin and had her repeat the names of each. Later the nurse again showed the three items and asked the patient to identify each. The patient was unable to identify the objects. The nurse assesses this as:
    1. apraxia.
    2. agnosia.
    3. concreteness.
    4. catastrophising.

16. Ms. N. has dementia associated with excessive alcohol use. The nurse caring for her asks, "Did you have a good night, last night?" The patient replies, "I had a lovely time. I went out to dinner at the Plaza Hotel, and then we danced for hours. I didn't get much sleep, that's why I'm tired today." The nurse is aware that the patient spent the night in the hospital. The symptom described can be assessed as:
    1. akathisia.
    2. confabulation.
    3. intellectualization.
    4. magical thinking.

17. The daughter of a patient with early-to-middle-stage Alzheimer's disease who is receiving home care is concerned about episodes of incontinence. What strategy should the nurse suggest?
    1. Limit fluids to 1000 ml daily.
    2. Discuss the use of an indwelling catheter with the physician.
    3. Put plastic coverings on the beds, upholstered chairs, and sofas.
    4. Take the patient to the bathroom every 2 hours when awake and use a bed pad at night.

18. The nurse caring for a patient with Alzheimer's disease can anticipate that the family will be most likely to need information about:
    1. antimetabolites.
    2. benzodiazepines.
    3. immunosuppressants.
    4. acetylcholinesterase inhibitors.

19. The nurse would attempt to reduce nighttime agitation for a patient with either delirium or dementia by:
    1. giving warm milk at bedtime.
    2. keeping a light on in the room.
    3. hanging pictures near the bed.
    4. placing a large-faced clock and calendar opposite the bed.

20. The expected outcome for the patient with a nursing diagnosis of disturbed thought processes is, "The patient will:
    1. be safe from injury."
    2. meet basic biological needs."
    3. achieve optimum cognitive functioning."
    4. maintain positive interpersonal relationships."

21. The Jones family has noted the following behaviors in their elderly mother: periodic indecisiveness, forgetfulness, mild transient confusion, occasional misperception, distractibility, and occasional unclear thinking. Where on the continuum of cognitive responses would this patient be?

    Adaptive responses Maladaptive responses

    1 2 3

    1. At point 1
    2. At point 2
    3. At point 3
    4. There is insufficient information to make a determination.

22. An elderly female patient is admitted with a tentative diagnosis of delirium, and a work-up is being conducted for occult infection. The patient repeatedly mistakes one of the nursing staff for her niece. The nurse documents that this patient is experiencing a disturbance in which of the following areas of functioning?
    1. Consciousness
    2. Attention
    3. Perception
    4. Cognition

23. An elderly patient with dementia paces the hallway and engages in wandering in the long-term care facility. The nurse documents that the patient is engaging in which of the following types of behaviors that is characteristic of dementia?
    1. Aggressive psychomotor behavior
    2. Nonaggressive psychomotor behavior
    3. Passive behavior
    4. Functionally impaired behavior

24. An adolescent patient is diagnosed with dementia. The nurse would suspect which of the following underlying conditions to be associated with this diagnosis because of the client's age?
    1. Head trauma
    2. Neurosyphilis
    3. Pick's disease
    4. Hypothyroidism

25. The nurse is working with a family that is in the prediagnostic phase of helping an elderly family member with Alzheimer's disease. The most important nursing intervention at this time would be to provide:
    1. a single-session family consultation to process information and facilitate communication.
    2. information about support groups and counseling.
    3. options to reduce caregiver stress.
    4. information and educational materials that help them understand their situation.

CHAPTER 24: CHEMICALLY MEDIATED RESPONSES AND SUBSTANCE-RELATED DISORDERS

1. Mr. W. is a 45-year-old man who is admitted to an alcohol detoxification unit. He has had no alcohol intake for 3 days. On admission he is noted to have tremors, anxiety, visual hallucinations, insomnia, suspiciousness, and disorientation accompanied by vomiting, temperature elevation, tachycardia, and diaphoresis. These signs and symptoms are characteristic of the syndrome known as:
    1. alcoholic hallucinosis.
    2. alcohol-induced psychosis.
    3. alcoholic seizure disorder.
    4. alcohol withdrawal delirium.

2. The nursing intervention of highest priority relative to alcohol withdrawal delirium is:
    1. application of restraints.
    2. reorientation of the patient to reality.
    3. identification of social supports.
    4. maintenance of fluid and electrolyte balance.

3. When a patient asks the nurse, "What do you know about AA?" the nurse should reply:
    1. "Controlled drinking is the goal of members."
    2. "The alcoholic strives to abstain for one day at a time."
    3. "A commitment must be made to permanent abstinence."
    4. "A member who feels compelled to drink is encouraged to do so in the group."

4. The wife of an alcoholic asks the nurse how to respond to him in a helpful way even though he disrupts the family life. The best response would be:
    1. "Search the house regularly for hidden alcohol."
    2. "Include him in family activities whether or not he is drinking."
    3. "Make him responsible for the consequences of his own behavior."
    4. "Help him avoid embarrassment by covering for him when he can't meet his obligations."

5. When planning teaching for a patient taking disulfiram (Antabuse), the nurse should explain the inadvisability of using certain over-the-counter substances. Given the following list, which substance could the patient select as safe to use?
    1. Antacids
    2. Mouthwash
    3. Cough syrups
    4. Aftershave lotion

6. A nurse is working the 3 PM to 11 PM shift in the ICU. He observes that sometimes patients do not respond to diazepam (Valium) injections. On further investigation, he discovers that the lack of response occurs after the medication has been administered by Ms. H., a day-shift nurse. One day when an evening shift nurse calls in sick, Ms. H. works a double shift. At 5 PM Ms. H. administers diazepam to a patient in a dose that is usually effective for the patient, but the patient remains markedly anxious. The nurse notes that Ms. H., however, seems slightly euphoric and uncoordinated and that her speech is slurred. The best action for the nurse to take is:
   1. immediately confront Ms. H. with the drug diversion.
   2. ask other nurses if they have observed anything unusual.
   3. personally supervise Ms. H. whenever she prepares medication.
   4. call the nursing supervisor and ask him or her to come to the unit to document and intervene.

7. A positive initial action for a health care agency to take for an impaired nurse would be:
   1. job dismissal.
   2. eliciting a promise to abstain.
   3. counseling by the head nurse.
   4. referral to the employee assistance program.

8. When a recovering impaired colleague returns to work, nursing professionals can be most helpful by:
   1. directly offering support.
   2. double-checking all the nurse's activities.
   3. assigning another nurse to watch the recovering nurse closely.
   4. avoiding mention of the problem unless the recovering nurse mentions it.

9. In the emergency room the nurse learns that Mr. G. has recently taken a large amount of PCP. The nurse should be ready to provide interventions for:
   1. acute psychosis, agitation, and violence.
   2. hypotension, sedation, and respiratory depression.
   3. heightened sensory perceptions, dizziness, and ataxia.
   4. paranoid thinking, hyperthermia, hyperactivity, and arrhythmias.

10. A young man has been admitted after PCP use that resulted in an acute psychotic state. He repeatedly removes his clothes and attempts to run in the hallway. A dose of a benzodiazepine has been ordered, but staff members have not been able to administer it. An appropriate intervention would be:
    1. provide an alternative activity to channel his energy.
    2. obtain an order for seclusion with close observation.
    3. perform a lavage to prevent continuing absorption of drug.
    4. assign a nurse to stay with him to reassure and "talk him down."

11. A new nurse on the chemical dependence unit mentions, "The drugs of abuse all seem to cause patients to become violent." The best reply would be that:
    1. violence is associated with abuse, rather than with withdrawal.
    2. some drugs, such as heroin, rarely produce violent behavior.
    3. the observation is astute and true because all users have antisocial tendencies.
    4. nursing behaviors toward the patients are more responsible for violence than the drugs.

12. At report the nurse learns that Ms. V. is in opiate withdrawal. For what objective data should the nurse be alert?
    1. Lacrimation, rhinorrhea, dilated pupils, and muscle spasms
    2. Somnolence, constipation, normal pupils, and hypothermia
    3. Tremors, hypertension, constricted pupils, and deep sleep
    4. Visual and tactile hallucinations, agitation, and grand mal seizure

13. Mr. T. sustained a fractured femur in an automobile accident while driving under the influence of drugs. "Tracks" are noted on his arms. The history obtained from family indicates that Mr. T. has "dabbled in drugs" for a number of years. The nurse notes that Mr. T. obtains little to no relief from the prescribed dose of narcotic analgesic. The failure to get pain relief may be related to:
    1. tolerance.
    2. habituation.
    3. substance abuse.
    4. onset of withdrawal symptoms.

14. An unconscious patient is brought to the emergency department. It is suspected that he has overdosed on heroin. Which vital signs would be most consistent with that diagnosis?
    1. BP, 70/40; P, 120; R, 10
    2. BP, 120/80; P, 84; R, 20
    3. BP, 140/90; P, 76; R, 28
    4. BP, 180/100; P, 72; R, 22

15. An unconscious patient is brought to the emergency department. It is suspected that he has overdosed on heroin. What drug can the nurse anticipate will be administered?
    1. Disulfiram
    2. Naltrexone
    3. Methadone
    4. Acamprosate

16. The nurse believes that one of her patients being admitted for surgery may have a drinking problem. To further assess this issue, the nurse should consider:
    1. using a screening tool such as CAGE or B-DAST.
    2. asking directly if the patient has ever had problems with alcohol.
    3. that all patients answer alcohol-related queries using denial and rationalization.
    4. ignoring the potential because it has no direct effect on the patient's surgery.

17. An appropriate long-term goal for a recovering alcohol or drug abuser would be, "The patient will:
    1. verbalize his or her addiction to significant others."
    2. state his or her intention to abstain from drug use."
    3. abstain from or reduce the use of mood-altering drugs."
    4. substitute a less harmful drug for the current drug of abuse."

18. A short-term goal for a woman addicted to sedatives and stimulants is, "The patient will:
    1. verbalize that she is dependent on drugs."
    2. discuss her addictive behavior with others."
    3. recognize the situations in which she uses drugs."
    4. understand the reasons she became addicted to drugs."

19. Short-term goals related to abstinence include all *except*, "The patient will:
    1. make a daily commitment to abstain."
    2. attend at least two support group meetings weekly."
    3. focus on improving the quality of the relationship with a significant other."
    4. contact a supportive person if he or she experiences an urge to use an addictive substance."

20. The following are goals for a patient being treated for alcoholism. In which order should these goals be approached?
    A. Developing alternative coping skills
    B. Attaining physiological stabilization
    C. Learning about dependence and recovery
    D. Abstinence and development of a support system
    1. A, B, C, D
    2. B, D, C, A
    3. C, D, B, A
    4. D, C, B, A

21. Some physicians recommend that, whenever possible, physical exercise should be a daily component of an addicted person's ongoing program of treatment. Meditation also may be recommended. The basis for these aspects of treatment is to make use of the body's:
    1. endocrines.
    2. endorphins.
    3. enkephalins.
    4. epinephrine.

22. A patient addicted to both alcohol and benzodiazepines tells the nurse she can control her drug use at any time she chooses. This statement can be assessed as:
    1. denial.
    2. repression.
    3. compensation.
    4. reaction formation.

23. Nurse W. is caring for a patient who may be withdrawing from barbiturates. In assessing the risk and planning interventions, Nurse W. should rely on the guideline that the longer the half-life of the drug:
    1. the shorter the withdrawal.
    2. the less intense the withdrawal symptoms.
    3. the sooner the patient will begin to crave the drug.
    4. the shorter the withdrawal and the more intense the withdrawal symptoms.

24. Nurse W. is beginning work on a unit that provides detoxification for patients addicted to drugs and alcohol. Care planning for patients undergoing detoxification to alcohol and sedative hypnotics is predicated on the treatment principle that says to:
    1. use medications to treat symptoms as they appear.
    2. avoid medicating a patient in "detox" to preserve liver function.
    3. substitute medication from the same drug class for gradual tapering.
    4. force fluids because sedative hypnotics and alcohol are detoxified mainly by the kidneys.

25. The police bring Mr. G. to the emergency department to be examined after an auto accident. He has slurred speech, ataxia, and drowsiness. He exhibits lability as evidenced by occasional angry outbursts. His blood alcohol level (BAL) is 0.40 g/dl. From the relationship between his behavior and his BAL, the nurse can make the assessment that the patient:
    1. takes disulfiram.
    2. rarely drinks alcohol.
    3. has ingested acamprosate.
    4. has a high tolerance to alcohol.

26. A nurse using cognitive-behavioral therapy to help a patient with substance abuse problems will:
    1. help the patient to develop self-control and social skills.
    2. support the use of emotion-focused coping mechanisms.
    3. focus on addiction as a disease requiring confrontational tactics.
    4. help the patient see that responsibility for substance use is shared with family and friends.

27. The view of relapse that will be most helpful for the nurse to transmit to the recovering substance abuser is relapse is:
    1. an error from which to learn.
    2. an indicator of treatment failure.
    3. an event with a physiological cause.
    4. the result of lack of environmental support.

28. A nursing diagnosis that would be considered universally appropriate for patients who abuse mood-altering drugs would be:
    1. confusion.
    2. imbalanced nutrition.
    3. ineffective coping.
    4. impaired environmental interpretation syndrome.

CHAPTER 25: EATING REGULATION RESPONSES AND EATING DISORDERS

1. When undertaking care for a patient with an eating disorder, the nurse should first:
    1. perform a complete patient assessment.
    2. obtain a history from the patient's family.
    3. examine his or her own feelings about weight.
    4. ask when the patient last ate and offer food.

2. The nurse determines that which of the following patients has the most severe form of maladaptive eating regulation response?
    1. A 15-year-old who overeats under stress
    2. A 16-year-old who engages in severe dieting
    3. A 14-year-old who skips a meal once or twice week
    4. A 17-year-old with night eating syndrome

3. The central concept around which a family education plan for preventing childhood eating problems is constructed is:
    1. promoting self-demand feeding for the child.
    2. distinguishing between physical and psychological hunger.
    3. scheduling meals because children do not recognize physical hunger.
    4. parental expectations of ideal intake as determinants of healthy eating habits.

4. Which information would be of greatest assistance to the nurse assessing patient motivation to change behavior associated with maladaptive eating regulation responses?
    1. Identify a person on whom you can rely for emotional support.
    2. Rate your desire for treatment on a scale of 1 to 10.
    3. Identify the advantages of giving up the maladaptive behavior.
    4. Identify the disadvantages of giving up the maladaptive behavior.

5. After assessing a female patient with anorexia nervosa, the nurse writes the following nursing diagnosis: imbalanced nutrition, less than body requirements related to refusal to eat as evidenced by being 25% below body weight for height. The expected outcome should be listed as:
    1. patient will exhibit fewer signs of malnutrition.
    2. patient will gain 1 to 3 pounds per week until the desired body weight is attained.
    3. patient will identify cognitive distortions about food, weight, and body shape.
    4. patient will restore healthy eating patterns and normalize physiologic parameters related to weight and nutrition.

6. The coping mechanism that the nurse will assess as being excessively and maladaptively used by patients with anorexia nervosa is:
    1. denial.
    2. projection.
    3. introjection.
    4. rationalization.

7. Care planning requires the nurse to recognize that the dynamic focus of the patient with anorexia nervosa is on:
    1. weight.
    2. control.
    3. anxiety.
    4. personal values.

8. The nurse has completed the assessment for T., age 15, who has a maladaptive response to eating regulation. Findings include: height, 5 feet 3 inches; current weight, 80 pounds with weight loss of 30% of body weight over the past 3 months; T, 96.6; BP, 68/40; P, 40; R, 20; poor skin turgor; lanugo; amenorrhea of 6 months' duration. Admits to restricting intake to 350 calories daily. Is a vegetarian. Dissatisfied with eating pattern as evidenced by patient statement, "I need to lose another 10 pounds to be at an ideal weight." These assessment findings are most consistent with the medical diagnosis:
   1. bulimia nervosa.
   2. anorexia nervosa.
   3. binge-eating disorder.
   4. personal identity disorder.

9. The nurse has completed the assessment for T., age 15, who has a maladaptive response to eating regulation. Findings include: height 5 feet 3 inches; current weight 80 pounds with weight loss of 30% of body weight over the past 3 months; T, 96.6; BP, 68/40; P, 40; R, 20; poor skin turgor; lanugo; amenorrhea of 6 months' duration. Admits to restricting intake to 350 calories daily. Is a vegetarian. Dissatisfied with eating pattern as evidenced by patient statement, "I need to lose another 10 pounds to be at an ideal weight." Patient states that she sees no need for treatment although her parents are upset. These assessment findings suggest that the best treatment setting for this patient would be:
   1. the hospital.
   2. an outpatient program.
   3. a day treatment program.
   4. at home with weekly nursing visits.

10. T., age 15, has a maladaptive response to eating regulation. Findings include: height 5 feet 3 inches; current weight 80 pounds with weight loss of 30% of body weight over the past 3 months; T, 96.6; BP, 68/40; P, 40; R, 20; poor skin turgor; lanugo; amenorrhea of 6 months' duration. Admits to restricting intake to 350 calories daily. Is a vegetarian. Dissatisfied with eating pattern as evidenced by patient statement, "I need to lose another 10 pounds to be at ideal weight." Diagnostic testing reveals serum potassium of 2.9 mEq/L and urine specific gravity of 1.028. Which of the following would be the highest priority nursing diagnosis for this patient?
   1. Imbalanced nutrition, less than body requirements
   2. Disturbed body image
   3. Deficient fluid volume
   4. Powerlessness

11. A first step in the creation of a therapeutic alliance between the nurse and a patient with a maladaptive response to eating regulation is:
   1. formulation of a nurse-patient contract.
   2. resolution of conflicts with family members.
   3. nurse and patient will agree on perception of patient's body.
   4. the means of stabilizing the patient's nutritional status will be specified.

12. A major difference in assessment findings between the patient with anorexia nervosa and the patient with bulimia nervosa is the patient with bulimia:
   1. is well-nourished while the anorectic is malnourished.
   2. denies hunger while the anorectic admits experiencing hunger.
   3. is often of near-normal weight while the anorectic is underweight.
   4. has a distorted body image while the anorectic has a realistic body image.

13. A short-term goal for a patient with anorexia nervosa is: Patient will select and eat a balanced diet. The nurse writes which of the following nursing interventions into the care plan that will foster attainment of this goal?
   1. Assist the patient to fill out the dietary menus to ensure a balanced diet.
   2. Encourage the patient to engage in compensatory exercise.
   3. Implement contracted consequences at 50% of the time if a meal is not completed.
   4. Allow patient to weigh self every time a meal is completely eaten.

14. Which of the following is a short-term goal that should be met first by the patient with anorexia nervosa undergoing nutritional stabilization?
   1. Schedules meals appropriately.
   2. Eats 100% of each meal.
   3. Selects food items from a menu appropriately.
   4. Cooks food under supervision.

15. What is the rationale for establishing a contract with a patient with an eating disorder at the outset of treatment?
   1. The patient and nurse form a coalition that is difficult for the family to disrupt.
   2. A team approach to planning therapy ensures that physical and emotional needs will be met.
   3. Patient involvement in decision making increases the sense of control and promotes cooperation.
   4. Permission for refeeding is essential because this measure has the potential for negative effects.

16. The nurse planning care for a patient with an eating disorder wants to be sure that research evidence supports practice. What type of therapy should the nurse select?
    1. Supportive therapy
    2. Behavioral therapy
    3. Cognitive-behavioral therapy
    4. Psychoanalytic group therapy

17. The nurse would conclude that a patient with an eating disorder is exhibiting a cognitive distortion after hearing the patient make which of the following statements?
    1. "I see now that I need to establish my own preferences and routines."
    2. "Bingeing cures my feelings of isolation and loneliness."
    3. "Controlling what I eat has been a way for me to exert control over my life."
    4. "I need to watch for hunger and fatigue as triggers for my eating disorder."

18. C., a 33-year-old single graduate student, is seeking treatment for bulimia nervosa. Her therapist decides to use cognitive-behavioral therapy and medication. For what medication can the nurse expect to develop a patient education program?
    1. An SSRI
    2. Lithium
    3. Acamprosate
    4. A benzodiazepine

19. C., a 33-year-old single graduate student, is a residence counselor. She has no friends because the students she supervises are much younger. Her schoolwork and residence duties leave her no time for socialization with others in her program. She began to binge in response to feelings of anxiety related to loneliness and later began purging. A goal is that she will use a constructive coping strategy to deal with anxiety in lieu of bingeing and purging. Which intervention addresses this goal?
    1. Role play use of assertiveness techniques.
    2. Teach progressive relaxation, imagery, or meditation.
    3. Explore ways the patient can feel in control of her environment.
    4. Encourage attendance at a support group for patients with eating disorders.

20. Which of the following questions asked by the nurse would be least helpful in evaluating the outcomes of a patient with an eating disorder?
    1. Have normal eating patterns been restored?
    2. Have the sequelae of malnutrition been corrected?
    3. Have neurotransmitter imbalances been corrected?
    4. Have biopsychosocial problems been resolved so relapse is less likely?

21. The nurse assesses that which of the following individuals is most likely to engage in binge eating behaviors characteristic of bulimia?
    1. A 22-year-old who weighs 225 pounds and is 5 feet 4 inches
    2. A 16-year-old who is 5 pounds overweight and cannot stick to a diet
    3. A 19-year-old who can lose up to 40 pounds but gains it back within a year
    4. A 17-year-old dancer who is slightly underweight who monitors caloric intake to maintain a stable weight

22. A patient is diagnosed with anorexia nervosa. The nurse who is assessing for comorbid psychiatric disorders should begin by looking for signs of which concurrent diagnosis that occurs most often?
    1. Phobias
    2. Depression
    3. Personality disorder
    4. Schizophrenia

23. The nurse would evaluate that a family education plan for preventing childhood eating problems has met the stated objectives if which of the following outcomes is evident?
    1. Parents serve 3 meals per day plus mid-morning, mid-afternoon, and bedtime snacks.
    2. Parents indicate an interest in learning about healthier eating patterns for their children.
    3. Parents can distinguish between psychological and physical hunger.
    4. Parents use food to reward especially good behavior, such as an excellent report card.

24. The nurse would assess for which of the following features in a patient diagnosed with anorexia nervosa without bingeing or purging?
    1. Is extroverted
    2. Abuses diuretics and laxatives
    3. Is sexually active
    4. Denies hunger

25. The nurse would assess for which of the following features in a patient diagnosed with bulimia nervosa?
    1. Is introverted
    2. Abuses diuretics and laxatives
    3. Is sexually inactive
    4. Does not experiences hunger

26. A patient with an eating disorder states, "Now that I've gained 4 pounds, I can't wear a skirt until I lose it again." The nurse documents that the patient is exhibiting which cognitive distortion related to maladaptive eating regulation responses?
    1. Magnification
    2. Superstitious thinking
    3. Personalization
    4. Dichotomous thinking

27. A patient with an eating disorder states, "I heard people laughing behind me in the check-out line at the department store. I bet they thought it was hysterically funny that I gained a pound in the last few days." The nurse documents that the patient is exhibiting which cognitive distortion related to maladaptive eating regulation responses?
    1. Magnification
    2. Superstitious thinking
    3. Personalization
    4. Dichotomous thinking

CHAPTER 26: SEXUAL RESPONSES AND SEXUAL DISORDERS

1. Ms. S. is upset because she has learned that her son is gay. She asks the nurse, "What causes homosexuality? Did I do something wrong?" The best reply would be:
    1. "It's thought that homosexuality is transmitted via the X gene."
    2. "The cause or causes of homosexuality have not been determined."
    3. "Many people consider homosexuality an expression of normal sexual behavior."
    4. "You sound as though you are expressing concern about both your son and yourself."

2. Mr. E. has come to the mental health clinic because he feels uncomfortable with his body. He relates, "I feel as though I'm really a woman trapped in this male body." This type of complaint is characteristically expressed by someone who is a:
    1. transsexual.
    2. transvestite.
    3. pedophile.
    4. homosexual.

3. Ms. A., a new graduate nurse, has been caring for a gay patient for the past week. She requests that her patient assignment be changed, saying, "I learned in school that homosexuality is not an illness, but every time I see my patient and his 'boyfriend,' I think it's really sick!" The nurse is experiencing the stage of the self-awareness process called:
    1. anger.
    2. anxiety.
    3. choosing values.
    4. cognitive dissonance.

4. Mr. B., a new nurse, tells his mentor, "When my patient, Mr. R., brought up the subject of resuming sexual relations with his wife after his surgery, I felt flustered and started to talk and talk. I realized I wasn't letting him express himself but I carried on diagnosing and analyzing." The nurse describes experiencing the stage of the self-awareness process called:
    1. anger.
    2. action.
    3. anxiety.
    4. cognitive dissonance.

5. Mr. Y., a 19-year-old patient, is hospitalized for an acute episode of schizophrenia. Today the nurse finds him in the lounge without any clothes on and telling everyone he is "the body beautiful." The most appropriate intervention for the nurse would be to:
    1. tell him to put on his clothes immediately.
    2. assist him to his room and help him get dressed.
    3. ignore the behavior to prevent the patient from receiving secondary gain.
    4. seclude him until he can regain control over his inappropriate, impulsive behavior.

6. Ms. D. is a 45-year-old woman who is seeking help controlling her newly diagnosed hypertension. The nurse plans to include questions about sexual health in the assessment. Which would be a good initial question relating to this topic?
    1. "Has your hypertension changed your sex life?"
    2. "How are you and your husband getting along sexually?"
    3. "I assume you don't have any problems with sex, do you?"
    4. "Can you identify any changes in your sexual activity since you learned about your hypertension?"

7. Mr. N. is a 32-year-old patient hospitalized for depression 1 month ago. Ms. C. has been his nurse therapist. The day before Mr. N. is to be discharged, he asks Ms. C. for a date. The most therapeutic response by the nurse would be:
    1. "That sounds nice, but I already have a boyfriend."
    2. "The hospital has a policy that does not allow professional staff to date patients."
    3. "I guess there would be no harm in meeting for coffee, if we know in advance that we're meeting just as friends."
    4. "It's sometimes difficult to sort out relationships. We've developed positive feelings in our working relationship, but it is a professional, rather than a social, relationship."

8. Mr. R., a patient being treated for cellulitis, tells the night shift nurse assigned to care for him, "I feel like you and I should get it on tonight. What do you say to closing the door and crawling into bed with me?" The nurse should respond:
   1. "You've got to be kidding."
   2. "You've gotten my attention. What is it you're feeling?"
   3. "Your suggestion is inappropriate and makes me very uncomfortable."
   4. "I wonder why you think I would be willing to have sex with you."

9. Mr. and Ms. K. come to the clinic for treatment of sexual dysfunction. The therapist obtains a detailed sexual history and decides to employ the Masters and Johnson model of therapy. The nurse who sees this in the record can rightly assume that treatment planning will include:
   1. examination of performance failures.
   2. enhancing warm feelings.
   3. exploring early sexual experiences.
   4. delving into early growth and development.

10. What factor is of concern during evaluation of effectiveness of sexual counseling or intervention?
    1. Patient satisfaction with treatment
    2. Patient reduction in use of fantasy
    3. Nurse completes sex education plan
    4. Patient behavior respects moral norms of the community

11. The nurse is asked to assess a 24-year-old patient who reports that she is unable to have intercourse because of involuntary contractions at the vaginal opening. The nurse can correctly assess this as:
    1. vaginismus.
    2. dyspareunia.
    3. arousal disorder.
    4. orgasmic dysfunction.

12. The nursing diagnosis that could be applied to a patient who is upset that she has developed vaginismus associated with fear of pregnancy, as well as a patient with diabetes who is concerned that he cannot attain an erection, is:
    1. ineffective sexuality pattern.
    2. sexual dysfunction.
    3. sexual arousal disorder.
    4. sexual aversion disorder.

13. The nurse is asked to consult with school nurse-teachers about what to teach to help students operationalize the concept of "say no to sex." One helpful method the nurse can suggest is:
    1. pretesting for accurate sexual knowledge.
    2. explaining why saying "no" is appropriate for teens.
    3. role playing being assertive in potentially difficult sexual situations.
    4. brainstorming examples of behaviors that promote good sexual health.

14. Which of the following statements made by a patient can the nurse evaluate as showing appropriate understanding of the particular sexual issue?
    1. "Oral intercourse is dangerous."
    2. "Sex during menstruation should be avoided."
    3. "Advanced age alone is not a deterrent to sexual function."
    4. "Alcohol ingestion enhances sexual pleasure and performance."

15. A nurse is caring for an attractive and interesting man of her own age. The nurse realizes she is beginning to fantasize about having a social and sexual relationship with him. A good way of dealing with these feelings is to:
    1. try to put them out of mind.
    2. share them with the patient.
    3. explore the patient's interest through slightly flirtatious behavior.
    4. seek consultation from an experienced and trusted peer.

16. Mr. B., a patient who has a new colostomy, tells the nurse, "This surgery is the end of my sex life." This revelation should lead the nurse to take the initial step of:
    1. making a referral to an ostomy self-help group.
    2. bringing the patient's partner into the discussion.
    3. helping the patient fully express fears and feelings.
    4. reframing the effect of illness on the patient's sexual functioning.

17. What is the rationale for seeking information about the effects of prescribed medications on the patient's sexual function?
    1. Sexual dysfunction may result from use of prescription medications.
    2. The question eases the transition to questioning about sexual practices.
    3. Patients are more comfortable talking about medications than about sex.
    4. The question provides an opening to question about nonprescription drug use.

18. To assess whether a patient is experiencing sexual dysfunction because of medication use, the nurse would inquire about the patient's use of which of the following types of medications?
    1. Diuretics
    2. Appetite suppressants
    3. Antihypertensives
    4. GI antiinflammatory agents

19. When a patient tells a nurse, "I think I'm impotent or something," what response by the nurse would be best?
    1. "That's a bummer."
    2. "How's your general health?"
    3. "What medications do you take?"
    4. "Tell me what you mean by impotence."

20. The nurse should write the expected outcome for a patient with maladaptive sexual response as: "The patient will:
    1. identify sexual questions and problems."
    2. implement one new behavior to improve sexual functioning."
    3. state comfort and satisfaction with gender identity and sexual orientation."
    4. obtain maximum level of adaptive sexual responses to enhance or maintain health."

21. A patient with a sexual response disorder reports hypersexuality. During the course of the interview, the nurse should inquire about a history of which of the following psychiatric disorders?
    1. Depression
    2. Mania
    3. Personality disorder
    4. Obsessive-compulsive disorder

22. A couple reports having rare to occasional variations in their sexual response patterns. The nurse should conclude that this couple has:
    1. no medically diagnosed health problem.
    2. sexual dysfunction.
    3. a paraphilia.
    4. a gender identity disorder.

23. The nurse is teaching a male patient about the use of sildenafil (Viagra) as treatment for an erectile disorder. The nurse explains that this medication should be taken approximately:
    1. 10 to 15 minutes before sexual activity.
    2. 1 hour before sexual activity.
    3. 4 hours before sexual activity.
    4. 8 hours before sexual activity.

24. A patient with gender identity disorder (gender dysphoria) tells the nurse that he wants to undergo a "sex change operation." Which of the following should the nurse share with the patient about the prerequisites for sexual reassignment surgery?
    1. The patient must be 25 years of age or older.
    2. The patient must live in the role of the preferred gender for at least 6 months.
    3. Two therapists must agree that the reassignment is appropriate.
    4. The patient must undergo approximately 5 years of psychotherapy after surgery.

25. An adult survivor of childhood sexual abuse is at risk for behavioral and social problems as sequelae. To determine whether the patient is experiencing social problems, the nurse would explore whether the patient:
    1. abuses substances such as drugs or alcohol.
    2. displays high-risk sexual behavior.
    3. experiences suicidal ideation.
    4. has become a victim of sexual violence as an adult.

CHAPTER 27: PSYCHOPHARMACOLOGY

1. Which of the following therapeutic nursing interventions would the nurse employ to reduce a patient's risk for the development of drug interactions?
    1. Ensuring adequate hydration and nutrition
    2. Formulating only one diagnosis on the multiaxial evaluation
    3. Eliminating all but the psychotropic medication that has been started until the patient's target symptoms subside
    4. Teaching the patient's family the psychotropic medication's side effects to avoid patient suggestibility

2. A 32-year-old female patient will be starting on fluoxetine hydrochloride (Prozac) therapy and taking 20 mg po every morning. Which nursing intervention would be most therapeutic for the nurse to teach her?
    1. "Make sure that you take your pulse before getting out of bed in the morning."
    2. "Try taking your medication with breakfast if you experience nausea."
    3. "You may need to reduce your fluids at night because of nocturnal urination."
    4. "You'll have to give up red wine, nuts, and any cheese except cottage and cream cheese while you're taking this medication."

3. Which of the following would the nurse ask a depressed patient who is complaining of nausea, palpitations, and "a terrible headache and chest pain" after physical examination reveals elevated blood pressure and temperature, dilated pupils, flushed head and face, and diaphoresis?
    1. "When did you last take your phenelzine (Nardil)?"
    2. "Did you take your amitriptyline (Elavil) earlier than you usually do?"
    3. "What natural foods have you had in the last 24 hours?"
    4. "Have you been drinking within the last 24 hours?

4. Which would be the most therapeutic nursing communication on the basis of the nurse's understanding of a depressed patient who says, "I need to stop taking my medication because it blurs my vision, and I'm making mistakes when I paint jewelry by hand?"
   1. "If you cannot take medication, perhaps a course of 6 to 10 ECT treatments would be best. These treatments are offered on an outpatient basis and usually work immediately."
   2. "You may need to take sick leave for 6 months until your depression abates."
   3. "I understand your concern, and I will ask the psychiatrist to change your medication. You need to be able to work to receive health insurance."
   4. "Do you recall my mentioning that blurred vision may occur but is only temporary and will resolve shortly? In the meantime, you might find magnifying glasses helpful in your work."

5. Which of the following would be the most therapeutic communication for a patient who has been taking an antidepressant for 2 months and who says to the nurse, "Now that my depression is over, I've stopped the Prozac and I won't need to see you any longer?"
   1. "Do you recall that we discussed the need for you to take the medication for up to 1 year before trying to taper off the drug? It took a long time for you to become depressed. Some patients require antidepressant medication over their lifetime."
   2. "You should not discontinue your medication without consulting your psychiatrist, because you will experience withdrawal symptoms and become more depressed than you were before."
   3. "It sounds like you're your own psychiatrist. I know you're trying to help yourself, but you need to follow the doctor's directions to the letter. Seeing me regularly ensures that any changes in your condition will be treated immediately."
   4. "You seem to be handling things very well. Call me if you have any questions and follow-up with your psychiatrist in a year."

6. Which of the following medications would the nurse expect to administer when observing that a patient seems to be fidgety, demonstrates motor restlessness, and jiggles his legs when asked to sit down?
   1. Olanzapine (Zyprexa)
   2. Molindone (Moban)
   3. Biperiden (Akineton)
   4. Thioridazine (Mellaril)

7. Which of the following instructions will the nurse teach the patient when collecting a 24-hour creatinine clearance for the performance of a prelithium workup?
   1. "Collect all urine when you wake up and for 12 hours thereafter, then discard all collected urine, noting the time. Begin to collect all urine and refrigerate it for the next 12 hours after your blood is drawn."
   2. "Discard your first morning urine on awakening and then begin to time and collect your urine. Keep it refrigerated in a clean 3-liter plastic container. Your blood may be drawn at any time during the collection."
   3. "Sign this consent form and then collect your urine for the next 24 hours after discarding the first urine of the morning and the refrigerating the clean 3-liter container between voidings."
   4. "Sign this consent form and collect your urine in a clean 3-liter plastic container for 24 hours."

8. Which of the following would the nurse suggest to a 26-year-old, depressed patient who has a past suicide attempt and who is starting to take amitriptyline (Elavil) 150 mg po at bedtime?
   1. "Would you be able to pick up your medication at the pharmacy each week?"
   2. "I'm going to order a 6-month supply to be filled by the pharmacist to save you money and time."
   3. "I'm going to insist that your wife dispense this medication to you."
   4. "Stop by the clinic each evening for your medication."

9. Which of the following would the nurse suspect when observing that a patient with schizophrenia is tapping his feet, smacking his lips, and blinking and contorting his face as he speaks to another patient?
   1. Neuroleptic malignant syndrome
   2. Tardive dyskinesia
   3. Torticollis
   4. Parkinson's syndrome

10. Which communication would be most therapeutic for an older adult patient treated successfully with clozapine (Clozaril) for 9 months who cancels an appointment with the nurse because of flu symptoms such as sore throat, fever, and tiredness?
    1. "I think you need to drink lots of juices and water and go to bed. Call me at the end of the week to reschedule your appointment."
    2. "I want you to go to the lab and get your blood work done. I'll call ahead and order it for today. Then come in and see me. The doctor may want to see you, too."
    3. "It's flu season all right. Two people have already called in with flu today. Get better soon and call me to reschedule when you're feeling better."
    4. "Oh my God! This is what we've been telling you to look for! I've been dreading it, and it is very serious. Go to the hospital at once."

11. Which would the nurse identify as being a potential problem when assessing a patient receiving an antipsychotic medication?
    1. "I am worried that I'm going to lose too much weight on this medication. I'm already too thin."
    2. "I'm a beach bum. I follow the sun—Florida in the winter and New England in the summer."
    3. "When I get married, I want to have four children, all twins—boys and girls."
    4. "My dad says that I'm the first person in my family to have any mental problems."

12. When a community health nurse visits a patient with schizophrenia who says, "I'm going to stop going to the clinic for my Prolixin shots because I think I'm okay now," which communication would be most therapeutic?
    1. "That's okay. Your mental status is fine, and our philosophy is to use the least amount of medicine that is needed to treat a problem."
    2. "You think you're okay now? Can you tell me more about your plan?"
    3. "You'll be sick again in just a week, but I guess I can't stop you."
    4. "Your doctor knows what's best for you. Just look at how well you're feeling now."

13. The nurse is assessing a patient who recently started taking an antipsychotic medication. Which of the following side effects could the nurse expect to observe?
    1. Constipation, decreased sweating, increased sensitivity to heat, and decreased moisture around the eyes
    2. Slurred speech, hand tremors, and severe occipital headache
    3. Sleeplessness, irritability, and muscle weakness
    4. Increased moisture around the eyes, vomiting, and severe frontal headache

14. Which of the following instructions will the nurse review when observing a patient with a thickly white-coated tongue who is taking fluphenazine (Prolixin)?
    1. "Remember to avoid foods high in sugar, brush your teeth and tongue frequently, floss, and gargle with mouthwash. Check your tongue for a thick white coating, and call the doctor if you observe it again."
    2. "Remember to avoid foods high in sugar, brush your teeth frequently, and gargle with mouthwash. Are you smoking? This can cause a white coating on your tongue."
    3. "Remember to avoid foods high in sugar, brush your teeth frequently, floss, and gargle with mouthwash. Are you taking any nasal inhalants? They can cause an infection on your tongue."
    4. "I know this looks troubling, but it is not a problem and will subside in 3 weeks."

15. A patient who is taking psychotropic medication is complaining of constipation. Which of the following dietary additions would the nurse plan with the patient?
    1. Drinking 6 to 8 glasses of water daily and eating green vegetables and bran
    2. Drinking 10 to 12 glasses of mineral water daily and eating liver and turnips once a week
    3. Taking a laxative and stool softener daily in addition to eating prunes and dates
    4. Using a retention enema every 4 days and increasing bran and vegetables in the daily diet

16. Which communication is the most therapeutic for the nurse to give a patient who is taking lithium and who says, "I'm planning to breast-feed my baby at the end of the month when I feel better."
    1. "Your medication would be excreted in your breast milk, so breast-feeding isn't possible. You will need to notify your physician before becoming pregnant again."
    2. "Breast-feeding will ensure your baby a natural immunity for a longer period of time and is perfectly safe with your medication."
    3. "This medication does not cross the placental barrier, so it is perfectly safe to breast-feed."
    4. "This medication causes extreme mood fluctuations, so you will need to watch carefully for postpartum depression."

17. What will the nurse include in medication teaching for a patient who will be starting a MAOI medication after ending treatment with sertraline HCl (Zoloft)?
    1. "Two weeks after stopping treatment with Zoloft, see me. The doctor will order a new medication for you. You will need to avoid eating all the foods on this list while taking the new medicine. Read it over, and if you have any questions, call me. We'll review your diet and medicine when we meet. You will need to obtain blood work next week."
    2. "After you have been off of Zoloft for a week, come see me. The doctor will order a new medication for you. This list includes all the foods you will not be able to eat while taking your new medicine. Read it over, and if you have any questions, call me. We'll review your diet and medicine when we meet, and I may have you obtain blood work tomorrow."
    3. "After 4 weeks off of Zoloft, come see me. I'll have the doctor order the new medication for you. This list includes all the foods you will not be able to eat when taking your new medicine. Read it over, and if you have any questions, call me. We'll review your diet and medicine when we meet, and I may have you obtain blood work in 2 weeks."
    4. "After 2 days off of Zoloft, come in to see me before going to work. I'll have the doctor order the new medication for you. This list includes all the foods you won't be able to eat when taking your new medicine. Read it over, and if you have any questions, call me. We'll review your diet and medicine when we meet, and I may have you obtain blood work tomorrow."

18. The patient who is on an antidepressant medication says to the nurse, "I've been getting dizzy since I started this drug. Do you think I should stop taking it?" Which communication would reflect the most therapeutic nursing intervention on the basis of the patient's problem?
    1. "It's important to change positions slowly and dangle your feet at the side of the bed before you get up. What time of the day do you take your medication?"
    2. "You'll have to stop operating the hydraulic equipment while you're on your medicine, and you should take naps during the day to relieve this problem."
    3. "This certainly should not be happening to you. Stop taking this medicine, and I'll notify your doctor to start another one immediately."
    4. "This medication does not cause dizziness. Are you taking any alcohol in any form? Have you experienced any ear infections recently?"

19. Which of the following assessment data would indicate to the nurse that the patient who is on a benzodiazepine is suffering from a medication side effect?
    1. Reduced irritability
    2. Physiological dependency
    3. Blurred vision
    4. Reduced nervousness

20. The patient taking a benzodiazepine says to the nurse, "I like this pill. It really helps me. If I get really anxious, I always take an extra one before it gets bad. Could I have another prescription? I'm running low."
    1. "This medication is very serious. It sounds as if you're getting addicted. It's time you stopped taking it. I'm going to call the doctor."
    2. "Let's review the way you use this medication. Have you been trying some of the measures that we discussed to help you control your nervousness?"
    3. "You are not taking the medication as the doctor ordered, and I think he will be angry with you and not order extra."
    4. "Well, you've been adjusting your medication well. You look well compared to the last time we met."

21. As a psychiatric nurse, you need to know how the body absorbs, distributes, metabolizes, and eliminates psychotropic medications to safely care for patients taking them. You need to continuously update your knowledge of:
    1. side effects of all medications
    2. pharmacokinetics
    3. the most current drug guide
    4. genomics

22. When a patient requires a higher dose of a medication to achieve the same therapeutic effect, the nurse must assess the patient for:
    1. withdrawal
    2. patency
    3. side effects
    4. tolerance

23. You are a psychiatric nurse working in a large city clinic. The population of individuals who are patients at the clinic is very diverse. You will remain current concerning cross-cultural perspectives so that the care you give will be safe and effective for your patients. You have a female, 29 years old, who is taking an antipsychotic medication. You will observe for side effects of the medication because you know that:
    1. women are at higher risk for tardive dyskinesia while taking conventional antipsychotic medications.
    2. women experience more severe side effects than men while taking atypical antidepressants.
    3. women are more susceptible to addiction than men.
    4. men are more susceptible to antipsychotic medications than are women.

24. You are a nursing student preparing for a psychopharmacology exam. Some of the content that you are expected to know includes the biological basis for psychopharmacology. More specifically, as a student who administers antipsychotic medication, you should be ready to explain which of the following neurotransmitters and how they are processed in the brain?
    1. Dopamine and GABA
    2. Monoamine oxidase inhibitors and serotonin
    3. Serotonin and dopamine
    4. Synaptic neurovesicles and neurodendrites

25. You are caring for a patient newly diagnosed with a psychiatric disorder. To do patient teaching, you will need to understand that which of the following information is essential for nurses who prescribe and monitor psychotropic medications and the effects of these medications on the patient?
    1. Clinical indicators, including results of diagnostic and lab tests
    2. Pharmacology algorithms
    3. Monotherapeutic symptoms
    4. Doses of all "atypical" psychotropic medications

CHAPTER 28: SOMATIC THERAPIES

1. A 41-year-old female patient scheduled for ECT treatment at 8 AM the next day asks the nurse, "Am I going to be able to eat breakfast before I go for ECT?" Which of the following responses by the nurse is most appropriate?
    1. "No, you may only have a liquid breakfast before the procedure along with your medications."
    2. "Yes, you can have a light low-fat breakfast along with your medications."
    3. "No, you can have nothing to eat or drink after midnight."
    4. "Yes, but we will have to wake you up early because it is important not to eat for 2 to 4 hours before the procedure."

2. The nurse is assisting in the preprocedure care of a patient in the treatment area just before ECT therapy. Which of the following nursing actions must be taken before the procedure is begun?
    1. The nurse shampoos the patient's hair.
    2. A 12-lead electrocardiogram is completed.
    3. A blood pressure cuff and oxygen saturation probe are applied.
    4. The nurse asks the patient to sign another informed consent form.

3. During the ECT stimulus, the nurse supports the patient's chin firmly against the bite block between the upper and lower teeth in the mouth. Which of the following provides the rationale for the nurse's use of a bite block?
    1. The device prevents tooth damage or gum laceration during electrical stimulus.
    2. The device prevents the patient from swallowing the tongue and developing TMJ.
    3. The device is unneeded (because the jaw relaxes when stimulated) but reassures the patient.
    4. The patient's jaw muscles relax, and the tongue may be swallowed.

4. Which would be the most therapeutic communication for the nurse to initiate in a meeting with a patient and his parents to discuss ECT treatments that are scheduled to begin three times a week on an outpatient basis?
    1. "What do you know about ECT treatment?"
    2. "ECT treatment is used very successfully for many conditions."
    3. "The risks of any other treatment are greater than those associated with ECT."
    4. "Do you have any questions about ECT treatment?"

5. Which of the following therapeutic nursing interventions would the nurse use just before ECT treatment?
    1. Have the patient void to prevent incontinence
    2. Insert a straight urinary catheter to ensure an empty bladder
    3. Administer diazepam 1 hour beforehand to prevent increased salivation
    4. Administer thiopental sodium (Pentothal) 30 minutes beforehand to prevent excessive salivation

6. Which of the following would indicate to the nurse that the patient experienced a brief generalized seizure while receiving bilateral ECT treatment?
   1. Motoric movement in the cuffed foot and EEG changes
   2. A motor seizure lasting 150 seconds
   3. A motor seizure lasting 200 seconds
   4. Motoric movement in both feet and an unchanged EEG

7. A depressed patient says, "Since I moved from Florida to New England I've been more depressed every time winter rolls around. I've never been in such a low mood. Is there anything I can do short of pills?"
   1. "Phototherapy or light therapy might be a possibility, because it has been effectively used by many people suffering from seasonal affective disorder (SAD). It must be administered by an expert."
   2. "If you have a biochemically based depression, you will need antidepressant medication if you want to be back to your old self."
   3. "I'm not clear about what you are saying. Can you tell me more about your depression?"
   4. "Well, if you want dramatic results, ECT works the fastest and requires only the general anesthesia that is used in minor surgery."

8. The patient says to the nurse, "I've been having excellent results with phototherapy, but as soon as I stop, my mood gets worse. Should I return to treatment and increase the dose?" Which of the following communications would be the most therapeutic on the basis of the nurse's understanding of light therapy?
   1. "That is one of the drawbacks with light therapy—depression comes back just as rapidly as therapy is stopped."
   2. "That is a strange reaction, but we know so little about light therapy that you may need to increase the dose."
   3. "I cannot account for your response to phototherapy. It is idiosyncratic, and you may need to take medication for your depression."
   4. "I think your response to phototherapy is really unusual, but the doctor will be best able to advise what to do. I'm going to place an emergency call to her."

9. Which of the following target behaviors would the nurse expect to observe in a patient scheduled for ECT treatment?
   1. Depressed patient who exhibits a sociopathic personality disorder
   2. Patient who is appears stuporous and is diagnosed with major depression
   3. Patient who has a dual diagnosis of cocaine and alcohol abuse
   4. Chronic schizophrenic patient who is functioning without psychotic behavior

10. Which of the following nursing interventions should be completed during the educational preparation of a patient who will undergo ECT therapy in 1 week?
    1. Tell the patient that the induced seizure will last for approximately 5 minutes.
    2. Tell family members that it is better not to accompany the patient to the hospital.
    3. Have the patient speak to a patient who has been successfully treated with ECT therapy.
    4. Explain that memory loss is due to small but permanent brain damage.

11. Which of the following behaviors would the nurse document as being an adverse event after ECT treatment?
    1. Elevated blood pressure immediately after ECT treatment
    2. Increased energy levels
    3. Increased appetite
    4. Recurrent nausea and headache

12. Which of the following pieces of equipment should be a priority to have available in the ECT recovery room area?
    1. Intubation tray
    2. Oxygen and suctioning equipment
    3. Chest tube insertion kit
    4. Straight catheter kit

13. Which interventions would be the most therapeutic for the nurse to implement for a patient just waking up after her first ECT treatment?
    1. The nurse says, "Hello, Ms. Smythe. You have just completed shock therapy. You'll be drowsy for a quite a while."
    2. The nurse silently checks the patient's blood pressure, temperature, pulse, and respirations.
    3. The nurse says, "Hello, Ms. Smythe. I'm your nurse at the hospital. You're doing fine, but you will feel somewhat confused for a short while."
    4. The nurse checks the patient's heart rate, blood pressure, temperature, pulse, and respirations.

14. A patient scheduled for an initial ECT treatment asks the nurse "Isn't the electrical current dangerous?" Which communication would be the most therapeutic?
    1. "The stimulus from the electrode is very minimal and of an extremely short duration. Also, the room and table are specifically set up for safety so you cannot be hurt."
    2. "The chance of electrocution is minimized, and you won't feel anything because you'll be anesthetized."
    3. "There's always a small chance of something going wrong, but no more so than with minor surgery."
    4. "You're worrying about being electrocuted, aren't you? Everyone thinks that, but it won't happen."

15. The depressed patient says to the nurse, "Since I've been on light therapy, I've felt a 99% relief from being down." Which of the following clinical manifestations of depression would the nurse expect this patient to have experienced?
    1. Suicidal ideation, early morning awakening, and appetite loss
    2. Depersonalization, hysterical personality disorder, and guilt
    3. Sleeping too much and afternoon and evening "let-down."
    4. Late insomnia, anxiety, early insomnia, and guilt

16. A recurrently depressed patient with anhedonia, early morning awakening, and sadness, asks the nurse "Do you think this sleep deprivation therapy would work for me?" Which would be the most therapeutic communication that would reflect the nurse's knowledge of sleep deprivation therapy?
    1. "Sounds helpful to me. Are you thinking that if you just stay awake, you'll be cured?"
    2. "Up to 60% of all depressed patients improve right after sleep deprivation, but the depression returns soon after patients return to sleeping even as little as 2 hours a night. Zoloft helped you the last time, yet you seem to be exploring other options."
    3. "You can't go without sleep forever, and that is what you need to do with that. What didn't you like about the treatment you received the last time?"
    4. "So, you're telling me you'd rather live with very little sleep for the rest of your life than take a pill that ends your depression and allows you to sleep?"

17. A depressed patient with a pacemaker says to the nurse, "I want to participate in those trials of transcranial magnetic stimulation (TMS) they're advertising here at the clinic. Will you recommend me?"
    1. "I cannot. These trials are far too experimental for a patient with your complex health problems."
    2. "Of course. Individuals who are willing to volunteer for these groundbreaking experiments are so courageous and much needed. Thank you for your commitment to help others and improve health care."
    3. "TMS may be effective for depression, but it isn't sufficiently safe for patients with pacemakers. Let's discuss other strategies you can try."
    4. "These trials have great risk attached to them, so I won't recommend them for any of our patients."

18. A patient's husband says during an ECT educational session "Isn't this a pretty risky treatment? I know pills haven't worked, but this seems barbaric to me."
    1. "Although no treatment is perfect, did you know that this therapy has the same risk as minor surgery and actually presents a lower risk than medication?"
    2. "What a good question. However, you've been misled by outdated information that stigmatizes ECT."
    3. "The psychiatrist would not order any treatment that would have any danger for your wife. I've seen many patients respond well to this treatment."
    4. "You're questioning your psychiatrist's judgment? This is something you will want to discuss directly with him."

19. The patient who has received three ECT treatments with no ill effects suddenly displays confusion and memory loss after the fourth treatment. Which of the following nursing interventions would be most therapeutic based on the nurse's knowledge of ECT effects?
    1. Call the psychiatrist and report this sudden alteration immediately.
    2. Administer a benzodiazepine by IM injection immediately.
    3. Orient the patient periodically and emphasize that memory loss is temporary.
    4. Orient the patient and inform the family that short-term memory loss has occurred and may be permanent.

20. Which would be the most therapeutic communication by the psychiatric nurse when a graduate nurse working split and rotating shifts says, "I love working, but lately I'm so depressed with no reason and there's no family history of depression. What should I do?"
    1. "It may be that your diurnal rhythms are disrupted from shift changes and that light therapy would lift your mood. Let's discuss who would be the best therapist for you to see."
    2. "As your friend I cannot advise you. You need to select a psychiatrist and see one immediately before this gets any worse. Remember, the longer you let it go, the worse depression becomes."
    3. "You know, as nurses, we never feel sorry for ourselves, because there's always someone who's worse off. This seems temporary and will disappear when you return to a stable work schedule. Meanwhile, install a sunroof in your car."
    4. "Just get into the sun a little more or use a tanning salon, and the depression will be relieved immediately."

21. A patient diagnosed with major depression tells the nurse, "At a family party I heard one of my cousins talking about sleep deprivation therapy as a treatment for depression. My doctor never mentioned this to me. Can you tell me a little bit about it?" Which of the following responses by the nurse is best?
    1. "It is true that this is a successful, scientifically based emerging therapy. Do you wish to speak to the physician about it?"
    2. "This therapy is not widely used at this time because the effects are not permanent and there is insufficient scientific evidence available on this treatment."
    3. "Sleep deprivation therapy is useful only when taking a monoamine oxidase inhibitor (MAOI) type of antidepressant in conjunction with sleep deprivation therapy."
    4. "Yes, the literature shows that this is a very promising therapy for a majority of patients with depression, and many clinical research studies are now underway to investigate this further."

22. The nurse should plan to do which of the following as part of the routine care for a hospitalized patient with depression who has just returned from having ECT therapy?
    1. Have a walker available for use if the patient is unsteady on the feet from residual effects of muscle relaxants.
    2. Measure vital signs once per shift.
    3. Check the gag reflex before offering medications and breakfast.
    4. Wake up the patient every 30 minutes to assess neurological status.

23. The nurse reviewing the medical records of inpatients on the psychiatric unit concludes that which of the following patients may benefit most from inclusion in a clinical trial of transcranial magnetic stimulation (TMS)?
    1. A 38-year-old with a mood disorder
    2. A 25-year-old with a personality disorder
    3. A 52-year-old with generalized anxiety disorder
    4. A 15-year-old with anorexia nervosa

24. A patient has been enrolled in a clinical trial of transcranial magnetic stimulation. The nurse ensures that which of the following items is available in the treatment area?
    1. A reflex hammer
    2. A blood pressure cuff
    3. Suction
    4. Earplugs

25. The nurse is planning a unit in-service with staff about vagus nerve stimulation (VNS) as an experimental treatment in the field of psychiatry. The nurse would conclude that patients with which of the following disorders would be most likely to benefit from this therapy, given current evidence?
    1. Sleep disorders
    2. Depression
    3. Anxiety disorders
    4. Addictions

CHAPTER 29: COMPLEMENTARY AND ALTERNATIVE THERAPIES

1. Nurses are in an ideal position to help patients understand how CAM therapies affect individuals. Nurses need to:
    1. remain current about important findings related to CAM therapies.
    2. be current with CAM information to help patients get the latest treatments.
    3. always warn patients about the dangers of using current energy and system therapies without consulting their primary care physician.
    4. recommend CAM therapies as often as possible, especially the herbal medicines, because of the relief they provide without the expense of prescribed medicines.

2. Patients with anxiety and depression use which of the following most often for treatment?
    1. Psychopharmacology
    2. CAM therapies
    3. Group therapy
    4. Individual psychotherapy

3. Which of these statements, if made by a patient, would indicate a need for further teaching?
   1. "I use garlic in all my cooking."
   2. "I swear by ginkgo biloba. It sets me up every day."
   3. "I'm using St. John's wort in addition to taking my antidepressant."
   4. "Have you heard of kola nut? It gives me such a lift in the morning."

4. Which patient statement is the best indication that the nurse's teaching about complementary and alternative therapies has been effective?
   1. "I don't think these 'new wave' treatments can help me at all."
   2. "Maybe acupuncture could cure my back problem."
   3. "These new treatments might make an effective adjunct to my medical therapy."
   4. "I'm going to discuss adding acupuncture to my plan with my doctor."

5. What is the best response for the nurse to give when a patient asks, "What do you know about massage therapy? A friend of mine says it helped her more than antidepressants."
   1. "While a few research studies do indicate that massage will help relieve depression and anxiety, it's effective for only a short time, and no studies have compared massage with medication."
   2. "I know very little, because there really is nothing out there in the way of research findings on the effectiveness of massage. It certainly can't hurt, and it might help you, so why not try it?"
   3. "The research has shown that massage is very beneficial, but it's a good question for you to ask your doctor. Why not have a good discussion with your psychiatrist today during her visit?"
   4. "I know very little, because there really is no research out there on the effectiveness of massage. However, many of these new therapies can do damage, so, 'when in doubt, don't.'"

6. Which of these steps is correct when carrying out progressive muscle relaxation (PMR)?
   1. Tensing and relaxing muscle groups from the middle of the body outward to the extremities
   2. Relaxing and tensing muscle groups from the middle of the body outward to the extremities
   3. Tensing and releasing muscle groups from the facial muscles and moving down to the muscles in the feet
   4. Relaxing and tightening muscle groups from the facial muscles and moving down to the muscles in the feet

7. You know that the patient needs more patient education when he states:
   1. "I want to use reflexology because I want to be able to better focus on the here-and-now."
   2. I want to try working with a chiropractor to see if I can experience better flexibility, especially in my lower back."
   3. "I think I will try the herbal medication that the nurse in the clinic is recommending."
   4. "I know that I will enjoy meditation from the information that the nurse has given me. I am supposed to start next week now that I have learned about what to expect."

8. When a patient asks the nurse about complementary and alternative (CAM) therapies, the nurse would teach that:
   1. therapeutic touch is the chief CAM therapy used by advanced nurse practitioners.
   2. it is important to check the provider's credentials and the most recent research about the therapy.
   3. even though there is little extant research evidence to support these therapies, they are generally harmless, so they can be tried without any adverse effects.
   4. medical practitioners usually are biased against these therapies because they have little research base for their claims.

9. When a patient is using St. John's wort, which information would the nurse provide?
   1. No research-based drug interactions have been reported.
   2. The herbal tea made with this herb can be taken concomitantly with antidepressants.
   3. Side effects are minimal, but dry mouth, photosensitivity, gastrointestinal symptoms, and dizziness can occur.
   4. The herbal product should be discontinued for 24 hours before starting an antidepressant.

10. When a patient asks if SAMe (s-adenosylmethionine) would be helpful for depression, which information would the nurse provide?
    1. "The research findings have demonstrated conclusively that SAMe is an effective antidepressant."
    2. "The few research findings we have demonstrate that SAMe is effective in the treatment of depression that is accompanied by anxiety."
    3. "SAMe has been found to be effective in the treatment of depression in a few research studies, but the long-term effects are not known."
    4. "SAMe is an element that may create harmful but still unknown effects in the human body."

11. Which of the following mind-body interventions would the nurse plan to include for a patient to facilitate the mind's capacity to affect bodily function and symptoms?
    1. meditation, hypnosis, prayer, art, music and/or dance therapy
    2. traditional oriental medicine, homeopathy, naturopathy, Ayurveda
    3. chiropractic, massage and body work, reflexology
    4. Qi gong, Reiki, therapeutic touch, electromagnets

12. Which information would the nurse provide to a client who asks about the benefits of CAM therapies in general?
    1. "They usually involve increased contact with your health care provider and more individualized care."
    2. "They usually are more costly than conventional therapies, but they have fewer side effects."
    3. "They usually produce hidden side effects because of their nonstandardized manufacture."
    4. "They can be used conveniently and as needed for short periods of time."

13. A client says, "My friend's girlfriend says she's cured her fear of flying since she started using relaxation combined with another holistic therapy. Do you think it would help my depression?"
    1. "Holistic therapies like relaxation can cure several types of phobias and anxiety-based disorders."
    2. "Holistic therapies like relaxation have been found to be more beneficial in a wide variety of anxiety disorders, phobias, and depression than conventional treatment."
    3. "What do you know about relaxation and holistic therapy? Let's talk about the findings of these research studies."
    4. "Have you discussed this with your doctor? As a nurse, I cannot recommend any treatment, and I know very little about holistic therapy."

14. A depressed patient asks the nurse "Do you think electroacupuncture would help me?" What information should the patient receive?
    1. "It has no research-based evidence to indicate that it would be helpful."
    2. "Do you think it would help you?"
    3. "Evidence-based research does indicate that it may be as effective in reducing depression as the tricyclic antidepressants and has a lower side-effect profile, but no research is available with the newer antidepressants."
    4. "Evidence-based research does indicate that it is as effective in reducing depression as the SSRI antidepressants and has a lower side-effect profile, but no research is available with the tricyclic antidepressants."

15. A patient who has a history of alcohol abuse complains, "I'm a regular in AA and I keep up with my therapy, but I wonder if there isn't something more that might help me." What information should the nurse provide to the patient?
    1. Evidence-based research has demonstrated that standard auricular acupuncture and biofeedback have reduced drinking days.
    2. There is no evidence-based research that complementary or alternative therapies reduce drinking.
    3. Evidence-based research has demonstrated that St. John's wort and kava have reduced drinking days.
    4. There is evidence that melatonin, a hormone produced by the pineal gland, has reduced the number of drinking days.

16. A patient says, "I told my doctor that my nurse practitioner performs therapeutic touch (TT) on me and it relaxes me. He said its just 'power of suggestion.' What do you think?" Which communication would be the most therapeutic nursing intervention?
    1. "Recent studies have demonstrated that TT promotes healing and well-being. It may be that TT works by altering immunoglobulin levels and reducing suppressor T cells."
    2. "I agree with the doctor. I do not approve of nurses engaging in interventions that have no evidence base for their practice."
    3. "You would do well to base your judgment on your own experience. TT cannot hurt you, so if you feel it helps, why not continue with it?"
    4. "That's a tough question. If I agree with your doctor, I'll be unsupportive as your nurse."

17. The patient asks the nurse, "My boyfriend says there's nothing wrong with my nerves that meditation can't cure. What do you think I should do? I'm always uptight and worrying about something." What information should the patient receive?
    1. To meditate, the patient would have to concentrate, and if she's too anxious, it won't work.
    2. Meditation is effective only when paired with yoga, and it has been most therapeutic for depression.
    3. Meditation is effective only when paired with psychodynamic therapy.
    4. Meditation is a relaxation technique that has been beneficial for generalized anxiety and panic disorder.

18. A patient with bulimia says, "My doctor says he's going to sign me up for guided imagery classes while I'm here. What do you know about it?" Which information should the client receive?
    1. "I don't really know much about it. But if it helps you to control your bingeing and purging episodes, I'm for it, aren't you?"
    2. "That is a good question and one that is best answered by the therapist who works with guided imagery in the clinic."
    3. "Hold onto your question until you meet with the therapist to do guided imagery. It's best if you hear it from the expert."
    4. "Although more research needs to be done, guided imagery has proved very effective in reducing the number of bingeing and purging episodes and also in helping patients soothe themselves after only 6 weeks of use."

19. Which information should the nurse provide to a client who says, "What kind of exercise should I do to raise my mood?"
    1. "A game of volleyball or softball three times a week is helpful."
    2. "You would find that horseback riding four times a week is helpful."
    3. "Walking half a mile at your own pace daily would be helpful."
    4. "Cardiovascular aerobic endurance, muscle strength, and flexibility training have been associated with helpful benefits."

20. Which information should the nurse provide to a patient who asks, "Can you tell me about eye movement desensitization and reprocessing (EMDR)? My wife thinks it would be helpful for my panic disorder."
    1. "It's based on rapid lateral eye movements paired with imaging of the traumatizing events. It has been found effective in a few studies of anxiety disorder."
    2. "It's the kind of treatment that, although effective, is not successful unless it's performed six to eight times each day for life."
    3. "It is based on relaxing and contracting the eye muscles, and it's most effective when paired with other cognitive-behavioral therapies."
    4. "It is based on spontaneous eye movements, and it's been proved most effective in the treatment of anxious depression."

21. A psychiatric nurse is working with a patient using therapeutic touch. The primary care physician for the patient states that he is concerned about which of the following ethical issues related to using CAM therapies?
    1. Placebo effect and lack of direct therapeutic effect
    2. Lack of medicinal effect and danger of dependency
    3. Safety and effectiveness
    4. Overuse and dependency by patient

22. A 56-year-old female psychiatric patient suffers from major depression. She has been attending a psychoeducational group at a downtown clinic, where she is learning life skills and becoming more informed about self-care. She asks you, the psychiatric nurse who is her case manager in the outpatient clinic, if she can be on some St. John's wort. She learned about the herbal medicine in the group. She now wants to try it because it's all natural. Your response to the patient would be:
    1. "Let's speak with your psychiatrist at your next appointment about trying the St. John's wort. He can decide whether you are able to try it."
    2. "I will find some information about the St. John's wort and how it could work with the medicine you take now, and then we can talk with the psychiatrist who prescribes your other medication at your next appointment."
    3. "You know that the medicine you are on now works well for you. You shouldn't change it if it works."
    4. "Talk to your psychiatrist at your next appointment about that."

23. A patient asks the psychiatric nurse whether light therapy would be beneficial for her depression. As you assess the patient's depression, you know that light therapy is used for:
    1. major depression with light deprivation
    2. seasonal affective disorder
    3. minor depression in spring
    4. postpartum depression

24. The FDA Consumer Advisory and Consumer Reports state that medical experts advise consumers to take precautions when using the herb kava. Kava when used in conjunction with other central nervous system medications:
    1. can be harmful, and kava may have addictive properties.
    2. may be fatal if taken in too large an amount.
    3. may produce a decrease in depression if used correctly.
    4. may be harmful to patients with asthma.

25. You are a psychiatric nurse in the alcohol and other drug outpatient clinics. A patient comes in for an intake assessment and says to you that she wants to stop drinking and taking heroin. You suggest that she make an appointment with the intake coordinator and ask whether she is aware of the variety of CAM treatments available today. She states that she would be happy to try CAM therapy. You will suggest which of the following CAM therapies used to treat addiction:
    1. Yoga
    2. Therapeutic touch
    3. Acupuncture
    4. Reiki

CHAPTER 30: PREVENTING AND MANAGING AGGRESSIVE BEHAVIOR

1. The adolescent patient comes up to the nursing station and says to the nurse, "I'm so glad you've come in. The head nurse ordered me to stay in my room all day just because I got into another fight!" Which of the following communications by the nurse would be most therapeutic?
    1. "I'm wondering why you've left your room, then. Please return to your room until your time-out is completed. I will talk with you then."
    2. "You've already broken your time-out by leaving the room. Please return to your room immediately. We can talk about this when your time-out is over. I cannot talk with you until then."
    3. "You're not going to split me from the head nurse. Get back in your room until your time-out is finished."
    4. "It sounds as if you haven't had a very good day. Return to your room and complete your time-out. It's over in 30 minutes, and I will speak with you in an hour."
2. The nurse is facilitating a social skills group on the inpatient unit for nursing staff assistants. Which of the following communications would the nurse identify as assertive?
    1. "I love my work and I always help others when I complete my work; it's a team effort."
    2. "I enjoy my work and I help others after I have spent sufficient time with my patients and feel my assistance is needed."
    3. "I enjoy my work and I always try to be helpful, but I am careful not to help malingerers."
    4. "I love my work, but I do mine and only my own work. Otherwise, I'd be worn out the rest of the day."
3. Which accurately evaluates the newly licensed nurse's communication to the charge nurse when the nurse says, "I'd like you to stop referring to me as 'the smart new degree nurse,'" and the charge nurse replies, "I was only teasing. You are being overly sensitive"?
    1. The nurse is overly sensitive and ought to have ignored the charge nurse's teasing until it was extinguished. Now the charge nurse will be more sarcastic than ever.
    2. The nurse is appropriately assertive, but the charge nurse will only belittle the nurse more now.
    3. The nurse is assertive, and responding that the nurse does not regard the charge nurse's comments as "teasing" would be an effective follow-up communication.
    4. The nurse is behaving aggressively because of the newness of being a graduate licensed nurse, and she owes the charge nurse an apology.
4. One morning, the head nurse asks the nurse to work overtime that evening for the fourth week in a row, saying, and "I know you've done a lot of overtime, but I'm in a bind. Can you help me out?" The nurse has planned to attend her daughter's recital that evening. Which of the following would be the most assertive response the nurse could give?
    1. "I cannot work tonight."
    2. "I'm sorry. This isn't a good time for me to help you. It's my daughter's recital, and the family has plans."
    3. "Well, my daughter's recital is tonight, but I can see you're in a bind, and I'm sure she'll understand."
    4. "Good grief! Am I the only one working for you? Get someone else—you're not going to take advantage of me anymore!"
5. The nurse is facilitating a social skills group for outpatients. Today, one patient monopolizes the group. After the group is terminated, the nurse meets for dynamic supervision with the psychologist who is observing the group from behind a one-way mirror. Which reflects an assertive communication by the nurse when the psychologist asks, "Why did you let that patient monopolize the group?"
    1. "Well, I didn't know what I was supposed to do. You could see how much the patient needed to control the meeting. I thought it would be good to let it be for today."
    2. "I didn't let the patient monopolize. I did not know if I ought to stop the behavior or let the patient talk. What could I have said to end the patient's monopolizing of the group?"
    3. "I felt that the patient needed to express his feelings and that the control was a rather tenuous one that required sensitivity and patience. I believe the other patients felt that, too, which is why they let him monopolize the group."
    4. "Honestly, I never do anything right to hear you talk. Why don't you lead the group and show me what I could be doing better?"

6. Which would be the most therapeutic nursing intervention by the nurse leader of a social skills group for recovering alcohol-troubled patients, who observes patients drinking nonalcoholic look-alike beer and wine coolers when decaffeinated coffee and soda are usually taken?
   1. Stop the group, tell the patients that they are behaving inappropriately, and ask them to throw the nonalcoholic beer and wine away.
   2. Stop the group and ask the patients who are drinking to leave and return next week without the nonalcoholic substances.
   3. Do not begin the group, ignore their behavior, and as you leave say, "I'll return next week to see if you're prepared to participate in this group."
   4. Begin the group and say to the members, "I see that you're drinking pseudo-beer and wine coolers in the group today. What is your understanding of the purpose of this group?"

7. The manic patient is being started on lithium. He is walking back and forth on the inpatient unit and interrupting other residents. In a loud, rather imperious voice, he says, "I have friends, and if you don't show me proper respect, you'll be sorry!" Which of the following therapeutic nursing interventions would the nurse implement first?
   1. Approach the patient and say, in a soft voice, "Mr. S., you will always have proper respect here. Let's sit over here and talk."
   2. Mr. S. is escalating out of control. The nurse will notify coworkers and security and place him in his room under constant observation.
   3. Approach the patient and say in firm voice of equal decibel level, "Mr. S., you are out of control. Go to your room immediately."
   4. Approach the patient and say, in a soft voice, "Mr. S., you seem to be escalating again. I've brought an injection that will calm you and slow your thinking."

8. Which would be the most therapeutic communication by the nurse who approaches a manic patient, John, demonstrating signs of escalation, after he complies with the request to sit and talk in an open alcove by the nurse's station?
   1. "You have been speaking loudly to your friends on the unit and interrupting. Are you having difficulty with your thinking right now?"
   2. "John. I cannot have you being disruptive on the unit. If you cannot follow the rules, I'll have to take steps to medicate you and place you away from everyone until you feel better."
   3. "John, do you know why I asked to speak with you? You seemed to be deeply troubled. I wondered if you would like an extra pill to calm you down faster?"
   4. "John, ever since you've been on this floor, you have been disrupting the place. Why can't you learn to get along with these people? They only want to help you."

9. Which of the following medications would the nurse expect the psychiatrist to order for an adolescent patient with a conduct disorder for aggressive behavior?
   1. Inderal
   2. Ritalin
   3. Lithium
   4. Dilantin

10. Which would be the most therapeutic communication by the nurse to a patient who threw a rock into a fast-food restaurant window (injuring no one) and who says, "I need to come to the hospital for a rest. It's so cold out. You better let me in, or the next time, I'll use a gun."
    1. "So if I admit you, you're going to behave?"
    2. "You seem very anxious to be hospitalized. Can you tell me more about your plan if I do not admit you?"
    3. "A gun? Do you have a gun? Where would you get one? Are you threatening to kill someone?"
    4. "Don't worry. Anyone who wants to be admitted to this place is certifiable. I'll see that you get your rest, all right."

11. Which would be the most therapeutic communication by the nurse to an adolescent patient who just completed a time-out for having slapped a manic, intrusive patient and says, "He started it, but I get punished. It's unfair"?
    1. "Don't expect me to take your side in this. You received punishment because you were violent. It doesn't matter who started it. Maybe you need another time-out before we talk."
    2. "Let's talk about that. Do you think you were asked to take a time-out because you 'started it' or because your response was out of control and violent?"
    3. "You make a good point. We need to punish the other patient, too. I believe in fair play. I'll assign him to his room."
    4. "Sounds to me as if you have really been picked on. I will have to chastise the staff for this. It was good that you accepted the time-out like a gentleman."

12. Which intervention will the nurse implement first after assembling a crisis team to manage a violent patient who has been medicated using physical restraint and is now being admitted to an inpatient unit?
    1. "I believe you're feeling very frightened right now. You will be going on an elevator to the second floor, where you can work with experts to solve your problems. We can walk to the unit. Will you help us to do this?"
    2. "You have been so violent that we are restraining you and will place you on the maximum security floor until you can pull it together. Try to cooperate with us. We don't want to hurt you."
    3. "I know that you're feeling very frightened, but we'll help you." A crisis team member says, "You'll feel calmer and have more controlled behavior." The admitting nurse says, "It's time to go to the unit." The first crisis team member says, "Do you feel you can do this without being violent?"
    4. "You are behaving very violently and have no self-control. We gave you medication to help you to control your behavior. Do you want us to carry you into the maximum security unit, or will you go quietly?"

13. Which communication by the nurse would be the most therapeutic for a patient whose contract to smoke (one cigarette every hour) has been postponed by unit emergencies when he says, "I've waited patiently for 2 hours, and now I want to smoke two cigarettes!"
    1. "You will have to wait. I only have two hands. Sit down and act like an adult. I am asking for a little consideration here. You know we haven't stopped for hours."
    2. "The orderly will take you to lunch with him, and you can smoke as many cigarettes as you like if you'll just wait patiently."
    3. "You are quite right. Thank you for being so patient. I will come right now and sit with you while you have a cigarette."
    4. "Please give me just a half hour more, and then I'll take as much time with you as you need."

14. Which communication would be the most therapeutic by the nurse for a newly admitted patient who says, on hearing about the token economy system, "I have a PhD, and I won't participate in a barter exchange for my human rights, and I'll be damned if you'll regulate my language"?
    1. "It seems as if you're having difficulty being here. Are you saying that you feel you don't have to abide by the same policies for living on this unit because you are well educated?"
    2. "Well, you just lost four tokens for swearing, and you haven't even earned any yet. That makes your score negative four."
    3. "Well-educated individuals are usually able to select from a large repertoire of vocabulary and have no need to swear. You have now lost four tokens. We'll talk when you are able to be more polite."
    4. "'Res ipsa loquitur—the thing speaks for itself.' That's the policy, and you now have minus four tokens."

15. What communication would be the most therapeutic by the nurse facilitator of a group in which John, a patient, starts talking out loud to himself and becoming agitated sitting in the chair in the inpatient community meeting where other patients appear uncomfortable and keep looking at the nurse?
    1. "John, it sounds as if your thoughts are troubling you. This isn't a good time for you to be meeting with us. I suggest you take a time-out."
    2. "What's happening right now? What are all of you going to do about John's behavior?"
    3. "Remember what we talked about in the assertiveness training group yesterday? Why do you all think you are being so passive?"
    4. "John, do you want to share your thinking with us in the group? Otherwise, I need to ask you to be quiet and listen today."

16. What therapeutic nursing intervention would be most appropriate by the nurse managing the unit where more than 10 violent outbursts resulted in forcible restraint in the last week, yet, on review, each violent event and all crisis management strategies were appropriately followed?
    1. None. The same policies should continue to be used on the unit.
    2. Schedule staff breaks at intervals that allow staff to leave the unit.
    3. Invite a team of experts to evaluate crisis management on the unit for a month to determine whether any procedures are being omitted.
    4. Schedule a multidisciplinary team education meeting and invite a distinguished expert who can help staff understand that they managed each crisis appropriately.

17. Which would the nurse identify as the rationale for placing a violent patient into seclusion in a quiet room?
    1. It restricts patients to a smaller space where they are safe from self-harm, have reduced sensory overload, and are distanced from self-other interactions that might be misinterpreted.
    2. It prevents the patients from harming themselves or others, reduces the need for proprioception, and provides a protective milieu at the risk of sensory deprivation.
    3. It is a roomy but carefully protected milieu that offers safety, permeability of sensory input, and only incrementally increased interpersonal relationships.
    4. It is an environment that offers safety by removing all sharps and potentially harmful objects and that allows for the testing of the patient's interpersonal control by gradually decreasing and/or increasing sensory input.

18. Which of the following would the nurse communicate to a patient whose physician orders, "Restrain to protect from violence to self and staff"?
    1. "You are being restrained because you have been biting yourself and others. Let the staff know if the restraints are uncomfortable, and they will be reapplied."
    2. "You have been restrained because you are violent and the staff is unable to deal with you. When you feel you can be cooperative, I will release you."
    3. "Your thinking is making you violent, and you're trying to bite us. Just think what could happen if you had AIDS. We do not like having to restrain you, so when you feel more in control, we will release you."
    4. "I know this feels terrible to you, but you are so violent that you may hurt yourself and the staff as well as other patients who are here. We won't keep you restrained for long—just long enough for you to control yourself."

19. Which communication would be the most therapeutic by the nurse facilitator during a staff discussion of secluding a patient with a history of violence during past unit stays when Mary, a nurse new to the unit says, "I think we acted prematurely because of the patient's past violence. We didn't spend enough time trying to talk the patient down," and John, a mental health worker says, "Okay, next time you be the 'angel of mercy' and we'll all watch and learn from you"?
    1. "Now, we're a team here. Perhaps Mary sees other possibilities."
    2. "You're only a mental health worker, John. Mary is a professional nurse who can use a variety of communication interventions."
    3. "Mary, I'd like to hear more specifically what you think we could have said or done, to talk the patient down."
    4. "Mary, you're new here. Trust the staff to make decisions based on sound, evidence-based practice."

20. Which would be the most therapeutic communication by the nurse for a patient who approaches the nurses' station and says, in a loud tremulous voice, "When is my doctor coming? He said he'd be in to see me first thing in the morning, and he's not here. Call him and tell him I'm waiting for him"?
    1. "Go and sit down for breakfast. It's only 7 AM. Your doctor will be in when he can get here."
    2. "Don't yell at me. I am a professional nurse. I want to help you, but I will not be verbally abused."
    3. "You seem very angry that your doctor has not come in yet. It's 7 AM, and your doctor will be in this morning, but not until a bit later, after rounds at the hospitals. He always leaves us so you have the most time with him."
    4. "Mr. Smith, it's 7 AM. Doctors don't make rounds until breakfast, early meetings, blood work, and x-rays are over. Why not shower and have breakfast on the unit today so you don't miss seeing the doctor?"

21. As a psychiatric nurse on a busy inpatient unit, you know that assertiveness is important as you interact with patients. You are finishing up with one patient when another patient approaches you and demands that you give him his medications immediately. Which of the following is the best response you can use with this patient?
    1. "I will get your medications as soon as I am finished with what I am doing right now, so go sit and wait for me in your room."
    2. "I will give you your medications as soon as I finish here. Don't keep asking me for your medications."
    3. "I will give you your medications as soon as I finish with what I am doing. You have not missed the time for your medications to work effectively."
    4. We need to talk about your behavior before I give you your medications. You must be patient and understand that you are not the only patient on the unit."

22. As a psychiatric nurse educator, you are preparing new employees to begin their employment on the nursing unit. You must convey to the new staff that attitudes and actions have a powerful effect on patient behavior. Which statement shows that staff members are beginning to understand and will try to contribute in a positive way to the well-being of the unit?
    1. "I understand that there are going to be days where the unit will be short staffed or busier than other days. As new members of the team, how can we contribute to keeping the stress level on the unit from escalating?"
    2. "I'm new, so I will try to keep out of the way when one of the more experienced staff members tries to keep control of the patients."
    3. "How do the physicians handle the situation when a patient begins to escalate?"
    4. "What do you expect us to do? We're new."

23. A newly admitted patient is in a manic phase and is speaking loudly and demanding attention. You tell the patient that you are concerned about his need to talk with you but you need to ask him to speak more slowly and softly. You also let him know that you are listening to him and will be happy to help him. You are demonstrating an example of:
    1. necessary aggression with a difficult patient.
    2. trying to keep your patience with a patient who is very hard to get along with.
    3. teaching the patient how to talk with a nurse.
    4. therapeutic use of self.

24. You are working in an outpatient psychiatric mental health clinic as a psychiatric nurse. You have a patient who comes into the clinic and insists that she see her psychiatric clinical nurse specialist immediately because she is in crisis. You would like to prevent a crisis with this patient; therefore you will:
    1. take the patient to an exam room and begin to assess her situation and needs.
    2. ask the patient to please take a seat in the waiting room until her nurse is free to see her.
    3. tell the patient that the nurse is not in the building yet, so she will need to wait in the waiting room with the other patients who are waiting for their caretakers.
    4. ask the patient to please sit in the waiting room and wait her turn or she will have to leave.

25. The inpatient unit is at full capacity. You have a patient who is beginning to pace and talk to himself. You will intervene with this patient by:
    1. asking him to sit in the day room and watch television with the other patients.
    2. telling him to go to his room and not come out until he can be sociable.
    3. asking him if he would like you to walk him to his room and sit with him for a few minutes.
    4. asking the nursing assistant to walk with him.

CHAPTER 31: COGNITIVE BEHAVIORAL TREATMENT STRATEGIES

1. A patient says, "I think I want a divorce. My husband doesn't love me! He came home a day late with a dozen red roses for my birthday, and he knows I only like pink roses. He never tries to make me happy." Which communication would be the most therapeutic response by the nurse?
    1. "Let me see if I understand you. You think you want a divorce from your husband because he forgot your birthday and brought the wrong color of roses a day late?"
    2. "You want to divorce your husband because he's been inconsiderate?"
    3. "I agree with you. All wives deserve much better treatment than that. What did your husband have to say in his defense?"
    4. "You want a divorce after 20 years of marriage because your husband forgets your birthday and the color roses you like?"

2. A patient says, "I've been sick a lot this last year, and I'm the oldest salesman there. Although I'm still the biggest seller, I think my boss wants me to leave. He changed to another health insurance last week." Which of the following responses by the nurse would indicate that the nurse is employing a cognitive behavioral assessment?
    1. "So you've been sick a lot. You're the oldest seller, but you're the best. You're only as old as you think you are, you know."
    2. "It seems to me that you are exaggerating. You're the oldest but still the best seller. It's important not to personalize what is probably a change to take advantage of a better health insurance deal."
    3. "You're saying several things. Although you're the oldest salesman, you're still the best seller, even though you've been sick a lot this year. You feel that your employer changed health insurance because of you and wants you to leave?"
    4. "It's hard to get up one day and find that you're the oldest person in any group. It's only natural that you'd be sicker than everyone else. Your boss is probably weighing your fine salesmanship record against the cost of changing insurance plans."

3. Which communication is the most therapeutic for a patient who tearfully says to the nurse, "I don't want to live without him. He's my husband, and I've dated only him since I was 15 years old. After 20 years of marriage, he left me for a woman half his age. Two of our 5 children are still in high school. I've never worked. How will I cope?"
   1. "You're a young woman who will manage well. I know several women your age who've actually done better after divorcing their husbands."
   2. "It always seems bleak when we lose someone we've loved. Don't worry, it will work out—we just need to think this through."
   3. "I am very concerned about you. You want to die because your husband left you and your children. It sounds like you're trying to solve all the problems you anticipate immediately. Let's focus on your feelings of hopelessness right now."
   4. "So he's having a midlife crisis and you are thinking of hurting yourself. Meanwhile, no one's thinking of your children, a commitment you both made."

4. A patient says, "I want my own private room. My roommate is always watching football on television with other guys on the unit. He probably thinks I'm gay because I don't like football." Which communication reflects cognitive behavioral assessment by the nurse?
   1. "You feel your roommate thinks you're gay because you don't like football and he spends his time watching football with the other guys? Will getting a private room change things?"
   2. "Don't you think your roommate might be more likely to think you're gay if you get a private room?"
   3. "It's hard to feel excluded. Isolating yourself is not the answer. Perhaps you might try watching football with the guys?"
   4. "Well, you must realize that most men like football, so it's only natural for them to think that you're gay."

5. Which of the following clinical manifestations would indicate to the nurse that the patient was employing relaxation training successfully?
   1. Decreased blood pressure, pulse, and respirations, and constricted pupils
   2. Decreased peripheral temperature, decreased blood pressure, and peripheral vasoconstriction
   3. Decreased pulse, peripheral temperature, and respirations, and peripheral vasoconstriction
   4. Decreased peripheral field, apathy toward environmental stimuli, and dilated pupils

6. Which of the following relaxation techniques will the nurse plan to use for a patient who complains of panic attacks that "come over me for no apparent reason" but who does not suffer from agoraphobia?
   1. Implosion therapy
   2. Interoceptive exposure
   3. Relaxation technique
   4. Progressive muscle relaxation

7. Which communication would indicate that the nurse is employing reframing with the children's father, who responds angrily and aggressively when his children confront their father with his abusive drinking behavior during a family meeting?
   1. "I wonder if you would like to take a time-out. We can resume in 10 minutes."
   2. "It is good that you can display anger. Now, tell us what it is you really want to say."
   3. "You need to join AA and offer this up to a higher power."
   4. "I wonder if you can feel the love and concern that prompted your children to come to this meeting."

8. Which teaching strategies are employed when the nurse asks a disruptive adolescent patient in the group to trade places with the group leader and then mimics the patient's disruptive behaviors?
   1. Shaping
   2. Role playing
   3. Positive reinforcement
   4. Modeling

9. The nurse is planning to teach the patient to meditate. Which of the following will the nurse plan for the patient's first meditation?
   1. Playing soft background music
   2. Ten-second tensing and relaxing of muscle groups
   3. Ten-second deep breathing and exhaling
   4. Providing a word or scene on which the patient can focus

10. Which of the following behaviors would the nurse target in a token economy?
    1. Altering cognitive dissonance
    2. Performing morning shower and dressing
    3. Reinforcing cognitive congruence
    4. Pairing desired behaviors with undesired behaviors

11. Which communication would be the most therapeutic for a patient who frequently loses her temper and says, "Is there anything I can do to stop mouthing off every time I get angry?"
    1. "Have you considered entering a social skills training program?"
    2. "I would highly recommend that you enter into therapy with a psychiatrist who is an expert in communications theory."
    3. "Patients who have trouble controlling their tempers are often helped by talking with a counselor."
    4. "Do you really want to stop mouthing off when you become angry?"

12. Which of the following would be the most therapeutic communication by the nurse for a patient who says, "When I married my husband, I thought he was perfect, but now I think he's the lowest of the low"?
    1. "I think you might want to reframe your thinking in a less perfectionistic way."
    2. "It seems as if you feel and think of people and things as being all good or all bad."
    3. "So, you now see your husband as a very bad person?"
    4. "It is good to be able to externalize the anger you feel and objectify it."

13. Which would be the most therapeutic communication by the nurse for a patient who says, "If I don't make the honor roll every term, a college will never want me"?
    1. "If that were the case, I might never have gotten into college."
    2. "I can understand your concern. The pressures are truly great to be accepted into college today."
    3. "You're correct. Only a consistent record of academic achievement will ensure college acceptance."
    4. "It sounds as if you believe that colleges should accept only students with perfect academic records."

14. Which communication would be the most therapeutic by the nurse for a patient who says, "They've been giving me the hardest assignment but making it look like I'm doing less than the others. The people I work with hate me, and I'll probably fail in my job"?
    1. "It seems like you're between a rock and a hard place. No job is worth that kind of stress. Why not change jobs?"
    2. "Let me see if I understand you correctly. While really the most difficult, your assignment appears light. You feel your coworkers won't see that it's hard, and they'll hate you. But mostly, you fear that you'll fail."
    3. "How can you have the hardest assignment yet your coworkers don't see that and hate you? And how can you be so sure that you'll fail in your job?"
    4. "Have you spoken about this to your boss? I think you should sit down and talk out your feelings. Perhaps you can come to a more agreeable situation."

15. Which communication is the most therapeutic by the nurse for a patient who says, "When I lost a ton of weight, everyone was so nice to me. Now that I've regained the weight, people don't want anything to do with me. They think I'm just a fat pig"?
    1. "It sounds as if your interpersonal relationships improved when you lost weight. Now that you have regained the weight, you feel people don't want to be with you?"
    2. "So, all you have to do is lose all the weight again and your relationships will improve?"
    3. "Yes, there is a stigma about obesity. People judge a book by its cover more often than not."
    4. "We have such a stigma about weight in America. In Europe, people are more respectful of the overweight."

16. Which question would indicate that the nurse is decatastrophizing with a patient who says, "I'm in the FBI, and there's not much I'm really afraid of, but I'm driving myself crazy worrying that I'll have another panic attack when I least expect it"?
    1. "Okay, let's talk about the worst case scenario. What if you're heading up a reconnaissance in the field and an attack occurs?"
    2. "It really feels to you as if you're going crazy with worry?"
    3. "You're not afraid of much, but these attacks cause you to be fearful?"
    4. "I can understand your consternation. But don't worry—these attacks go away as quickly as they appear."

17. The nurse teaching a group of parents about positive and negative reinforcement in shaping behavior would use which of the following as an example of a positive reinforcer?
    1. A parent who kisses a child who is crying to make the crying stop
    2. An adolescent who runs away from home because of trouble in school
    3. A parent who praises a child for cleaning his or her bedroom
    4. An adolescent who drives within the speed limit to avoid getting a ticket

18. The nurse is explaining the technique of extinction to parents who are seeking to reduce the frequency of unwanted behaviors in their children. The nurse would mention which of the following as an example of this type of strategy?
    1. Ignoring a temper tantrum
    2. Losing an allowance for not keeping a clean room
    3. Sending children to their rooms after fighting with each other
    4. Not allowing children to play with friends because homework is not completed

19. The nurse is explaining the technique of response cost to parents who are seeking to reduce the frequency of unwanted behaviors in their children. The nurse would mention which of the following as an example of this type of strategy?
    1. Ignoring a temper tantrum
    2. Losing the ability to watch television until homework is completed
    3. Grounding a child for a month after a poor report card
    4. Making a young child sit in a corner after fighting with a younger sibling

20. A patient is considering treatment options and is talking with the nurse about cognitive behavioral therapy. The nurse shares that an important characteristic of cognitive behavioral therapy is:
    1. collaboration with the patient through every phase of treatment.
    2. emphasis on the subjective experiences of the patient.
    3. an approach to treatment that often results in a cure for the problem.
    4. the authoritarian role assumed by the therapist in the therapeutic relationship.

21. The nurse instructing a group of patients in the sequence of progressive muscle relaxation tells the group to tense and relax which of the following areas first?
    1. Eyes
    2. Toes
    3. Hands
    4. Mouth

22. The nurse determines that a patient with a fear of insects has mastered the first step in a systematic desensitization process if the patient is able to:
    1. rate anxiety produced by various insects on a scale of 1 to 10.
    2. relax the muscles of the body.
    3. look at a picture of an insect in a book.
    4. touch a clear glass bottle containing an insect.

23. The nurse would most likely employ techniques of social skills training for a patient with which of the following problems?
    1. Obsessive-compulsive disorder
    2. Binge eating
    3. Anxiety
    4. Poor impulse control

24. Which of the following strategies for assisting patients to learn new behavior is considered by some to be unethical?
    1. Aversion therapy
    2. Token economy
    3. Contingency training
    4. Shaping

25. A patient contemplating cognitive behavioral therapy asks the nurse what the nurse's role in therapy would be? Which of the following items would not be included in the list of activities cited to the patient?
    1. Providing direct care
    2. Participating in planning the treatment program
    3. Assisting in psychotherapy sessions
    4. Teaching family members how to use cognitive behavioral techniques

CHAPTER 32: THERAPEUTIC GROUPS

1. The nurse is screening a patient for a therapeutic group. Which of the following communications would be implemented during a screening interview?
    1. "I know that it is difficult to talk with someone about your hopelessness."
    2. "Can you share with me how you'll gain from this group?"
    3. "You identified how lost you feel at his leaving. Can you tell me more about feeling lost?"
    4. "Have you ever participated in a therapeutic group before?"

2. Which of these nursing interventions would be the most therapeutic communication in the orientation stage of the initial phase of a therapeutic group?
    1. "I'd like to review the goals that this group has agreed on."
    2. "Tom, you think that John is going through the same feelings that you experienced?"
    3. "Tom, your sharing with John what happened to you seems to have helped several others, too."
    4. "So people are beginning to realize that if Tom has been so successful, they can be, too?"

3. Which of these nursing interventions would the nurse employ in establishing the contract for a therapeutic group?
   1. "One of the things I would like to emphasize is that what is said in this group needs to remain here in the group."
   2. "Tom, you were saying that you feel you have come a long way during this group. Can you tell us more about that?"
   3. "This group is very quiet today. Is there any reason for this?"
   4. "Yesterday, we identified that people who are open can be vulnerable. I suggested that each of you record one time you felt vulnerable."

4. One patient in the group, John, has been doing all the talking and says, "I feel like I'm the only one who says anything in here." When no one in the group responds, which of the communications by the nurse facilitator would be the most therapeutic?
   1. "John, the reason you feel this way is because you do all the talking."
   2. "Can anyone in this group answer John?"
   3. "Hello out there... Well, John, it looks like you're the only one working in this group."
   4. "John, it is true that you've done all the talking in here today."

5. Which of these outcomes would be most appropriate for a patient in a therapeutic group who says, "I need to drop out of this group, because I don't think I'm getting enough from it"?
   1. The patient stays in the group and works out problems.
   2. The patient leaves the group and enters individual therapy.
   3. The patient stays in the group and enters long-term psychotherapy.
   4. The patient leaves the group and enters one that provides more one-to-one time.

6. A group member says, "Why don't you say something? You know, it's not just me, there are others in this group who feel that you could do more in here." Which of these nursing interventions would be most effective?
   1. "So, you and others here feel that I should speak up more?"
   2. "You feel that if I were to speak up, I would be doing more in this group?"
   3. "If I understand you correctly, you and others in this group feel I should 'say something' and 'do more in here'?"
   4. "You sound pretty enraged. Are others feeling that way, too?"

7. Which of these observations would indicate to the nurse facilitator that some members of the therapeutic group are demonstrating resistance?
   1. Expression of disappointments
   2. Trying to please the leader
   3. Shared silence in the group
   4. Facing discoveries about self

8. One member of the group suddenly says, "I'm leaving town. I've been offered a better job, and I want to create new memories with new friends." Which of the following nursing interventions would be the most therapeutic facilitation of this member's termination from the group?
   1. Thank the member for sharing and quickly move on to another issue
   2. Provide time for the members to say goodbye to each other
   3. Reflect that the member seems to be abandoning the group
   4. Help the other members to share their anger at the member's abrupt termination

9. After facilitating a therapeutic group, the nurse leader documents patient issues that arose on their patient charts. Which of the following observations would the nurse leader include in a group session note?
   1. Group growth response such as "group think"
   2. Themes that emerged in the group
   3. Countertransference that fosters group cohesion
   4. Identification of responses by each member of the group

10. The nurse is co-leading a therapeutic group with a psychiatric resident. Which of the following statements, if made by a group member, would indicate the need for further teaching?
    1. "I wish that the resident was a woman and you were a man. Then the women in the group would have more power for a change."
    2. "I realize that sometimes I react to you both like I do to my parents."
    3. "Are you two married or dating outside of this group?"
    4. "I'm glad there are two of you so both sides can be considered."

11. Which of the following nursing interventions would the nurse employ to help reduce group resistance?
    1. Distribution of clear group guidelines and review of them individually and in the orientation stage of the group
    2. Using pretesting and posttesting in each group session
    3. Accepting all referrals to the group without any restrictive barriers
    4. Allowing members to come in late or to be absent without comment

12. The nurse who facilitates a group for parents of schizophrenic children joins a bimonthly peer support group for advanced practice psychiatric nurses. Which of the following communications would indicate that the nurse is using this group appropriately?
    1. "I am feeling so inadequate for this group. The Johnsons reported that their son was found on the street last week and had died overnight from the cold."
    2. "I didn't know that you were married, Beth. How many children do you have?"
    3. "I didn't know that your sister was diagnosed with schizophrenia. Is that why you have so little to say to me?"
    4. "If you want to measure your success by how much money you make, nursing is not the profession for you."

13. Which length of time would be appropriate for the nurse to allocate for a Prolixin medication group for chronic schizophrenic patients?
    1. 20 to 40 minutes
    2. 10 to 15 minutes
    3. 45 to 60 minutes
    4. 60 to 120 minutes

14. Which of these statements, if made by a patient, would indicate to the nurse that the patient is demonstrating a maintenance role?
    1. "I guess the reason I'm chronically late is that I don't particularly value what we do in here. I mean, who believes this stuff really works outside this group?"
    2. "I know that I struggle to be on time, too. Can we agree to try to be on time and that we will start this group after waiting 5 minutes?"
    3. "Now, just a minute. I thought we agreed last week to talk about things troubling us that occurred last week."
    4. "I think that Beth is absolutely right about our rules. After all, we agreed on them when we entered this group."

15. A group member states, "John was making fun of me to another person not in our group last night." John says, "Meg, you personalize everything. I wasn't talking about you at all." Which of these communications by the nurse leader of a group would be the most therapeutic?
    1. "Meg, I don't think you're personalizing this. We talk about very personal things openly in this group. We're all in this together. I'd hate to think John was talking about what I said in here to someone not in this group."
    2. "John, perhaps you are trivializing Meg's concerns. What do others think?"
    3. "It sounds like John and Meg are seeking assistance from us. Do we all agree that what's discussed in this group by each of us personally needs to stay in the group?"
    4. "Well, I can envision times when John might share something he learned from the group in a very generic way, but I would tend to feel that, first, John, you are being aggressive to Meg and minimizing her feelings, and second, John, you are breaching confidentiality."

16. Which of these nursing communications would be most therapeutic when a group member challenges the nurse leader's authority?
    1. "You feel that I have no right to be the leader of this group? Who do you think should be the group leader, if not me?"
    2. "So you're saying, 'who made me the leader?'"
    3. "Let's take a vote. Who here wants to be the group leader? Let's put their names on the board and vote."
    4. "Sometimes you feel you are subject to my authority? Does anyone else feel this way? Because the fact is, I am the leader."

17. The nurse is attending an educational conference that is describing the use of the Internet to implement a group. Which of these outcomes should receive priority when planning to conduct an educational group for members seeking to improve their assertiveness?
    1. Group members developed trust and were able to practice communicating assertively.
    2. Group members reduced the diversity of assertive responses over a 4-week period.
    3. Group members were able to leave at any time they so designated.
    4. Group members were able to maintain anonymity during their participation in the group.

18. A patient who is new to an activity group in which members are working on a quilt for the hospital raffle says, "The only way I'm going to last in this group is with Velcro." Which of the following would be the most therapeutic communication by the nurse leader after the members stop laughing?
    1. "Perhaps someone could teach Jean to do the quilt stitching?"
    2. "If you think your sewing is bad, just look at my stitches."
    3. "Oh, we don't care about the stitching—the important thing is being with us in the group."
    4. "That's okay. You can just sit and talk with the rest of us."

19. Which of the following nursing interventions will the nurse implement during a brief therapy group?
    1. Determine with members the underlying cause of the chief problem
    2. Assist group members to view their behavior and the underlying dysfunctional personality
    3. Identify what can be accomplished now to change problem-solving skills to more adaptive ones
    4. Teach members to become co-teachers of the group

20. What outcome would be important for a nurse facilitator to include in a plan of care for a support group for parents of children with ADHD?
    1. Parents will be able to parent all children in the family with equality.
    2. Parents will be able to talk with other parents and share feelings.
    3. Parents will be able to assist hyperactive children to modify their behavior.
    4. Parents will be able to discipline all children with equal negative reinforcement.

21. You are a psychiatric nurse who is part of a multidisciplinary team. Other team member roles include a psychologist, a social worker, a psychiatrist, and the rehabilitation counselor. The benefit of having this team approach to patient care in the inpatient unit is:
    1. having more people to do the work on the unit.
    2. to provide more opinions about treatment outcomes of the nursing care plan.
    3. for pooling of resources for more efficient use of available resources.
    4. to make more effective decisions about nursing care.

22. A patient in a psychotherapy group states, "I'm tired of your whining all the time. Why won't you just try to stick with the topic we are trying to discuss?" You will know that a responding member of the group is beginning to understand the process of the group when he states:
    1. "You are hard to be in this group with because you say what you mean without thinking about it. I learned from you because I used to do the same thing. Now I am trying to think a little more about what to say before I say what I think and hurt someone."
    2. "You are always criticizing me. Don't talk to me like that."
    3. "I understand that you have a hard time talking with people. I do too."
    4. "Why do you always say nasty things that will hurt people's feelings? Maybe you could be more like the rest of us and think before you talk."

23. Which of the following groups would be most appropriate for a nurse-led educational group that would meet eight times with 10 to 12 members weekly for 50 minutes per week?
    1. Smoking cessation group
    2. Parents without partners
    3. A medication group
    4. Living with schizophrenia

24. A primary task of an effective group leader is to observe and analyze the communication patterns within the group. Which of the following documentation by the nurse leader indicates that the group was demonstrating an appropriate pattern of interaction during the group process?
    1. Each group member spoke during the group today. All members communicated about the same amount of time.
    2. The members discussed the fact that the number of chairs set up in the room exceeded the number of group members. Members felt that the extra chairs should be taken out if they were not going to be used because the group members felt this would make the group setting more cohesive.
    3. Group members shared today while the group was in session.
    4. One member was missing today, but the group members who were present did achieve a great deal of the group's work.

25. When the group leader is evaluating the group process, which of the following would best describe an unresolved issue that should be further discussed at a future group meeting?
    1. An individual termination that occurred during the most recent group session but was not acknowledged by group members
    2. The seating of the two new members who will be present at the next session of the group
    3. The resolution of the goals already accomplished
    4. The group leader's role now that the group has been meeting for 4 weeks

CHAPTER 33: FAMILY INTERVENTIONS

1. Which of the following refers to the mutual support, time, energy, resources, and advancement of awareness about psychiatric illness to improved family services?
    1. Family aid in the community
    2. Family advocacy
    3. Suicide prevention advocacy network
    4. Community Advancement Agency

2. A nurse has recently begun to work at a community mental health clinic. Which of the following is a priority for this nurse, who is working with a family also new to the community mental health clinic? The nurse needs to:
   1. have a social worker present for the family to help them acquire services in the community to help them make the adjustment to the community.
   2. determine similarities among the family and the other families at the clinic.
   3. examine her own sociocultural contexts, and recognize similarities and differences with patients and families in the clinic.
   4. help the family to meet other families in the community who have members with mental illness as well.

3. A nurse is assessing a family to try to distinguish functional versus dysfunctional characteristics. The dysfunctional target symptoms include which of the following?
   1. The adolescent who is a member of a gang
   2. A 13-year-old female who is pregnant
   3. The spouse who maintains peace at any price and feels self-righteous when she discovers her husband is having an affair
   4. A young adult who is working full time as a laundry worker

4. The diagnosis of parent-child relational problem is indicated on which DSM-IV-TR axis?
   1. I
   2. II
   3. III
   4. IV

5. A nurse is working in an inpatient psychiatric unit with a 16-year-old male patient. The nurse knows that, according to the risk and protective factors model, this young patient is at risk for psychiatric problems because of which of the following risk factors identified as part of his intake assessment?
   1. His mother is divorced and remarried.
   2. He has two siblings, half brothers, in the home where he lives with his mother and stepfather.
   3. He admits to alcohol and marijuana use at least weekly with his older brother.
   4. He admits that some of the other 16-year-olds in his high school class were involved with the robbery of a convenience store last week.

6. An adolescent is visiting the school nurse because of a large bruise on his forehead, which he indicates he got when he "ran into a door last night at home." As the school nurse, you would do a more thorough assessment with this youth because:
   1. you will use the risk and protective factors model to determine whether this youth will identify other risk factors.
   2. you need to report the parents to the department of social services for child abuse.
   3. you suspect that this child is from an extremely poor home and is therefore abused.
   4. you believe that this child has been fighting in school.

7. An indicator that a family will not be appropriate to receive family therapy is:
   1. the family is unable to find an appropriate therapist who is covered by their insurance.
   2. a family member's primary care physician does not give a referral to the patient.
   3. one of the parents in the family does not want to participate.
   4. the parent who is insured is not willing to participate in a weekly family therapy session.

8. You are the admission and discharge nurse in an inpatient psychiatric unit. The patient you are admitting to the unit, a 17-year-old high school senior who is ready to graduate from high school and move on to college, states that he is in the hospital because he and his father have been arguing all the time for the last few months and he just can't stand the yelling anymore. The patient told his mother that he wanted to kill himself, and his mother brought him to the emergency room, where he was assessed by a crisis worker and referred to the inpatient unit. Because of the history and current condition of the patient and the family dynamics, you believe that which type of therapy will be recommended for this young man?
   1. Short-term individual therapy
   2. Family therapy
   3. Group therapy
   4. Individual therapy while the patient is in the inpatient psychiatric unit

9. An important component of family therapy is:
   1. to be sure all members attend every session of family therapy.
   2. to consider the length of time that the family will meet and the frequency of the meetings.
   3. to be clear about targets for therapeutic change.
   4. to be sure that all members of the family are willing to participate.

10. An essential component of family therapy is:
    1. change in behavior of the children in the family
    2. change
    3. accountability for timeliness
    4. equal participation of all members

11. While working with a family, a therapist may decide that, because the presenting problem is with a child, the therapist may meet with:
    1. the child only.
    2. the child and one of the parents.
    3. the child, the parents, and the sibling closest in age to the child.
    4. the parents only.

12. It is useful for a therapist who is completing a family assessment to:
    1. gather information from all nuclear and extended family members.
    2. meet with one family member at a time to gather unbiased information about the family members.
    3. construct a family genogram to capture history, structure, and genetics related to psychiatric disorders and health.
    4. visit the family home to gather information by observing the nuclear and extended family members interacting.

13. A family participating in family therapy includes the mother, father and three children. The child identified as having a difficult time coping is the middle child, who is an 11-year-old male child. The other two siblings are female, 13 and 8. All family members are participating in family therapy weekly. The members probably will be encouraged by a family therapist to:
    1. give support to the identified patient and help him make necessary changes in behavior to become a more congruent family member.
    2. participate in therapy sessions by identifying the daily difficulties that the patient has initiated.
    3. be active participants not only in therapy sessions but also in suggested activities between therapy sessions, so that family and patients can increase their knowledge and improve their coping skills.
    4. come only to the sessions when the therapist recommends that the member participate in the therapy.

14. A psychiatric nurse is asked to conduct a training session for high school guidance counselors in a city district office. For their target population, what type of program would these guidance counselors most likely set up within the high school setting?
    1. Family dynamics for teens and their younger siblings
    2. Parenting skills for potential parents in the community
    3. Coping skills for families with stressful family environments
    4. Competence building for parents of teens

15. Which of the following would indicate that a group is a culturally focused family support group?
    1. Survivors of Suicide
    2. Alcohol and Drugs—a teen peer support group
    3. Mood Disorders and Who They Affect—way of life and treatment
    4. Support for Your Blood Pressure

16. Of the following, which should be used to assess changes in parent-child interactions as part of a family intervention?
    1. Family interventions should begin with the least important measures.
    2. Direct observations
    3. Detailed questions early in the interview
    4. Interviews should begin with the most sensitive issues.

17. Studies of family therapy effectiveness:
    1. have been regularly monitored for many years.
    2. cannot be performed without breaching confidentiality.
    3. are new.
    4. interrupt family dynamics during the interview.

18. To conduct research based on family intervention, the researcher would be focused on the family as a unit or system to better understand:
    1. the extended family dynamics.
    2. each individual's role in the family.
    3. the research process for family intervention.
    4. family functioning.

19. A guideline known as the Prevention Enhancement Protocol System (PEPS) is a process that synthesizes a body of knowledge on specific prevention topics. The PEPS document is based on the belief that the family is the first line of defense to help with the prevention of:
    1. psychiatric mental health illness in children
    2. family miscommunication
    3. substance abuse
    4. delinquency in the family

20. You are working with a 16-year-old male who is having difficulty talking with his parents. He believes that they are too strict, and he states that he, "just wants to do what all other kids my age are doing." You are referring him to a therapist who uses functional family therapy (FFT). The treatment goal of FFT is:
    1. to help the family come closer by having them meet at least biweekly to begin the process of modification of communication.
    2. to modify interaction and communication patterns to foster more adaptive family functioning.
    3. to bring the family of a suicidal teen together to help prevent future attempts at suicide.
    4. to educate the family members about developmental behavior modification.

21. One of the major goals identified in marital therapy is:
    1. support from families of origin.
    2. the couple maintaining a balanced number of mutual friends.
    3. the couple maintaining good communication skills.
    4. the couple planning when they will have their children.

22. A patient is being discharged to home today, where he lives with his wife of 5 years and his two small children. The patient was hospitalized in the locked psychiatric unit for the initial treatment of, and beginning recovery from, bipolar disorder. His discharge plan includes family therapy and ongoing weekly psychoeducational group meetings and prescribed medication. Psychoeducational and marital therapy are recommended because they both focus on:
    1. the patient and the relationship.
    2. keeping the wife informed of the ongoing progress of treatment.
    3. helping both the husband and wife to help the patient.
    4. communication and problem solving.

23. Skills building may include relapse-prevention drills and disorder-related conflict skills for families in which an adult member is experiencing schizophrenia or a mood disorder. Along with skill building, the patient is usually receiving:
    1. individual therapy for work skills.
    2. pharmacotherapy.
    3. work skill hardening training.
    4. psychoeducational skills for improving relationships.

24. A couple presents at their primary care physician's office. They identify the reason for the visit as their need for help because their 16-year-old daughter committed suicide 1 week ago. The couple has two other children, a son, 10 years old, and another daughter, 13 years old. As the psychiatric nurse to which the couple is referred, your initial goal is to:
    1. introduce them to a bereavement counselor.
    2. begin the intake assessment to determine the couple's needs.
    3. ask their physician to prescribe a mild sedative for each of the parents.
    4. sit with the couple and ask them to express their feelings and plans for helping their other children with grieving.

25. As a psychiatric nurse working with families, an effective use of humor can:
    1. help family members forget the pain that they are feeling in their difficult family situation.
    2. help the therapist feel more at ease with family members during counseling sessions.
    3. bring family members closer together by getting the members to talk about difficult issues while at the same time reinforcing their affection for one another.
    4. bring family members back to therapy week after week although they are continuously dealing with difficult people in their lives.

CHAPTER 34: HOSPITAL-BASED PSYCHIATRIC NURSING CARE

1. Which of these patients would the nurse expect to be considered for admission to an inpatient hospital?
    1. A patient who jokingly says, "If I don't win the contest, I plan to jump off the bridge."
    2. An adolescent patient whose family states they "can do nothing with her."
    3. A young adult patient, jilted by her fiancée 3 months before the wedding, who says, "My heart is broken."
    4. A 52-year-old married mother of three children who says, "If my husband doesn't spend more time at home with me, I'm suing him for a divorce."

2. Which of these outcomes would the nurse set for a hospitalized patient who requires symptom management?
    1. The patient will increase sleeping time from 1 hour to 6 hours during the night.
    2. The patient will be able to identify potential side effects from psychotropic medication.
    3. The patient will participate in the tree decorating on the unit today.
    4. The patient will be able to engage in mutual goal setting with the nurse.

3. When a newly admitted patient is assessed as being highly suicidal today, on what will the discharge plans focus?
    1. Stabilization
    2. Institutionalization
    3. Symptom remission
    4. Diagnostic evaluation

4. Which of these nursing interventions would be most appropriate when assisting a patient who has been transported to the hospital admissions unit by police for wandering barefoot and naked on the street in freezing weather?
    1. Establishing trust in the one-to-one relationship
    2. Performing a rapid multidisciplinary diagnostic evaluation
    3. Managing care in an unrestricted setting
    4. Speaking softly and clearly so that the patient can concentrate

5. A very confused and highly disheveled patient who was found wandering the street naked and barefoot in freezing weather is admitted to the inpatient unit. Which priority nursing action would best promote the stabilization of illness?
   1. Place patient on frequent observation to assess lethality
   2. Employ the most restrictive care at first
   3. Place patient on weight scale to monitor any fluid loss
   4. Place patient on 24-hour intake and output to monitor any fluid and electrolyte imbalances

6. The activity room is "trashed" while the director and nurse are handling an emergency on the inpatient unit. Which of the following communications would be the most therapeutic nursing intervention when the mess is first discovered?
   1. "This room is off-limits for 2 weeks. I am most distressed with this intolerable behavior."
   2. "It seems that there is a great deal of feeling in this group today. Perhaps someone would like to share the problem while we all clean up the room?"
   3. "Look at this place. It looks like a cyclone hit it. Are you humans or animals? Straighten this place up at once."
   4. "This is certainly a mess. Can anyone tell me what caused this while I straighten it up?"

7. When the nurse tries to intervene with a flirtatious, manic patient who is embarrassing patients on the unit, the patient says, "You have a nice body, nurse." Which of the following communications would be the most therapeutic nursing intervention?
   1. "Please go to your room. You're being inappropriate to me and others this morning."
   2. "I know your thoughts are very rapid right now. Let's walk to your room where you can rest for a half hour."
   3. "Did you ever hear the saying, 'You can look but not touch'?"
   4. "Do not speak to me or others like this. It is not appropriate and will cause embarrassment for you and others."

8. When a patient loses a pool game on the unit, he starts acting out. Which of the following interventions by the nurse is the most therapeutic?
   1. Talking with the patient about his behavior when thwarted and exploring what the appropriate consequences would be
   2. Setting limits on the behavior immediately, in front of other patients, to communicate that the unit rules must be for everyone
   3. Saying to the patient, in front of the other patients, to be democratic, "Well, you certainly are acting like a child."
   4. Saying, "The rules here are for everyone. If you cannot control your temper, you may need to leave."

9. The patient follows the nurse around the unit and asks, "What do you think I should do, nurse?"
   1. "You need to think for yourself. I can't do that for you."
   2. "You're asking me what to do? I think you should ask yourself what would be best."
   3. "One of the things I've observed is your incredible dependency on me. Is this the way you behave all the time?"
   4. "Let's discuss this when we meet today. In the meantime, I would like you to think about some options that you may have."

10. When the nursing staff from the incoming and outgoing shifts has open report on the inpatient unit, which of the following concepts underlies this approach?
    1. Therapeutic community
    2. Democratic society
    3. Proletarian milieu
    4. Egalitarian community

11. A patient who is to have one cigarette every hour with staff supervision begins to ask if it is time for a cigarette after only half an hour has passed. Which of the following actions by the nurse would be most therapeutic?
    1. Providing the patient with a paper of hourly times and asking staff to check it after each time is used so that the patient can gain more control of behavior
    2. Saying firmly to the patient, "Someone will come to be with you while you smoke every hour on the hour."
    3. Saying, with empathy, to the patient, "It is difficult to curb any addiction, especially smoking."
    4. Providing the patient with cigarettes and placing him or her on an honor system to promote trust and inner control

12. Which of the following would be the best initial approach for the nurse to take when the patient says to the nurse, "I don't seem to be sleeping any better since I came here"?
    1. Check the patient's current sleeping pattern and compare it with the admission sleep pattern with the patient.
    2. Give the patient a warm glass of milk at bedtime.
    3. Teach relaxation techniques to the patient.
    4. Start a running program for the patient.

13. After teaching a patient on the inpatient unit to use a map to take a bus in the community, which of these groups would the nurse recommend for follow-up?
    1. Community resource group in the day hospital
    2. Substance abuse group on an outpatient basis
    3. Prolixin medication group at the outpatient clinic
    4. Running club at the YMCA

14. Which observation should be included to the supervisor by the shift nurse who is assigned to run an inpatient unit with only one mental health worker?
    1. "If you cannot find sufficient staff, I will have to leave this unit, because it is unsafe, and I would risk my license."
    2. "I cannot run this floor with such a short staff safely. How soon will you have more help?"
    3. "If you don't provide extra staffing, I'm quitting right now."
    4. "Having two people staff this unit is unsafe. Can you obtain help or pitch in yourself? I am limiting care to priority needs only until you can send help. My written report will document my actions."

15. For which of these patients should the nurse plan when the admitting psychiatrist calls the unit nurse manager and asks, "Do you have a crisis bed available?" A patient who:
    1. wants inpatient alcohol withdrawal
    2. plans to kill himself
    3. has a history of violent outbursts
    4. is homeless and wanting hospitalization "for the winter"

16. The multidisciplinary team is meeting with the family of a client who recently attempted suicide to discuss discharge for the following morning. Which of the following statements by a family member might constitute criteria for delaying discharge?
    1. Husband says, "I'll be taking long weekends from now on to spend more time with her."
    2. Daughter asks, "Does mom know that I lost my baby that day I found her on the floor?"
    3. Son says, "If mom thinks I'm going to make a fuss over her, she's wrong."
    4. Mother says, "What can we do to help her get back on her feet?"

17. After teaching the soon-to-be-discharged patient about the partial hospitalization program, which of these client outcomes would the nurse evaluate as evidence of a favorable response? Patient says to her husband:
    1. "I think that the partial hospital program will be a good interim rest for me."
    2. "The partial hospital program will be a good support to me as I adjust to being home and meet up with everyday problems."
    3. "I'm looking forward to the partial hospital program, because I can gather my thoughts there and think about what I want to do."
    4. "I know that partial hospitalization seems like a baby step, but it guarantees my adjustment to being home and will prevent readmission to the hospital."

18. Which of these nursing interventions would be most effective when assisting a young adult patient who is alienated by other patients who are offended by his poor hygiene and the resultant body odor?
    1. Having two mental health workers shower and clean the patient every morning
    2. Teaching good hygiene and planning daily showers and shampoos for the patient
    3. Assessing the patient's understanding of good hygiene and mutually planning strategies to address personal grooming
    4. Instructing the patient that daily hygiene is mandatory on this unit for all patients

19. The nurse observes that a patient with an ileostomy and who has been in a seclusion room is covered in feces. Which of the following nursing interventions would be most successful to encourage a patient to comply with bathing?
    1. Say to the patient, "We are going to help you to bathe and freshen up."
    2. Say to the patient, "Would you like to clean up and change your clothes?"
    3. Do nothing and wait for the patient to request a shower and fresh change of clothes
    4. Sit with the patient and demonstrate no personal response to fecal spoiling

20. The nurse would determine that medication teaching was successful for a patient starting on lithium if the patient says:
    1. "I will need to get monthly blood levels while I'm on my medication."
    2. "I know that I will need to reduce exercising to three times a week."
    3. "I will discontinue my medication if I experience fine hand tremors."
    4. "I will continue my medication unless I increase my activity level or catch a cold."

21. Today, most psychiatric nurses work in inpatient or partial-hospitalization settings. Therefore the nurses must acquire and maintain a broad scope of practice knowledge and expertise to carry out the components of psychiatric care to patients in these settings. To do this, the nurse must:
    1. utilize all of the patient's skills in a hospital setting.
    2. understand the structure and process of hospital-based psychiatric nursing care.
    3. accept the need for cost savings and short-term stay.
    4. learn to accomplish discharge planning for the patients on the inpatient unit.

22. You are a psychiatric nurse working in a partial-hospitalization program based in a community health care system. Which of your primary responsibilities would be ongoing and directed at primary psychiatric care for your patients?
    1. Helping patients acquire the skills for performing ADL self-care
    2. Making sure that patients take their prescribed medications on time
    3. Assessing and identifying medical issues that may be contributing to their psychiatric condition
    4. Helping patients to acquire the skills necessary to become more independent after discharge

23. The patient is being discharged from the inpatient unit to a partial-hospitalization program. Which of the following is a primary nursing care responsibility for the nurse admitting the patient to the program?
    1. Gather all pertinent demographic information.
    2. Do a nutritional assessment with the patient.
    3. Perform a patient-centered intake assessment, show patient the unit, and introduce him to the other patients and staff with whom he will be working daily in the program.
    4. Educate the patient about the activities in which he will be expected to engage daily, including times, places, and the person to whom he is responsible to report daily.

24. As the psychiatric nurse, one of your responsibilities is patient teaching. To address the educational needs of the patients in the unit, you want to develop a teaching plan that incorporates which of the following components?
    1. Repetition of information and opportunities for practice
    2. Artwork and music therapy for reducing anxiety while learning
    3. Specific instructions for attainment of outcomes using patient projects
    4. The giving of short-time-span allowances for completing activities

25. The shorter length of stay in all psychiatric care settings has increased the burden on family and caregiver roles when psychiatric patients are discharged to their care. You are setting up a teaching group for family members of patients with schizophrenia who need to be closely monitored in their medication administration and side effects. Your priority teaching for this group of caregivers will concentrate on:
    1. how to prepare and administer the patient's medication to prevent noncompliance.
    2. the daily family/caregiver responsibilities and methods to manage and control the patient's behavior.
    3. how to recognize and manage symptoms of their illness, potential for relapse, management of desired effects, and potential side effects of medications.
    4. activities of daily living, with a concentration on bathing and nutrition.

CHAPTER 35: COMMUNITY-BASED PSYCHIATRIC NURSING CARE

1. According to the report from the New Freedom Commission on Mental Health, which of the following health care methodologies is believed to be most effective?
    1. A physician's office located in a shopping mall
    2. A stand-alone community mental health clinic with a wide range of multidisciplinary services
    3. A hospital emergency room with minimum waiting time
    4. An inpatient specialty hospital located in the center of a large metropolitan community neighborhood

2. You are a psychiatric nurse working in a community mental health clinic. Your fifth area of service, based on the Community Mental Health Centers Act of 1963, includes a focus on:
    1. inpatient services.
    2. partial hospitalization.
    3. mental health services to all despite income.
    4. primary prevention.

3. As a result of changes in funding, the Community Mental Health Centers Act in 1975 required that community mental health centers still offer necessary services to people with serious mental illness. Which of the following would be the least important service and might be the first service cut from the centers because of budget constraints?
    1. Screening admission services to inpatient services
    2. Aftercare services
    3. Preventive care
    4. Transitional housing services

4. A long-term psychiatric patient is living in a refrigerator box in an alley behind a city housing project. He has scheduled follow-up appointments at the community mental health clinic. The patient stays at the local homeless shelter when the weather is cold but otherwise lives in that alley. This patient was deinstitutionalized, which:
   1. is part of the Mental Health Reorganizational Program of 1970.
   2. includes the transfer of patients from long-term institutionalization to live in the community.
   3. is a system developed to provide funding for the homeless population.
   4. is a part of a prisoner early-release process initiated to help short-term prisoners become more productive individuals in the community.

5. Deinstitutionalization was not immediately successful because:
   1. there was not enough money available to care for the psychiatric mental health patients at the homeless shelters currently in place.
   2. patients had to be readmitted to state hospitals because of the lack of adequate community services.
   3. policy makers had released sufficient funds, which were not utilized appropriately.
   4. there were not enough visiting nurses available to care for the homeless psychiatric patients.

6. A special federal initiative led by the National Institute of Mental Health (NIMH) began to fund programs for:
   1. the hospitalized severely mentally ill.
   2. the Department of Mental Health.
   3. community mental health support systems.
   4. local community housing centers.

7. As a psychiatric nurse, you are responsible for visiting a community group home which houses three adult patients with severe psychiatric illness. The primary nursing responsibility to the patients is:
   1. assessment of human, physical health, and psychiatric treatment needs of the patients.
   2. performing regular visits to be sure that caretakers in the home are performing their daily assignments in the care of the patients.
   3. assuring that patients are not being neglected or abused.
   4. overseeing all day-to-day operations of the home.

8. In the 1999, in the *Olmstead v. L.C.* decision, the U.S. Supreme Court held that the unnecessary institutionalization of people with disabilities is discrimination under the Americans with Disabilities Act. From this we understand that confinement in an institution:
   1. labels individuals and is therefore discriminatory.
   2. diminishes the everyday life activities of individuals.
   3. prevents individuals from making their own decisions.
   4. prohibits the individuals from choosing their preferred work and workplace.

9. A nurse who is a case manager for three psychiatric patients in a residential home has the primary responsibility to:
   1. oversee the daily scheduling and services in the residential home.
   2. provide their primary contact to psychiatric treatment and monitor their medication administration.
   3. help the clients coordinate their ADLs and psychiatric treatment.
   4. link service systems to the consumer and coordinate the service components so that the patient can achieve successful community living.

10. Two contradictory goals of case management are increasing:
    1. access to services and limiting costs.
    2. community living and access to care.
    3. access to normal living and limiting costs.
    4. access to community living and monitoring medication.

11. According to a survey conducted by *Parade*:
    1. 76% of Americans believe that something should be done about homelessness in this country.
    2. homeless individuals usually are found mostly in large cities all over the country.
    3. most Americans do not believe that homelessness is a visible problem.
    4. 70% of Americans think that homeless people are violent.

12. A psychiatric nurse decides to try to work with some of the homeless individuals in the community. Which would be one of the key components of focused treatment that has been successful for working with homeless individuals?
    1. Leaving finger foods in a visible, well-lit location daily
    2. Frequent and consistent staff contact through assertive outreach
    3. Sitting in the city park every day at the same time so that the homeless individuals will see them and eventually approach them
    4. Volunteering at the soup kitchen

13. Rural suicide rates:
    1. are not calculated individually as are urban rates.
    2. cannot be determined with accuracy.
    3. are very low in this country.
    4. have surpassed urban suicide rates over the past 20 years.

14. You are assessing a new inmate in the state prison where you are the psychiatric nurse. You know that you carefully screen new inmates for mental illness because:
    1. the rate of serious mental illness among inmates is three to four times greater that that of the general U.S. population.
    2. the number of newly diagnosed mentally ill individuals is high among newly incarcerated inmates.
    3. it is a part of your intake assessment.
    4. nearly 70% of new inmates are diagnosed with mental illness.

15. As the psychiatric nurse, you are part of a team of multidisciplinary professionals who design and implement programs for the inmates that concentrate on:
    1. depression.
    2. physical and sexual abuse and substance abuse.
    3. personality disorders and substance abuse.
    4. depression and anger issues.

16. As a community mental health nurse, you are part of a multidisciplinary Assertive Community Treatment (ACT) team. One of the primary concentrations of care is:
    1. medication support.
    2. voluntary outpatient counseling.
    3. providing housing and job opportunities for patients as they are discharged from an inpatient facility.
    4. relapse prevention.

17. The National Alliance of the Mentally Ill (NAMI) believes that which of the following agencies offers the most comprehensive treatment for severely mentally ill individuals across the country?
    1. The Multisystemic Therapy Model
    2. The Rural Mental Health Model
    3. The Program of Assertive Community Treatment
    4. The National Mental Health Treatment Program

18. The primary goal of a multisystemic therapy (MST) is:
    1. to preserve the family.
    2. to prevent a parent in a family from being incarcerated.
    3. to counsel the family members about drug and alcohol use.
    4. to help parents to understand the effects of a parent's alcohol and drug abuse on the family.

19. You are visiting a female patient in her home. She tells you that she never wants to go back to that hospital again. As a psychiatric home care nurse, you respond to this patient by assuring her that:
    1. you will do all that you can to help her stay at home and have the care that she needs but cannot promise that she will never go to the hospital again, but if she does, you will work with the hospital team throughout her stay.
    2. she doesn't ever have to go to the hospital again because you will provide all the care she needs in her home.
    3. sometimes she will need to be rehospitalized because of her mental health disease, but that you will work with her throughout her stay in the inpatient setting.
    4. any inpatient hospitalization that she needs in the future will be very short now that she is receiving home psychiatric care.

20. As a psychiatric community home care nurse, you are aware that psychiatric home care programs have proven to be very effective in meeting the needs of the psychiatric patient in a cost-effective manner. You also know that Medicare home health reimbursement, which has a major effect on programs, has:
    1. limited the growth of psychiatric home care programs.
    2. increased the number of psychiatric home care programs.
    3. had no recent effect on the number of psychiatric home care programs.
    4. a plan to increase the number of psychiatric home care programs.

21. As a psychiatric nurse, you know that the patient understands the advantage of home care when he states:
    1. "At least when I get care at home, I get better treatment by all the people who come to my house and help me to stay out of the hospital."
    2. "I have better services than in the locked unit of the hospital. The food at home is better too."
    3. "I am so happy now that my nurse who takes care of me at home works with the nurses in the hospital so I don't have to go to the unit so often or stay so long like I used to."
    4. "Now I can stay working and still get what I need to take care of my schizophrenia."

22. Which of the following patients would benefit from in-home psychiatric nursing services?
    1. A psychiatric patient diagnosed with schizophrenia who still experiences hallucinations and is taking medication for treatment of his schizophrenia
    2. A patient diagnosed with bipolar disorder successfully being treated with psychotherapy and medication who also has a medical diagnosis of diabetes
    3. Patients with repeated admissions or crisis-unit admissions
    4. A patient newly diagnosed with HIV

23. As a psychiatric home care nurse, one of the greatest challenges that you face daily as you care for patients is:
    1. assessing home care needs of the patient.
    2. documenting care to reflect the skilled service given.
    3. implementing all the care each patient needs.
    4. assessing family situations accurately.

24. Forensic nursing has two very different and sometimes conflicting goals. The goals include:
    1. providing care to inmates and their family in the community
    2. providing individualized patient care and providing custody and protection of the community
    3. providing family care to patients in a patient care facility and helping police and corrections with custody and abuse care of victims
    4. providing care in a respite setting and providing emergency care with a crisis team

CHAPTER 36: CHILD PSYCHIATRIC NURSING

1. When assisting a child to develop the ability to delay gratification, it is important for the nurse to do which of the following?
    1. Play with the child during unstructured play time.
    2. Teach parents to assign a point system for daily expected activities.
    3. Encourage the child to express feelings in all situations.
    4. Model the ability to just sit around and think about things in general.

2. Which of these assessment findings would clearly indicate that the child has a conduct disorder?
    1. Nonattendance at school
    2. Depression
    3. Disturbed sleep
    4. Hurting animals

3. What outcome would be most appropriate for a child who has a nursing diagnosis of conduct disorder?
    1. The parents will demonstrate effective parenting skills and end conflicts with their child.
    2. The child is diagnosed with a learning disability.
    3. The child will steal only occasionally.
    4. The father will reduce verbal abuse of children and wife.

4. What is the best approach for the nurse to take when a mother complains that her daughter will not "tie her own shoes even though she can do it"?
    1. Say, "Let your daughter go with her shoes untied. She'll soon tire of tripping over her shoelaces."
    2. Respond, "What kind of pressure are you placing on her to tie her own shoes?"
    3. Ask, "What strategies have you tried to encourage her to tie her own shoes?"
    4. Say, "It sounds as if your daughter is seeking attention. How much quality time do you spend with her each day?"

5. What is the most appropriate action for the nurse to take when parents ask for help with their child, who has been caught drawing sexually explicit pictures in her school textbooks?
    1. Say, "I have to ask whether either of you has molested your child or been overly explicit with her."
    2. Ask, "What did your daughter say to you about the incident?"
    3. Ask, "Who are the men, women, or close friends in her social world?"
    4. Say, "Who is the social worker assigned to your case? I will need your permission to speak directly with her or him and your daughter."

6. Which communication would be the most therapeutic when a boy confides to the nurse, "Our priest tried to play with me—you know, fondle me—after church. My parents will be upset if they find out. I'll be to blame. Everybody thinks he's great"?
    1. "You feel your parents will blame you rather than this man?"
    2. "Can you describe more specifically what the priest did?"
    3. "This is the typical picture of a perpetrator who holds spiritual office."
    4. "Would you like me to talk to your parents for you? I intend to talk to your priest and his bishop."

7. Nursing care for a child with attention deficit/hyperactivity disorder (ADHD) should include which of these measures?
    1. Foster care
    2. Institutionalization
    3. Stimulant drug therapy
    4. Cognitive processing games

8. Which of these nursing observations would indicate that a child has difficulty tolerating frustration?
    1. Mother says, "Jimmy just can't seem to finish anything he starts."
    2. Child says, "I guess I understand what he was feeling as I look back now."
    3. Father says, "He never stands up for himself. Even when he knows he's right, he'll cave in to someone else."
    4. Mother says, "He never believes me when I tell him he looks fine. He thinks he's ugly."

9. What is the best indication that a child is able to relax and play?
    1. A child who sits quietly on the unit and claims to be relaxing when the staff asks him what he's doing
    2. A child who seems to enjoy participating in activities such as cleaning his room and learning graphics on his father's computer
    3. A child who enjoys unstructured play every day and can list several group sports at school and church that he enjoys
    4. A child who always has to be reminded to clean his room because he's always playing games

10. After teaching a child to play a board game, which of these patient outcomes would the nurse evaluate as evidence of a favorable response?
    1. The child takes second place in the game and congratulates the winner.
    2. The child excuses himself or herself to run off to play hide and seek after 15 minutes of playing the game.
    3. The child takes second place in the game and wants an immediate rematch.
    4. The child invites another child to join the game after play has begun.

11. Which of these therapeutic nursing interventions would be most effective when assisting a child to learn to express his feelings verbally without hurting others?
    1. Fantasy play
    2. Role playing
    3. Game playing
    4. Subliminal messaging

12. Which of the psychotropic medications would the nurse expect to include in a care plan for an adolescent with a history of conduct disorder and violent behaviors?
    1. Antipsychotic medications
    2. Antianxiety agents
    3. Antihistamine medications
    4. Antidepressant medications

13. Which of these nursing interventions would be the most effective but least restrictive intervention that is safe and possible for an aggressive and self-destructive child?
    1. Restraining both arms and legs
    2. Secluding the patient in a room with the door closed
    3. Chemically restraining the patient
    4. Secluding the patient with a time-out

14. Which of these nursing interventions would be most effective when assisting a child with ADHD to learn to use good hygiene measures each morning?
    1. Add a new activity, such as brushing teeth, to the morning care routine as the child masters each graduated task.
    2. Have the child watch daddy and mommy groom and dress each morning.
    3. Dress the child slowly and let him or her practice by redoing everything afterward.
    4. Stay with the child and talk him or her through each activity every morning.

15. When giving a history, a child reports refusing to go to school because "my stomach aches in the morning." A nurse should identify this as potentially being related to which of the following?
    1. Sociopathy
    2. Anxiety disorder
    3. Gastrointestinal ulcerations
    4. Early truancy

16. When a child complains of feeling "like I just want to blow his head off," what action should a nurse take initially?
    1. Report his statement to parents, police, and school authorities.
    2. Say, "Tell me more about what you mean by that."
    3. Say, "You're feeling angry with him right now, aren't you?"
    4. Report his statement to the parents and the school counselor.

17. When parents report that their child has been medically cleared but continues to complain of headache, reduced appetite, and poor school performance this last semester, what would the psychiatric nurse do initially?
    1. Draw a family genogram.
    2. Talk with the child and her teachers together.
    3. Hold a family intervention that includes the child's teachers and classmates.
    4. Perform a culturally congruent comprehensive examination, including a mental status, on the child.

18. When planning care for a child who has an anxiety disorder, which of these measures would the nurse include in the treatment plan?
    1. Support from the child's teacher
    2. Identification of the mother's anxiety and depression
    3. Provision of individual relaxation training
    4. Admission of the child to a private residential facility

19. Which of the following would be most appropriate to determine a child's ability to established trusting relationships?
    1. Does the child enjoy making friends?
    2. Does the child seek to be liked by everyone?
    3. Does the child tolerate refusal appropriately?
    4. Does the child tolerate loss and failure appropriately?

20. When conducting a biopsychosocial assessment of a child, which observations would a nurse consider when planning immediate care?
    1. The biological development of the child
    2. The effect of medical illness on the child
    3. The family, school, and social support systems available to the child
    4. The child's mastery of specific ego competency skills

21. The precise etiology for ADHD is unknown, but there are factors directly linked to its development in children. Of the following behaviors, which would indicate that the child probably suffers from ADHD?
    1. A first-grade child who does not like to read a first-grade reading book in the seventh month of the school year, does not interact well with other students in his class, but loves to play kickball in the schoolyard for recess
    2. A second-grade child who is on detention for the third time during the third month of the school year and loves to read second-grade books
    3. A second-grade child who is withdrawn and isolated most school days. He can read a third-grade storybook
    4. A fourth-grade child who loves to daydream during class and does not enjoy reading

22. Which of the following characteristics would indicate that a child has many resiliency factors?
    1. The child is able to win a physical battle with another child of his size and weight.
    2. The child whose father is an abusive parent but who finds positive role models from other sources in his life.
    3. The child who is able to survive his childhood and become a parent despite experiencing frequent episodes of rage and an ongoing low self-esteem as a child.
    4. The child who experienced frequent episodes of physical abuse.

23. Which of the following statements by a child who is being interviewed by the psychiatric nurse about school, play, and friends would indicate that the child is probably experiencing symptoms of depression?
    1. "I don't like to play outside too much, I've got so much homework lately, and my parents want me to be a good student. But it's hard, and I don't do too good with school stuff."
    2. "I have some friends at school but there's no one my age that lives in my neighborhood."
    3. "I've got friends, but they pick on me all the time, so I don't play with them a lot. They are all bigger than me, too. Sometimes we play good but not all the time."
    4. "I don't know."

24. The nurse is meeting with a 12-year-old about his progress with medication and treatment. He is feeling that he is better able to cope with his anxiety now that he is taking an antipsychotic medication and is meeting weekly with a behavioral therapist. Which of the following statements by the young man would indicate a need for a change in goals?
    1. "I went to the school dance last week. I didn't dance, but I didn't leave either. I stayed until the end. Next time I'm going to try to talk with some of the kids."
    2. "I'm so glad I went to the ball game last week with my friend. We sat way down in the front and met a couple of other guys from school that were there. I didn't feel too out of place either."
    3. I'm going to call one of the kids in my class next week so we can play ball or something."
    4. I wish the other kids in my school would include me in their game of kickball. I would play if I could."

25. The psychiatric nurse who works with school-age children who have low self-esteem because of their psychiatric mental health disorders will help the children by:
    1. giving frequent, positive feedback for small goal accomplishment.
    2. giving frequent positive statements about how incredible the child is.
    3. setting major goals on which the child can work so that the child can have accomplishments to improve self-esteem.
    4. have the child participate in a peer self-help group.

CHAPTER 37: ADOLESCENT PSYCHIATRIC NURSING

1. Which would be the best response by a nurse when an adolescent relates a mutual masturbatory experience and says, "I think I'm a homosexual"?
    1. "Many heterosexual adolescents experiment with homosexuality."
    2. "Isn't it important to be happy with your sexuality, whatever it may be?"
    3. "Do you think you could be bisexual? Tell me about your sexual behavior in detail."
    4. "Many homosexual men begin to experiment at your age."

2. An 18-year-old girl says to the school nurse, "I saw my boyfriend put a gun in his locker. He's so depressed about not getting into his father's alma mater that I'm worried about him." Which would be the best action for the nurse to take?
   1. Call the principal and request a locker search without breaching confidentiality.
   2. Accompany the girl to the principal's office to tell what she has seen.
   3. Call the police immediately and ask them to evacuate the school for a "bomb threat."
   4. Have the girl call her boyfriend's parents to come and help him.

3. Which would be the best approach for the school nurse to take on the 1-year anniversary date of a rampage murder that killed three adolescent students?
   1. Plan a convocation for students, family, and teachers to mourn and grieve.
   2. Recommend that the principal cancel school for private observances around the town.
   3. Plan a forum of commemoration for faculty, students, and family with grief counselors and experts on violence prevention.
   4. Insist that the principal conduct business as usual to avoid reinforcing attention to the violence.

4. Which of these adolescent behaviors would indicate to the nurse that the youth had entered the third stage of substance abuse?
   1. The adolescent is abusing alcohol on the weekends.
   2. The adolescent was caught smoking hash in the school bathroom.
   3. The adolescent admits to being curious about the alcohol in his parents' bar.
   4. The adolescent has begun selling dope at school to support his habit.

5. Which of these nursing interventions would be most effective when assisting an adolescent who is in stage three of substance abuse?
   1. Recommend a drug-free self-help group and family therapy.
   2. Provide drug education and drug-free activities for the adolescents.
   3. Recommend hospitalization at a drug abuse center to help the adolescent withdraw.
   4. Provide anticipatory guidance to help the adolescent to develop drug-free alternative choices.

6. When using the cognitive theoretical view to take a history of an adolescent, the nurse would ask which of these questions?
   1. "So you're feeling that, since your mother started to work, you get all the housework but none of the adult benefits at home?"
   2. "So you are beginning to learn that there may be other ways to look at politics than what your parents believe?"
   3. "You're saying that you feel you should have a brassiere because your friends are wearing one?"
   4. "You're telling me that you seem to fall in and out of love very easily?"

7. Which communication would be most therapeutic for a parent who says to the school nurse about her 15-year-old, "Lately, he reads everything about Hitler and watches the History Channel when it shows the concentration camp footage. What do you make of it?"
   1. "I don't know if I make anything of it. Are there any other behavior changes?"
   2. "I don't know if I make anything of it. What are you thinking?"
   3. "Why don't I see him and talk with him and let you know what I find?"
   4. "I'll be happy to talk with him, but anything I learn is confidential."

8. Which is the most appropriate initial action for a school nurse to take when a parent calls to say her son "got a tattoo on his forearm" and that he won't be returning to school because she's "going to educate him at home, away from this vice"?
   1. Report the mother's comments to the school guidance counselor.
   2. Invite the parent to come in to meet with the nurse and the guidance counselor.
   3. Educate the parent that, in artistic circles, a tattoo is considered "body art."
   4. Inform the parent that many students get them today.

9. When the teacher reports that a 16-year-old student has begun failing in his class and is isolating himself from his friends during laboratory sessions, how should the nurse respond?
   1. "The symptoms of adolescent depression can look very different from those of adult depression."
   2. "Have you set limits on his behavior and called for an immediate family intervention?"
   3. "Would you like me to examine his mental status and talk with his parents?"
   4. "Have the others been bullying him in your class? You know, sometimes a teacher can cause school failure by inappropriate teasing that the student's peers then continue."

10. Which of these would be the most therapeutic communication for an adolescent who tries to hang himself in the school bathroom?
    1. "Can you tell me why you thought you had no other option but to kill yourself?"
    2. "If you wanted to die, why not hang yourself at home, where no one would find you?"
    3. "If you really wanted to die, you wouldn't have tried to hang yourself here, where you could be rescued."
    4. "Most attempts to try to die are really cries for help. How do you feel I can help you?"

11. Which is the most effective nursing intervention when a teacher brings in a textbook that has been defaced with sexually explicit drawings by an 11-year-old and asks, "Do you think that this student is being molested at home?"
    1. Direct the teacher's attention to the adolescent's behavior as a cry for help, and try to keep the teacher from drawing premature conclusions.
    2. See the adolescent immediately, and call social services for placement in a foster home.
    3. Ask the teacher what the adolescent said about the drawings, and direct attention away from content and to the behavior and its indication.
    4. Tell the teacher to hold the student, and call the parents to report the behavior.

12. Which is the most therapeutic nursing intervention when a teacher brings in an intoxicated 12-year-old adolescent who was found in the school bathroom drinking vodka?
    1. Let the adolescent "sleep it off" in the nurse's office, and call the parents and an alcohol counselor for a family assessment and intervention.
    2. Report the adolescent to the police, and let him sleep it off in the "drunk tank" in jail.
    3. Call the parents and tell them that the adolescent is being sent home in a taxi and is suspended for a week.
    4. Suspend the adolescent for a month and have him transported home in a police car.

13. Which of these nursing interventions would be most effective when assisting an adolescent whose best friend recently committed suicide?
    1. Arrange for crisis intervention for the adolescent for the year.
    2. Establish a trusting relationship, and periodically assess the adolescent for depression.
    3. Perform a lethality assessment on the adolescent weekly.
    4. Perform an ongoing mental status and lethality assessment and a body search for weapons randomly every month.

14. Which of the following questions by parents to the nurse who is lecturing on adolescent suicide would indicate no need for further teaching?
    1. "My son's great-great-grandfather committed suicide, or so they think. Do you think that places him at higher risk?"
    2. "My son has been taking karate and boxing to channel any aggressive drive. Does that mean he won't be violence-prone?"
    3. "My daughter is wearing all black and has painted her nails to match. Do you think she's at risk for violence?"
    4. "My daughter has been listening to hard rock music. Don't you think this could trigger violence in her?"

15. Which of these interventions would be most effective when a male adolescent says, "You're so smart. Tell me what I'm supposed to do. My parents are Gestapo agents all the time. They never let me do anything or go anywhere with my friends?"
    1. Maintain a balanced stance with the adolescent, but mentally plan to teach parents gradual delegation of responsibilities.
    2. Ask the adolescent to provide specific times and situations in which the parents acted like "Gestapo agents."
    3. To establish trust, tell the adolescent that you will "put pressure on" the parents or anyone else who is aggressive with him.
    4. To determine the extent of the countertransference, ask the adolescent why he thinks the nurse is so smart.

16. When the school nurse observes that a 16-year-old adolescent girl complains of feeling sick and goes home or calls in sick with no medical basis every Friday since her parents separated, which of these actions should the nurse take?
    1. Ask the student what is happening on Fridays.
    2. Call the girl's parents to determine their view of her behavior.
    3. Ask the school counselor to invite the student's parents for a family meeting.
    4. Suspend the girl from school until she agrees to attend school on Fridays.

17. Which of the following behaviors by an adolescent would indicate the need for further teaching when the nurse therapist begins to terminate treatment?
    1. The adolescent says, "I'm ready to get started on my own, but I'm just a little worried. Can I call if I need to talk?"
    2. The adolescent says, "I thought we had two more sessions together."
    3. The adolescent says, "I never thought I'd be sorry to stop coming here!"
    4. The adolescent says, "I don't think I'm ready to stop coming here yet."

18. Which communication would be most therapeutic when an adolescent says, "I need to tell you something very important, but first you have to promise not to tell anyone else"?
    1. "I will always maintain your confidence unless what you tell me might be dangerous to you or others."
    2. "As you've already heard from your friends, I can be trusted not to tell what anyone else says to others."
    3. "What do you think I'm here for? I have taken an oath to maintain the confidentiality of all my patients."
    4. "I am very discrete when it comes to my patients telling me about serious concerns."

19. Which of these interventions would be most therapeutic for an adolescent who refuses to go to the gym after his pediatrician called two freckles under his nipples "undeveloped accessory breasts"?
    1. Dismiss the freckles and send the student back to the gym to play basketball.
    2. Call the boy's pediatrician and ask him to visit and reassure the youth.
    3. Be sensitive to the youth's self-consciousness while reflecting the reality that he has two freckles and not breasts.
    4. Have an intervention with the pediatrician, the student, his parents, and the gym teacher.

20. Which intervention would be most therapeutic when a father drags his son by the scruff of his neck to the nurse's office at school and says, "I caught him trying to run away from school again"?
    1. Refer the adolescent and his father to the juvenile authorities.
    2. Inform the father that he is close to physical abuse of his son and conduct a comprehensive assessment of the adolescent.
    3. Conduct a comprehensive assessment of the adolescent and his father to assess their interaction and relationship and to try to discover why the son keeps running away.
    4. Say to the father and his son, "Let's talk about what's going on."

21. A parent reports that the adolescent sometimes acts like an adult and at other times acts like a child. The nurse reassures the parent, explaining that this represents an expected attempt to cope with changes in which of the following?
    1. Sexual behavior
    2. Social role
    3. Identity
    4. Peer pressure

22. The nurse is working with an adolescent and her parents about issues related to independence in the adolescent. The mother states, "When I was young, I would never have even thought of answering my parents back or being disobedient." The nurse gains insight from this comment that the adolescent's mother was probably raised in a home with which of the following parenting styles?
    1. Authoritarian
    2. Traditional
    3. Democratic
    4. Laissez faire

23. The nurse would be most concerned about the risk of suicide in which of the following adolescents?
    1. A 13-year-old girl with poor school performance
    2. A 14-year-old male exhibiting hostile behavior
    3. A 17-year-old female with alcohol abuse
    4. An 18-year-old male with relationship problems

24. Which of the following strategies by the nurse would be least helpful to the adolescent who engages in cutting as a form of self-mutilation?
    1. Encourage the adolescent to identify feelings rather than act them out.
    2. Encourage the adolescent to select and wear clothing that will hide the injuries.
    3. Teach the adolescent to use distraction techniques, such as snapping a rubber band, when destructive feelings arise.
    4. Teach the adolescent techniques to reduce impulsivity, such as counting to 10.

25. An adolescent patient who is just beginning individual therapy with the advanced-practice nurse says, "I don't really need to be here. It's my parents who have the real problems, not me." The nurse interprets that the patient is most likely exhibiting which of the following?
    1. Arguing
    2. Limits testing
    3. Resistance
    4. Embarrassment

CHAPTER 38: GEROPSYCHIATRIC NURSING

1. Which would be the best approach for a geropsychiatric nurse to take when initially assessing a mentally ill older adult patient?
    1. Case management
    2. Primary level
    3. Individual, culturally congruent, comprehensive care
    4. Elderly interdisciplinary treatment team

2. Which of these nursing communications would be most effective for teaching an older adult patient about aging through a biological theoretical framework?
   1. "So you see, it's a matter of adding free radicals to your system."
   2. "Some speculate that aging is programmed within DNA and can't be reversed, but a healthy lifestyle and preventive health care can prevent wearing out."
   3. "All we have to do is increase the collagen that is causing flexibility to delay aging."
   4. "The key is in the immune system, and once we solve the problem by gradually adding error cells, we extend youth."

3. Which would be the best approach for a nurse to take when assessing the self-care needs and activities of daily living (ADL) of an elderly adult?
   1. Interact with the elderly patient to determine his or her ability to bathe, toilet, eat, and dress.
   2. Observe the level of grooming and dress of the elderly patient.
   3. Ask the elderly patient how daily toileting and bathing are performed.
   4. Ask the elderly patient's son if his father independently cares for himself and enjoys socializing.

4. Which of these nursing interventions would be most effective when assessing an older adult patient's ability to maintain adequate nutritional intake?
   1. Administering all medications as ordered
   2. Performing a comprehensive health assessment
   3. Stocking up on the patient's preferences for sweets
   4. Asking the patient to determine a 7-day nutritional recall

5. Which observation should be included in the nurse's note for an older adult patient who is taking several prescribed medications?
   1. Experiencing early morning confusion
   2. Taking sugarless hard candy for dry mouth
   3. Dangling at the side of the bed before getting up
   4. Experiencing slight recent memory loss

6. Which of the following would not be included in a nursing care plan for an older adult patient who has sundown syndrome?
   1. Minimizing daytime sleep
   2. Increasing mild activity such as walking
   3. Protecting the patient from sunlight
   4. Increasing social interaction with staff and others

7. Which communication is most therapeutic when a daughter, the primary caregiver for her mother with Alzheimer's disease, says, "Sometimes I hate my mother for living this long and dad for dying and not caring for her"?
   1. "Can you tell me what you do to cope with these negative feelings?"
   2. "It's normal for a caregiver to feel negative emotions as well as stress and strain."
   3. "Don't worry. The fact that you can talk about your angry feelings means you will never be abusive to your mother."
   4. "Do you ever say these things directly to your mother or any of your family?"

8. Which of the following behaviors by an older adult patient who has recently moved to a retirement community would the nurse evaluate as absence of relocation stress syndrome?
   1. Increased confusion
   2. Increased distrust
   3. Decreased weight
   4. Decreased withdrawal

9. Which of these assessment findings would indicate that the older adult patient has the functional ability of mobility?
   1. Presence of postural hypotension
   2. Wears sandals most of the time
   3. Dresses and feeds self without assistance
   4. Takes calcium for osteoporosis

10. Which of these nursing communications would be most effective in teaching an older adult patient about aging through a sociocultural theoretical framework?
    1. "It's a natural result of growing older that your level of activity would not be as great as before."
    2. "It's important to maintain the same level of socialization in your older years as you did when younger, even though the type of activity may be refined to accommodate growing older."
    3. "It's important to maintain the sameness of your environment to reflect your enduring competencies even though you're an older adult."
    4. "Look to the ways in which your family of origin functions. If they are inadequate, you will be, too, as you age."

11. When an older adult patient is being moved from a psychiatric inpatient unit to a nursing home, which of these treatment measures should be given priority by the nurse?
    1. Have the patient visit the nursing home before actually moving.
    2. Administer a sedative-hypnotic to the patient before the patient moves.
    3. Place the patient's shaver in his new room after it is checked electrically.
    4. Remove all medications from the patient's system until the move is completed.

12. When a 68-year-old adult male patient with a history of a suicide attempt in his youth complains of feelings of uselessness, which nursing intervention would be most therapeutic?
    1. Perform an immediate lethality assessment.
    2. Plan strategies to provide continued assessment of lethality.
    3. Avoid asking the patient if he is planning suicide to eliminate potential lethality.
    4. Conduct an examination of cognitive abilities.

13. Which is the best approach for the nurse to take when an older adult patient is grieving over the loss of a loved one?
    1. Assess for past coping skills, the presence of support systems, and evidence of prolonged grieving.
    2. Provide anticipatory guidance to the patient, explaining that prolonged grieving is a normal part of loss to aging.
    3. Provide anticipatory guidance to the patient that includes increasing socialization for a short period of time until mourning is over.
    4. Assess for evidence of being at peace with one's own mortality.

14. When an older adult patient refuses to eat some meals, does not take some medications, and is secretive, the patient should be carefully assessed for which of the following?
    1. Depression
    2. Paranoia
    3. Disorientation
    4. Confusion

15. An older adult patient with a diagnosis of depression says, "Yesterday, I had a heck of a time recalling where I had parked my car in the shopping center. Am I getting Alzheimer's disease?" Which would be the best approach for the nurse to take?
    1. Refer the patient for diagnostic testing.
    2. Reply, "When people are very busy or depressed, they can forget simple things like where they parked the car. Nevertheless, I will report your concerns to the doctor."
    3. Reply, "It certainly sounds as if you have some memory deficit for recent events. I'll notify your doctor."
    4. Allay the patient's concern, saying, "I do this all the time myself."

16. When planning care for a 68-year-old, divorced, recently retired, depressed patient whose only son has moved 3000 miles away, which intervention should be initially implemented?
    1. Provision of travel brochures about the state where her son resides
    2. Assessment of environment
    3. Provision of retirement community brochures for facilities in the state where her son now lives
    4. Assessment of the extent of family and social support systems

17. Which of these assessment findings would indicate to the nurse that the older adult patient is at risk for falls?
    1. A 92-year-old, stoic man who moves to a retirement community after fracturing a hip
    2. A 68-year-old woman who moves in with her son and daughter-in-law and who will baby-sit their 3-year-old while they work during the day
    3. A 75-year-old man who uses a cane at night and when out of doors
    4. An 80-year-old man who marries a 77-year-old woman and moves in with her

18. Which patient profile would place an older adult patient at highest risk for falls?
    1. A 76-year-old single woman who still works the night shift part-time at a 24-hour convenience store and who wears eyeglasses and a hearing aid
    2. A 55-year-old widowed man who begins taking an antidepressant at bedtime
    3. A 65-year-old diabetic woman who exercises regularly
    4. A 70-year-old retired farmer who cares for his incontinent wife at home

19. Which of these nursing interventions would be most effective when evaluating the physiological health status of an older adult?
    1. Obtaining a complete medication profile, including over-the-counter medications
    2. Asking the patient, "How do you think your physical health has been overall?"
    3. Obtaining the patient's old chart from a prior hospitalization
    4. Asking the patient's family, "How do you think your elder family member is doing physically?"

20. Which of these nursing communications would be most effective in teaching an older adult patient about aging through a psychological theoretical framework?
    1. "When your life focuses on adolescence, aging is reduced by a youthful mental status."
    2. "If your family feels your personality has changed radically during the last year, perhaps the physician will want to order some testing to ensure your physical health is unchanged."
    3. "The best way to prepare for a 'good death' is to systematically review your life and any behaviors you feel might interfere with this process."
    4. "You are in the last stage of development in your life, and you will want to correct anything that dissatisfies you."

21. The nurse is interviewing a 77-year-old female patient. When the nurse asks, "Can you describe the events that led you to move to this assisted living center?" the patient looks perplexed and does not respond. What would be the most appropriate communication for the nurse to make next?
    1. "We can talk about this at a later time if you wish."
    2. "You do not need to answer; I can get this information from your medical record."
    3. "What led you to sell your house and move here?"
    4. "You seem to have some issues with moving from your home to assisted living. Would you like to talk about them?"

22. The nurse would determine that which of the following older adults is at greatest risk for falls based on medication profile?
    1. A 69-year-old patient who takes an over-the-counter sleep aid on the average of once per week
    2. A 78-year-old patient who takes psyllium daily as a bulk-forming laxative
    3. A 75-year-old patient who takes calcium daily
    4. A 73-year-old patient taking a beta-blocker and an angiotensin converting enzyme inhibitor daily for high blood pressure

23. Which of the following interventions by the nurse would be best when trying to create a therapeutic milieu for an older adult patient?
    1. Use soothing music, non-glare lighting, and the patient's personal articles
    2. Use bright colors and the patient's personal articles, and plan frequent activities
    3. Periodically rearrange the furniture for variety, but remove environmental barriers
    4. Create a stable physical environment, but vary the daily routine to prevent boredom

24. A mildly confused older adult patient states, "I am in the Mojave desert." The nurse who is using validation therapy with the patient would make which of the following responses?
    1. "Can you tell me about a time in your past when you were in a desert?"
    2. "Are you feeling hot or thirsty?"
    3. "You are in a rehabilitation nursing center because you need assistance with your care."
    4. "Your medical record shows that you have hyperthyroidism, which is probably responsible for any confusion you have about being in the desert."

25. The nurse evaluating the outcome of family education about expected age-related changes would need to reinforce the teaching if a family member made which of the following statements?
    1. "It is normal for my mother to take longer to complete daily activities because of age."
    2. "I should expect my mother's gait to change a little because of arthritis."
    3. "Depression is to be expected because of losses associated with getting older."
    4. "I shouldn't worry about my mother waking up at night once in a while."

CHAPTER 39: CARE OF SURVIVORS OF ABUSE AND VIOLENCE

1. Which would be the best approach for a nurse to take when a young adult patient is verbally abusive?
    1. Teach the patient how to communicate assertively.
    2. Ask the patient who the model for verbal abuse was.
    3. Identify the patient's verbal abuse, and set standards for future dialogue.
    4. Remove privileges from the patient until communications become more acceptable.

2. Which of these nursing communications would be most effective in teaching a patient about abusive behavior?
    1. "So when your husband says he needs other women because you aren't sexually satisfying, you believe him?"
    2. "You say that your son has been pulling the neighbor's pigtails and you are worried he's becoming violent and abusive like your brother?"
    3. "You say that you placed your son on an allowance but that you also want to regulate everything he spends and saves?"
    4. "I noticed that when your mother paid you a compliment, you seemed skeptical."

3. Which would be the best approach for a nurse to take with a battered wife?
    1. Teach the battered wife how to avoid provoking her husband.
    2. Assist the battered wife to seek a divorce through an attorney.
    3. Help the battered wife to identify her situation and options and to obtain support.
    4. Teach the battered wife that she is safe while she's carrying the batterer's child.

4. Which of these nursing interventions would be most effective when using an empowerment model of intervention with a battered woman?
   1. "You have left your husband many times only to return. Tell me how you view this last time as being different."
   2. "Last time we talked, you thought your children would miss their father, but you now think they seem happier and almost relieved with your separation."
   3. "So you're having doubts and want to return to your husband even though you know that he broke your arm and precipitated your miscarriage?"
   4. "I support you returning to your husband until you decide that 'enough is enough.'"

5. When giving care to a patient who suffers from rape trauma syndrome, which of these measures would the nurse include?
   1. Structure a plan of decision making for the patient.
   2. Help with obtaining a medical care provider.
   3. Enroll the patient in a community group after discharge.
   4. Teach the patient to confide carefully to loved ones and to health professionals.

6. Which of these steps is correct when trying to overcome negative attitudes when caring for a patient from a violent family?
   1. Nurse explores his or her own attitudes and values toward survivors of violence.
   2. Nurse identifies the dysfunction in the violent family.
   3. Nurse says to the family that negative attitudes are the underlying cause of their violence.
   4. Nurse suggests that the family members can increase their understanding by studying survivors' books.

7. Which communication is most therapeutic when a young, newly married, adult woman says, "My husband never lets me out of his sight. He doesn't want me to do anything without him and is always accusing me of cheating on him. What can I do?"
   1. "What do you want to do about this abusive situation?"
   2. "You feel that you would like to end this struggle for power and control?"
   3. "Sounds as if you're behaving very seductively to engender your husband's jealousy."
   4. "Don't give your husband anything to be upset or suspicious about."

8. Which of the following behaviors would the nurse expect to observe in a patient who commits psychic rape?
   1. The perpetrator gives money to the patient after raping her.
   2. The perpetrator seduces the patient by plying her with wine, flowers, and music.
   3. The perpetrator threatens the patient to submit or else she will be beaten.
   4. The perpetrator harasses the patient and tells her, "I don't want it from you anymore. You've lost it—not that you were ever that good."

9. Which of these assessment findings would indicate that the patient who has been raped is in the acute stage of sexual assault?
   1. Patient is very demanding and controlling in manner.
   2. Patient is extremely confused, restless, and fearful.
   3. Patient uses profanity to describe experiences.
   4. Patient is phobic about being left alone serveral weeks after the attack.

10. Which of the following nursing communications would be most effective in teaching a patient who says, "When I was clearing out the late doctor's file, I found my chart, and it records lots of visits and that I was being physically and sexually abused by my father, who was an alcoholic. How could it happen and I don't remember it?"
    1. "It is well established that many people forget episodes of childhood abuse. Thirty-eight percent of people who visited the hospital ER don't recall it 20 years later."
    2. "You can't. Your old family physician was probably just being hysterical because your dad had a drinking problem and you were prone to accidents and urinary tract infections."
    3. "You know that more reported instances of delayed memory have been recanted. It seems they are the products of therapists' overactive imaginings."
    4. "Some experts believe that delayed memories are the result of alterations in the function of neuromodulators. This is your case."

11. When a patient who is a battered wife recants her testimony to prevent her husband from being imprisoned, to which of these treatment measures should the nurse give priority?
    1. Terminating the relationship until the patient takes legal action against her husband
    2. Teaching the patient about groups that can assist her husband to relearn new ways to cope
    3. Continuing the relationship with the patient, but avoiding the topic of battering
    4. Telling the husband that you will report the violence to the police

12. A nursing colleague says, "This patient was admitted with complaints of being raped, but just look at the sexy dress she was wearing." Which of these nursing interventions would be most therapeutic?
    1. Remind your colleague that it's rape whenever the woman is forced after saying "No."
    2. Suggest to your nursing peer that you care for the patient because you can be tolerant.
    3. Say to your nursing colleague, "You are acting very biased about the patient's dress."
    4. Say to your nursing colleague, "Sounds as if you feel that wearing a sexy dress is tacit permission to be raped."

13. Which is the best approach for the nurse to take when an adolescent patient whose boyfriend raped her during an argument says, "It's no use reporting it. No one will ever believe me, because we were sexually intimate for some time"?
    1. "You will want to report this to your parents."
    2. "It's a very common occurrence, and reporting it would only bring embarrassment."
    3. "You're correct in your decision-making. It only results in negative publicity and embarrassment for you and your family."
    4. "If you said 'no,' you have a right to expect your partner to respect your wishes. You will want to prevent the reoccurrence of this situation and get help for both of you."

14. When a nurse observes a patient being struck by her husband during an argument, which of these actions should the nurse take?
    1. Ask the husband to stop, and then leave the room and call the police.
    2. Step between the spouses and insist that they take a time-out.
    3. Tactfully leave the spouses to provide them with privacy.
    4. Tell the husband that the police are on their way and that they will put him in jail.

15. An older adult patient who is living with her daughter and who exhibits bruising for the second time on her upper outer arms bilaterally says, "Please don't say anything. It's not my daughter's fault. I just bruise easily." Which would be the best approach for the nurse to take?
    1. Visit with the daughter and her mother and observe their interaction together before documentation.
    2. Report the elder abuse and inform the patient and her daughter of your intention.
    3. Inform the patient and her daughter of your intention to document and report findings to obtain assistance for both while continuing to observe their interactions for further signs of elder abuse, such as rough handling and impatience.
    4. Document and report findings only when they are substantiated by further indications of elder abuse.

16. When assessing a patient who has witnessed abuse, which findings would the nurse not expect to observe?
    1. A 16-year-old white female with no memory of sexual assault by her father and who is truant from school and who smokes marijuana on a daily basis
    2. An 11-year-old Hispanic female with multiple somatic complaints without a physical basis, who has been in two violent fights at school, and who says she caused her father to break her arm
    3. A 15-year-old Asian male who says of a fight at school, "John kept calling me 'four-eyes,' so I decked him. I shouldn't have done it, and I apologized. We learn to use our skills for defense only."
    4. A 17-year-old black female with a long history of delinquency who says, "Sure, I took his laptop computer. The jerk left it out in his office."

17. Which of these assessment findings would indicate to the nurse that the patient has not experienced family violence?
    1. "I remember that my mother would haul off and whack me when I annoyed her."
    2. "My husband is ashamed that I had to get a job to supplement our income."
    3. "My husband says he's not attracted to me since I gained 10 pounds."
    4. "My daughter does her best for me. I am just such a burden to her and her family."

18. Which of these nursing communications best reflects the nurse's use of an empowerment model with a battered woman?
    1. "Let me share with you my knowledge of what happens to abused women."
    2. "I know you feel that he'll change, but the research does not validate your thinking."
    3. "It's up to you to end the violence. No one can set limits on him but you."
    4. "Let's consider what you believe your options are in terms of your relationship with him in light of what we've talked about."

19. Which of these nursing interventions would be most therapeutic for a spouse who says, "When I called the police, my husband was shoving me around and kicking me, but I don't want to report him. He just lost his temper with me because I spent too much money"?
    1. "I can understand that you don't want to press charges, but your husband needs help."
    2. "You tell your husband that if he beats you up again, I'll report him to the police."
    3. "You feel your husband was justified in his abuse of you because you overspent?"
    4. "Your husband abuses you when you overspend. So he'll stop if you stop provoking him?"
20. Which of these nursing communications would be most effective in teaching an affluent patient who says, "It's ridiculous for our son to accuse his father of abuse. He's a prominent doctor, for goodness sake"?
    1. "You believe that abuse does not exist in financially and professionally affluent families?"
    2. "It is true that abuse is rarely identified in financially and professionally affluent families."
    3. "I know your husband from working with him in the emergency room. He has always been supportive and kind to his patients, but that can be misleading."
    4. "Abuse is more common among financially and professionally affluent breadwinners."
21. You are the nurse educator at a large health care center. You are orienting new psychiatric nurses who will work with victims of abuse. You want to be sure new nurses understand abuse in families and explain that which of the following are the most "at-risk" individuals for abuse?
    1. The mother of a 13-year-old child and her father, 59
    2. An elderly tenant whose landlord is her caretaker, a male college student who is quiet and shy and who keeps to himself, and the partner in a heterosexual relationship
    3. An elderly woman who lives with an abusive son, his wife, and their two children
    4. A school-age child who wears glasses, keeps to himself, and is a student at an inner city school in a poor neighborhood
22. You are working with a 29-year-old white female whose husband has repeatedly physically abused her over the last 3 years. Her injuries are extensive, and she says she does not want to return to the marital situation. Which statement would be indicative of the woman's belief in dysfunctional family values?
    1. "I just can't stay with this guy or I'll do something to him while he is sleeping and end up in jail."
    2. "I know that he knows that I'm having an affair. I was brought up to believe that you never cheat on your husband no matter how bad it gets. I know this is all my fault because I'm not a good wife."
    3. "My mother told me he was not good. I guess she was right."
    4. "I'm not going to go back to him this time. I'm done with being his punching bag."
23. Which statement would indicate the use and abuse of power in a violent family situation?
    1. "I was yelling and swinging a knife in the air. I didn't mean to do anything with it. He didn't have to take the knife away from me. He overreacted."
    2. "I didn't get the kids to the park this afternoon because I was watching my soap opera. Why did he get all upset and leave the house and slam the door. He has no right to get mad at me. I should have some time to myself; you know, he's always working or out with the kids or somewhere."
    3. "I can't believe I did it again. I thought he would like this. I just wanted to try a new recipe. I will not do that again. He was right. He works all day and should come home to a good meal that he can enjoy."
    4. "All I did was tell him I need some money. I can't understand why he can't just give me what I need. I married him and now I stay home and take care of his house and kids, and he can't even give me enough money to go shopping a couple of times a week for myself."
24. You are the nurse in the ER admitting a woman with multiple head, neck, and face injuries. She states that she fell down the cellar stairs at her home. She then states that she was lucky her husband was home to take her to the hospital. "He's such a good husband." As her nurse you will:
    1. look for old injuries and begin to assess her for abuse.
    2. have the husband stay with her because he is so supportive of her.
    3. have the husband wait in the waiting room and go out to the nurses' station and call the police.
    4. confront the husband about the suspicions you have concerning abuse.
25. You are a school nurse who is concerned about changes in the administration and cutbacks recently implemented by the school board to save money. You are concerned because you know that the school administration, faculty, and student body are demonstrating a change as well. Which of the following risk factors would be of primary concern in this situation?
    1. People in the community verbalizing the need for more school funding
    2. Talk in the school by faculty about "unfair treatment of faculty and staff"
    3. Increase in the number of student absences since the budget cuts began
    4. An increase in students' use of illegal drugs and student behavior that is more impulsive

CHAPTER 40: PSYCHOLOGICAL CARE OF PATIENTS WITH LIFE-THREATENING ILLNESS

1. A nurse is beginning to work with a patient who is waiting for test results that will indicate whether the patient has cancer. Which of the following communications would be most helpful at the beginning of this therapeutic relationship?
   1. "I'm sure this must be a difficult time. It may be helpful to focus on the fact that many more people are surviving cancer with the development of new drugs and other therapies."
   2. "This is a time of uncertainty for you and your family. While talking with you, I sense that you are quite anxious and in disbelief. Is this how you feel?"
   3. "I am trying to imagine how you feel. If you spend this time making sure all your affairs are in order, it will give you more of a sense of control over the situation."
   4. "How sad and frightened you must feel. Do you have any family or friends that are good support systems to you?"

2. The nurse who is working from an evidence base for practice concludes that which of the following patients with a life-threatening illness is most likely to complete an advance directive?
   1. An 80-year-old white man with Alzheimer's disease
   2. A 67-year-old white woman with severe asthma
   3. A 44-year-old black man with severe congestive heart failure
   4. A 54-year-old Latino woman with skin cancer

3. A 64-year-old female patient has just been diagnosed with an inoperable brain tumor. Which of the following patient statements about her concerns does the nurse conclude is expected at this time?
   1. "Well, all of us have to die someday. I'll have to see a lawyer about a will and I'll need you to tell me more about advance directives."
   2. "I don't feel ill enough to have cancer. Can I be retested at a different hospital?"
   3. "My daughter is expecting twins in 3 months, and I am supposed to help her with them. What if I become a burden to her instead of a help?"
   4. "If that is the case I would like to look into nursing home placement or hospice care right away."

4. A patient with liver failure rings the call bell and says to the nurse, "The lunch is cold, and my sheets are wrinkled. You never seem to have enough help, because it takes so long to get my call bell answered." Which of the following should the nurse do initially?
   1. Listen quietly but attentively until the patient has finished speaking.
   2. Correct each problem the patient has identified immediately.
   3. Say to the patient, "I'm sorry; you know the staff is really doing the best they can."
   4. Ask the patient, "How many minutes has it been since you rang the call bell?"

5. A patient diagnosed with amyotrophic lateral sclerosis says to the nurse, "I've been looking on the Internet to get more information about this disease. Which of them has the most reliable information?" Which of the following sites would the nurse recommend?
   1. Centers for Disease Control (CDC)
   2. National Institutes of Health (NIH)
   3. Occupational Safety and Health Administration (OSHA)
   4. Food and Drug Administration (FDA)

6. The nurse who is advocating for an anxious patient newly diagnosed with a life-threatening illness would ask the physician for an order for which of the following types of medications commonly prescribed for this purpose?
   1. Selective serotonin reuptake inhibitor
   2. Tricyclic antidepressant
   3. Monoamine oxidase inhibitor
   4. Benzodiazepine

7. R. underwent surgery for cancer and now needs follow-up chemotherapy. He reports little appetite, fatigue, and trouble with concentrating and sleeping. The nurse would place highest priority on responding to which of the following statements by the family member?
   1. "We are so concerned about him. He hardly eats or sleeps anymore. Can something be done?"
   2. "We can't wait for the chemotherapy to start. He worries about any remaining cancer starting to grow between the surgery and the chemotherapy."
   3. "We are not surprised he is so depressed. It ought to be expected after all that he has been through, and he should get back to normal after the chemotherapy."
   4. "We are not surprised he is depressed after all he is going through, but is there some medicine that can help him right now?"

8. The nurse enters the room of a 42-year-old female patient newly diagnosed with multiple sclerosis and notes she is crying quietly while lying in bed. Which of the following communications by the nurse would be most appropriate?
   1. "You are crying. Can you talk to me more about your feelings, such as being sad or depressed?"
   2. "Crying is a normal response to a diagnosis such as yours. I hope you will get over it after your plan of care has been fully developed."
   3. "Oh, you are crying! Shall I call the physician to order some medication for you?"
   4. "I can understand why you would cry. I imagine most people would feel that way after being given your diagnosis."

9. The daughter of a critically ill patient has been either with the patient or in the hospital waiting room for the past 2½ days, and has not been eating or sleeping properly. The family member is becoming somewhat short-tempered and is starting to make small criticisms of the care being provided. Which of the following communications from the nurse to the patient's daughter would be most appropriate at this time?
   1. "I can see that you are feeling short-tempered, which is not unusual under the circumstances. However, it is not good for your father's state of mind to hear you complaining."
   2. "It must be difficult for you to be here day after day, not eating well or sleeping properly, in addition to worrying about your father's condition. Is there someone who can help you out and stay here for a night so you can get some sleep?
   3. "Many people have been in the same situation that you are in now. It really would be best for you in the long term to go home for a few days and get some sleep and proper nutrition. I'll give you the unit phone number so you can call us when you wish."
   4. "How much sleep have you had in the last few days? Perhaps you should eat and get some rest. You will be of little help to your father if you are so tired you can't think properly."

10. The nurse is working in the pediatric intensive care unit and is assigned to pediatric patients who are experiencing pain. The nurse would select the Wong FACES Pain Rating Scale for use in which of the following children?
   1. A 6-month-old patient with failure to thrive
   2. A 12-month-old patient with a burn injury
   3. A 2-year-old patient with injuries after an auto accident
   4. A 3-year-old patient with sickle cell disease

11. A patient receiving palliative care is being treated with large doses of narcotic analgesics to control pain. To minimize the side effects of this medication the nurse ensures that there is an order for which of the following types of medications?
   1. Stool softener
   2. Antiemetic
   3. Non-opioid analgesic
   4. Bronchodilator

12. A patient undergoing chemotherapy is experiencing anxiety-induced anticipatory nausea and vomiting. The nurse could assist this patient by requesting an order for which of the following preferred medications?
   1. Lorazepam (Ativan)
   2. Hydroxyzine (Vistaril)
   3. Chlorpromazine (Thorazine)
   4. Promethazine (Phenergan)

13. A patient with advanced acquired immunodeficiency syndrome (AIDS) is experiencing hiccups. Which of the following noninvasive measures would the nurse employ before requesting a medication order?
   1. Slow, deep breathing
   2. Rapidly drinking a glass of water
   3. Eating a high-protein snack
   4. Covering the head with a paper bag

14. The nurse should use which of the following measures first to reduce dyspnea in a patient with end-stage chronic obstructive pulmonary disease?
   1. Administer a dose of an ordered PRN bronchodilator.
   2. Encourage the patient to use an incentive spirometer.
   3. Assist the patient to cough and deep breathe.
   4. Elevate the head of the bed.

15. The son of a terminally ill patient tells the nurse, "My dad's doctor says I should begin thinking about end-of-life care." The nurse interprets that this most likely means that the patient will not likely live more than:
   1. 1 month
   2. 3 months
   3. 6 months
   4. 1 year

16. A patient with cancer that has metastasized to the brain and liver says to the nurse, "I've been reading about some of the cancer research, and I am still hoping for a cure in the next few months." In formulating a response to the patient, which of the following should the nurse consider first?
   1. The purpose that would be served in confronting the patient's denial
   2. The educational level of the patient and his ability to understand research
   3. The prognosis of the patient
   4. The need for a consultation with a psychiatrist

17. The family of a patient who is terminally ill and unresponsive has acknowledged that the patient's condition will not change and asks about palliative care. The nurse explains to the family that palliative care includes:
    1. comfort measures and medications to treat pain and prevent stomach ulcers.
    2. hygiene and intravenous fluid volume replacement.
    3. pain medication, hygiene, and range-of-motion exercises to prevent contractures.
    4. nasogastric tube feedings, all current medications, and hygiene.

18. A patient with mental retardation has no family and becomes critically ill with severe pneumonia. Which standard should the health care team utilize as the best method for decision making in planning care for this patient?
    1. Patient's Bill of Rights
    2. Informed consent
    3. Substituted-judgment standard
    4. Best interests standard

19. A patient with end-stage renal disease does not want further aggressive treatment, but does not want to withdraw current treatment. The nurse would help the patient to understand that this typically includes maintaining:
    1. dialysis and full code status.
    2. nutrition and hydration but removal of dialysis.
    3. nutrition, hydration, and dialysis.
    4. comfort measures only.

20. When a critically ill patient makes a decision to withhold further treatment, the nurse discusses the types of treatments that would not be ordered in the future. The nurse would include in the discussion the information that which of the following types of medications would be withheld?
    1. Antibiotics
    2. Antiemetics
    3. Non-opioid analgesics
    4. Opioid analgesics

21. The nurse has explained hospice services to a patient with metastatic cancer. In evaluating the teaching, the nurse determines that the patient needs further information if the patient states that one of the services provided in hospice care is:
    1. symptom management.
    2. chemotherapy.
    3. psychosocial and emotional support.
    4. nutritional counseling.

22. The nurse is working with the family of a terminally ill 11-year-old child with leukemia. The nurse shares with the parents that the sibling of what age will have an attitude toward death that is more factual than emotional because of developmental factors?
    1. 16 years
    2. 12 years
    3. 8 years
    4. 5 years

23. A child who was struck by an automobile while riding a bicycle sustains life-threatening injuries and is subsequently diagnosed with brain death. The parents refuse organ donation, despite the potential benefits of this process for both the donor family and the recipient. Which of the following is the best action by the nurse?
    1. Refer the matter to the hospital's ethics committee.
    2. Ask the physician whether a court order to do so would be indicated.
    3. Say nothing and support the parents to the fullest extent possible.
    4. Gently share with the parents that they could be making a mistake they will later regret.

24. A 22-year-old female nurse is working with a seriously ill 23-year-old female patient recovering from a motor vehicle accident. The nurse understands that she is having difficulty maintaining professional boundaries based on their age. Which of the following actions should the nurse take initially?
    1. Seek guidance from another experienced nurse or the unit manager.
    2. Provide excellent care but keep conversation to a minimum.
    3. Arrange to have a nurse's aid complete as much care as possible within the scope of practice.
    4. Discuss with the nursing supervisor the possibility of transferring to a different nursing unit.

25. A patient who is terminally ill expresses a wish to "hurry up and end it all." In exploring reasons for this wish, which of the following should the nurse assess first?
    1. Guilt and fatigue
    2. Pain and depression
    3. Self-esteem and hope
    4. Competency and pain

ANSWERS TO TEST BANK

CHAPTER 1

1. Answer: 3
Rationale: Nurses were trained as resource persons, teachers, leaders, and counselors who cared for psychiatric patients. Answers 1, 2, and 4 are incorrect.
Cognitive Level: Comprehension
Nursing Process: NA
NCLEX: Psychosocial Integrity
Text Page: 5

2. Answer: 2
Rationale: Early nursing education made a distinction between physical and emotional needs, and nurses were taught in either a general hospital or a psychiatric hospital.
Richards maintained that nurses should be competent to assess both physical and emotional needs.
Cognitive Level: Comprehension
Nursing Process: NA
NCLEX: Safe, Effective Care Environment: Management of Care
Text Page: 2

3. Answer: 2
Rationale: Maxwell Jones published *The Therapeutic Community* in 1953. It encouraged making use of the patient's social environment as a means of providing therapeutic experiences.
Cognitive Level: Application
Nursing Process: Planning
NCLEX: Psychosocial Integrity
Text Page: 5

4. Answer: 3
Rationale: In 1962, Peplau's article identified the heart of psychiatric nursing as fulfillment of the role of counselor or psychotherapist.
Cognitive Level: Comprehension
Nursing Process: NA
NCLEX: Safe, Effective Care Environment: Management of Care
Text Page: 5

5. Answer: 4
Rationale: Psychiatric nursing is concerned with individuals, families, groups, and entire communities. The other statements listed are false.
Cognitive Level: Application
Nursing Process: NA
NCLEX: Safe, Effective Care Environment: Management of Care
Text Page: 6

6. Answer: 3
Rationale: Answers 1 and 2 are not true answers, while Answer 4 is incorrect because advances in the psychodynamic model of psychiatric care were made by psychiatrists and psychologists, not by psychiatric nurses.
Cognitive Level: Analysis
Nursing Process: NA
NCLEX: Psychosocial Integrity
Text Page: 6

7. Answer: 3
Rationale: Addressing an individual using his or her title and surname implies dignity and worth and conveys respect.
Cognitive Level: Analysis
Nursing Process: Implementation
NCLEX: Psychosocial Integrity
Text Page: 7

8. Answer: 3
Rationale: This principle best addresses the aide's comment that the patient's behavior is "senseless" by explaining that all behavior has meaning that can be understood when the patient's internal frame of reference and the context of the situation are known.
Cognitive Level: Analysis
Nursing Process: Implementation
NCLEX: Psychosocial Integrity
Text Page: 7

9. Answer: 1
Rationale: The role of the psychiatric nurse today is multifocused. The psychiatric nurse must have a broader perspective on NCLEX, psychiatric needs, personal needs, financial needs, and legal needs that encompass the patient's quality of life.
Cognitive Level: Analysis
Nursing Process: NA
NCLEX: Safe, Effective Care Environment: Management of Care
Text Page: 8

10. Answer: 3
Rationale: Because only Answer 3 is a true statement, it is the only statement that supports the concept that psychiatric nursing, as a specialty, is vulnerable.
Cognitive Level: Analysis
Nursing Process: NA
NCLEX: Psychosocial Integrity
Text Page: 7

11. Answer: 4
Rationale: Students who have the opportunity to work in a psychiatric mental health setting benefit because of the opportunities to work directly with a specific population of patients with psychiatric mental health illnesses. In acute care, medical-surgical units, general outpatient clinical settings, or long term-care settings, students can only care for the patients served in the setting and hope that they will acquire some knowledge about the psychiatric mental health disease process and how it affects patients. Unfortunately in these settings, the chances for learning about advances in the field of psychiatry or behavioral health would not be available.
Cognitive Level: Application
Nursing Process: NA
NCLEX: Psychosocial Integrity
Text Page: 6

12. Answer: 2
Rationale: Answer 2 is correct because delegation includes the domains of management and direct care. Collaboration includes communication and management; teaching includes direct care and communication; and coordination includes direct care, communication, and management.
Cognitive Level: Analysis
Nursing Process: NA
NCLEX: Safe, Effective Care Environment: Management of Care
Text Page: 10

13. Answer: 3
Rationale: Management is a direct care activity. Figure 1-3 depicts this graphically.
Cognitive Level: Analysis
Nursing Process: NA
NCLEX: Safe, Effective Care Environment: Management of Care
Text Page: 10

14. Answer: 3
Rationale: Collaboration is defined as the shared planning, decision making, problem solving, goal setting, and assumption of responsibilities by people who work together cooperatively and with open communication.
Cognitive Level: Analysis
Nursing Process: NA
NCLEX: Safe, Effective Care Environment: Management of Care
Text Page: 9

15. Answer: 3
Rationale: State law is the primary determinant of the roles nurses may assume in any state.
Cognitive Level: Analysis
Nursing Process: NA
NCLEX: Safe, Effective Care Environment: Safety and Infection Control
Text Page: 10

16. Answer: 4
Rationale: All aspects of care for patients are important, but because of the reform in health care systems, patient triage and management of care become primary responsibilities for an efficient, cost-effective system.
Cognitive Level: Analysis
Nursing Process: Assessment
NCLEX: Safe, Effective Care Environment: Management of Care
Text Page: 9

17. Answer: 3
Rationale: The answer is number 3. All other answers are incorrect.
Cognitive Level: Knowledge
Nursing Process: NA
NCLEX: Safe, Effective Care Environment: Management of Care
Text Page: 10

18. Answer: 2
Rationale: It is important to prove that psychiatric nursing contributes to positive outcomes in the prevention of illness, the promotion of health, and the provision of cost-effective treatment of psychiatric disorders. Without such information, the specialty of psychiatric nursing may be discounted by users and others.
Cognitive Level: Analysis
Nursing Process: NA
NCLEX: Safe, Effective Care Environment: Management of Care
Text Page: 11-12

19. Answer: 2
Rationale: Alternative treatment settings have emerged throughout the continuum of mental health care, and hospitals have responded by creating integrated clinical systems that provide inpatient care, partial hospitalization, day treatment, residential care, home care, and ambulatory care as part of the parent organization. Psychiatric nurses provide care in each of

these settings as well as in community-based treatment settings such as shelters, schools, and HMOs.
Cognitive Level: Application
Nursing Process: NA
NCLEX: Safe, Effective Care Environment: Management of Care
Text Page: 8

20. Answer: 1
Rationale: Psychiatric nurse leaders need to be change agents who work not only in the profession but also with other interdisciplinary colleagues to advance the care of patients with psychiatric disorders.
Cognitive Level: Application
Nursing Process: NA
NCLEX: Safe, Effective Care Environment: Management of Care
Text Page: 12

21. Answer: 4
Rationale: The only act that is genuine is Answer 4, the Community Mental Health Centers Act of 1963.
Cognitive Level: Comprehension
Nursing Process: NA
NCLEX: Psychosocial Integrity
Text Page: 5

22. Answer: 2
Rationale: The psychiatric nurse uses knowledge from the psychosocial and biophysical sciences and theories of personality and human behavior. From these the nurse derives a theoretical framework on which nursing practice is based.
Cognitive Level: Analysis
Nursing Process: NA
NCLEX: Psychosocial Integrity
Text Page: 6

23. Answer: 4
Rationale: To help a new nurse into a psychiatric setting, there should be a supportive environment that has open and honest communication, as well as respect and recognition of the nurse's contributions, and a safe and gradual introduction of duties and responsibilities.
Cognitive Level: Application
Nursing Process: NA
NCLEX: Psychosocial Integrity
Text Page: 11

24. Answer: 3
Rationale: Answers 1, 2, and 4 are concentrated on other disciplines. A nurse's support group would concentrate on the advancement and support of nurses and the discipline of nursing.
Cognitive Level: Analysis
Nursing Process: NA
NCLEX: Psychosocial Integrity
Text Page: 11

25. Answer: 4
Rationale: For a psychiatric nurse to be politically active, helping others to become involved in their local area is a good step toward political awareness. Answer 1 would be health care related rather than political action. Answer 2 would not have a direct correlation with psychiatric mental health issues, and Answer 3 would be beneficial to the community that the crisis center serves but not a direct political action.
Cognitive Level: Analysis
Nursing Process: NA
NCLEX: Health Promotion and Maintenance
Text Page: 12

CHAPTER 2

1. Answer: 4
Rationale: Social and therapeutic relationships both involve the giving of information, emotional investment, and personal satisfaction. These aspects all have differences, but they are minor in comparison with the difference in responsibility that exists between social and therapeutic relationships. In the therapeutic relationship, the nurse has both ethical and legal responsibilities to the patient; these responsibilities do not exist in the social relationship.
Cognitive Level: Analysis
Nursing Process: Implementation
NCLEX: Psychosocial Integrity
Text Page: 16

2. Answer: 1
Rationale: Quadrant 1 is the open quadrant; it includes the behaviors, feelings, and thoughts known to the individual and others. The smaller an individual's quadrant 1, the poorer the communication of that individual. The goal of increasing self-awareness is to enlarge the area of quadrant 1 and reduce the size of the other three quadrants.
Cognitive Level: Application
Nursing Process: Planning
NCLEX: Psychosocial Integrity
Text Page: 17

3. Answer: 3
Rationale: Nursing students have many new experiences that provide opportunities for self-learning. Nurses should focus on and discuss the feelings related to these experiences. Instructors and peers can help students by facilitating self-awareness during these discussions; self-awareness contributes to authenticity.
Cognitive Level: Analysis

Nursing Process: Implementation
NCLEX: Psychosocial Integrity
Text Page: 18

4. Answer: 1
Rationale: The highest level of value clarification is acting in a pattern. Adopting two "special children" is affirmation of a pattern. Acting follows choosing and prizing in the sequence of value clarification.
Cognitive Level: Analysis
Nursing Process: Implementation
NCLEX: Psychosocial Integrity
Text Page: 19

5. Answer: 2
Rationale: The feelings that nurses have serve an important purpose. They are valuable clues about the patient's problems, and they are barometers for feedback about the nurses themselves and their relationships with others.
Cognitive Level: Application
Nursing Process: Implementation
NCLEX: Psychosocial Integrity
Text Page: 19

6. Answer: 2
Rationale: Self-exploration leads to the development of self-awareness, and it is essential that the nurse be self-aware to learn to deal with anxiety, anger, sadness, and joy in helping patients through the health-illness continuum.
Cognitive Level: Application
Nursing Process: Implementation
NCLEX: Psychosocial Integrity
Text Page: 20

7. Answer: 1
Rationale: Self-examination is a task of the preinteraction phase of a relationship. This is especially important if the value systems of the nurse and patient are known to be different.
Cognitive Level: Application
Nursing Process: Planning
NCLEX: Psychosocial Integrity
Text Page: 20

8. Answer: 4
Rationale: In the preinteraction phase, the nurse and the patient have not yet met. The nurse prepares for the initial contact by performing self-assessment, gathering available data about the patient, reviewing the goals of a therapeutic relationship, and considering what he or she has to offer the patient.
Cognitive Level: Analysis
Nursing Process: Implementation
NCLEX: Psychosocial Integrity
Text Page: 21

9. Answer: 3
Rationale: Conditions for termination are part of the nurse-patient contract negotiated during the introductory/orientation phase of the relationship. In a social relationship, termination is open-ended.
Cognitive Level: Application
Nursing Process: Implementation
NCLEX: Psychosocial Integrity
Text Page: 21

10. Answer: 1
Rationale: Tasks of the introductory phase of the nurse-patient partnership are to establish a climate of trust, understanding, acceptance, and open communication and to formulate a contract with the patient.
Cognitive Level: Application
Nursing Process: Planning
NCLEX: Psychosocial Integrity
Text Page: 21

11. Answer: 3
Rationale: It is appropriate to acknowledge the angry or otherwise negative feelings of a patient who has not voluntarily sought treatment. Feeling understood by the nurse paves the way for a therapeutic relationship.
Cognitive Level: Application
Nursing Process: Implementation
NCLEX: Psychosocial Integrity
Text Page: 21

12. Answer: 4
Rationale: When a patient initially offers psychiatric symptoms as the reason for admission, the nurse will want to ask for clarification and elaboration to better understand the life experiences of the patient. Understanding fosters empathy, empathic remarks lead the patient to feel understood, and this understanding paves the way for the therapeutic nurse-patient partnership.
Cognitive Level: Application
Nursing Process: Implementation
NCLEX: Psychosocial Integrity
Text Page: 22

13. Answer: 4
Rationale: Testing behavior serves the purpose of exploring the nurse's consistency and intent.
Cognitive Level: Analysis
Nursing Process: Planning
NCLEX: Psychosocial Integrity
Text Page: 22

14. Answer: 2
Rationale: Establishing the reality of separation is difficult for both the nurse and patient. Patients often respond to impending termination with increased anxiety; they may experience negative feelings associated

with earlier terminations, and they may regress to previous, less adaptive behaviors in the hope of postponing termination.
Cognitive Level: Application
Nursing Process: Implementation
NCLEX: Psychosocial Integrity
Text Page: 23

15. Answer: 4
Rationale: Resistance is the patient's reluctance or avoidance of verbalizing or experiencing troubling aspects of himself or herself. This is often caused by the patient's unwillingness to change when the need for change is recognized. However, all of the behaviors mentioned are possible ways of expressing resistance. Superficial talk and "having nothing to talk about" are behaviors that novice nurses understand as expressing resistance, and the other behaviors listed, although they do occur, are less easily associated with resistance.
Cognitive Level: Analysis
Nursing Process: Implementation
NCLEX: Psychosocial Integrity
Text Page: 23

16. Answer: 2
Rationale: The relationship can become stalled if the nurse is not prepared to deal with the impasse. The nurse may use the techniques listed in Answer 2 by saying something like: "I sense that you're struggling with yourself and wanting to explore your relationship with your mother but that you're not yet wanting to experience the pain it may bring."
Cognitive Level: Application
Nursing Process: Implementation
NCLEX: Psychosocial Integrity
Text Page: 23

17. Answer: 2
Rationale: Perception is the identification and interpretation of a stimulus based on information received through the senses. In this instance the patient has incorrectly interpreted the shadows as a face on the wall.
Cognitive Level: Application
Nursing Process: Implementation
NCLEX: Psychosocial Integrity
Text Page: 26

18. Answer: 3
Rationale: Incongruent communication occurs when the verbal content and the nonverbal level of communication are not in agreement.
Cognitive Level: Application
Nursing Process: Implementation
NCLEX: Psychosocial Integrity
Text Page: 27

19. Answer: 3
Rationale: The nurse's statement can be construed as critical. The parent ego state consists of all the nurturing, critical, and prejudicial attitudes, behaviors, and experiences learned from other people, especially from parents and teachers.
Cognitive Level: Application
Nursing Process: NA
NCLEX: Psychosocial Integrity
Text Page: 28

20. Answer: 4
Rationale: In this interaction, the two parties are communicating from adult ego state to adult ego state. Communication flows smoothly between the sender and the receiver.
Cognitive Level: Application
Nursing Process: Implementation
NCLEX: Psychosocial Integrity
Text Page: 28

21. Answer: 1
Rationale: This is an example of the "Why don't you? Yes, but..." game. On the surface the game involves two adults solving problems; in reality, one person is using the child ego state to show what a bad parent the other person is.
Cognitive Level: Application
Nursing Process: Implementation
NCLEX: Psychosocial Integrity
Text Page: 29

22. Answer: 4
Rationale: Clarification involves the nurse attempting to put into words the vague ideas or thoughts that are implicit or explicit in the patient's conversation.
Cognitive Level: Analysis
Nursing Process: Implementation
NCLEX: Psychosocial Integrity
Text Page: 30-31

23. Answer: 4
Rationale: Sharing perceptions involves asking the patient to verify the nurse's understanding of what the patient is thinking or feeling. The nurse can provide information and then ask for feedback.
Cognitive Level: Analysis
Nursing Process: Implementation
NCLEX: Psychosocial Integrity
Text Page: 32

24. Answer: 3
Rationale: Suggesting is the presentation of alternative ideas. It is useful in the working phase of the relationship, when the patient has analyzed the problem and is exploring alternative coping mechanisms. At that

time, nurse suggestions will increase the patient's perceived options.
Cognitive Level: Analysis
Nursing Process: Planning
NCLEX: Psychosocial Integrity
Text Page: 33

25. Answer: 2
Rationale: Confrontation is an expression by the nurse of discrepancies in the patient's behavior.
Cognitive Level: Analysis
Nursing Process: Implementation
NCLEX: Psychosocial Integrity
Text Page: 38

26. Answer: 2
Rationale: Confrontation, when posed as an observation of incongruent behavior, can be used infrequently during the orientation phase of the relationship, but it is more useful during the working stage to expand the patient's awareness and to help him or her move to a higher level of functioning.
Cognitive Level: Analysis
Nursing Process: Planning
NCLEX: Psychosocial Integrity
Text Page: 38

27. Answer: 1
Rationale: Immediacy involves focusing on the current interaction of the nurse and the patient in the relationship.
Cognitive Level: Analysis
Nursing Process: Implementation
NCLEX: Psychosocial Integrity
Text Page: 39

28. Answer: 4
Rationale: Dependent reaction transference is characterized by submissive, ingratiating behavior, regarding the nurse as a godlike figure, and overvaluing the nurse's characteristics and qualities.
Cognitive Level: Application
Nursing Process: Implementation
NCLEX: Psychosocial Integrity
Text Page: 43

29. Answer: 1
Rationale: Countertransference is a therapeutic impasse created by the nurse's specific emotional response to the qualities of the patient. This response is inappropriate to the content and context of the therapeutic relationship or inappropriate in the degree of intensity of emotion.
Cognitive Level: Application
Nursing Process: Assessment
NCLEX: Psychosocial Integrity
Text Page: 43

CHAPTER 3

1. Answer: 1
Rationale: Interpersonal therapists believe that behavior evolves around interpersonal relationships, so their assessments will focus on the identification of interpersonal difficulties.
Cognitive Level: Application
Nursing Process: Assessment
NCLEX: Safe, Effective Care Environment: Management of Care
Text Page: 53

2. Answer: 3
Rationale: The emphasis of supportive therapy is to improve behavior and subjective feelings of distress rather than achieve insight or self-understanding. The methods used draw from as many different models as needed.
Cognitive Level: Application
Nursing Process: Implementation
NCLEX: Psychosocial Integrity
Text Page: 56

3. Answer: 3
Rationale: In the interpersonal model, behavioral deviations are seen as rooted in the needs for satisfaction and security. In the given situation, the patient's need for security is threatened, and anxiety is created.
Cognitive Level: Application
Nursing Process: NA
NCLEX: Psychosocial Integrity
Text Page: 52

4. Answer: 3
Rationale: The emphasis of supportive therapy is on improving behavior and subjective feelings of distress. Answer 3 is a realistic immediate goal that may be addressed by supportive nursing measures and medication, whereas Answers 1, 2, and 4 may require more time to achieve.
Cognitive Level: Application
Nursing Process: Planning
NCLEX: Psychosocial Integrity
Text Page: 56

5. Answer: 3
Rationale: In accordance with the medical model, the physician identifies the illness and prescribes specific therapy. Providing a safe environment and monitoring patient response to therapy requires the interventions listed in Answer 3.
Cognitive Level: Application
Nursing Process: Planning
NCLEX: Safe, Effective Care Environment: Management of Care
Text Page: 57

6. Answer: 4
Rationale: Transference is a psychoanalytical concept that refers to feelings the patient develops toward the therapist that are unrelated to the therapist's current behavior or characteristics. Transference can be used to explore previously unresolved conflicts.
Cognitive Level: Application
Nursing Process: Implementation
NCLEX: Psychosocial Integrity
Text Page: 51

7. Answer: 4
Rationale: Psychoanalysts trace disrupted behavior in the adult to earlier developmental stages in which psychological energy (libido) has become fixated in an attempt to deal with anxiety.
Cognitive Level: Application
Nursing Process: Implementation
NCLEX: Psychosocial Integrity
Text Page: 51

8. Answer: 1
Rationale: Interpretation involves explaining dream symbolism to patients and exploring the significance of the issues that are discussed or avoided during therapy.
Cognitive Level: Application
Nursing Process: Implementation
NCLEX: Psychosocial Integrity
Text Page: 52

9. Answer: 4
Rationale: The psychoanalytical model makes use of interpretation and focuses on working through previously unresolved conflicts.
Cognitive Level: Application
Nursing Process: NA
NCLEX: Psychosocial Integrity
Text Page: 51

10. Answer: 2
Rationale: Existential therapists focus on the person's experience in the here and now, the search for authenticity and reduction of self-alienation.
Cognitive Level: Application
Nursing Process: Assessment
NCLEX: Psychosocial Integrity
Text Page: 55

11. Answer: 4
Rationale: Unconditional acceptance helps the patient speak openly to the therapist. The patient-therapist relationship serves as a model of adaptive interpersonal relationships that can be generalized to people outside of the therapeutic situation.
Cognitive Level: Application
Nursing Process: Implementation
NCLEX: Psychosocial Integrity
Text Page: 53

12. Answer: 3
Rationale: Szasz believes that culture is useful in defining mental illness, prescribing therapy, and determining the patient's future. He believes that social deviance is often labeled mental illness, and that people are responsible for their own behavior.
Cognitive Level: Application
Nursing Process: NA
NCLEX: Psychosocial Integrity
Text Page: 54-55

13. Answer: 4
Rationale: The social model considers the social environment as it affects the person and the person's life experience. Answers 1, 2, and 3 focus on intrapsychic processes and interpersonal experiences.
Cognitive Level: Analysis
Nursing Process: Implementation
NCLEX: Psychosocial Integrity
Text Page: 54

14. Answer: 2
Rationale: In psychoanalysis, the patient is active and the therapist is described as a "shadow" person who listens and only occasionally interprets behavior.
Cognitive Level: Application
Nursing Process: NA
NCLEX: Psychosocial Integrity
Text Page: 51

15. Answer: 1
Rationale: Supportive therapy calls for the therapist to be active and directive.
Cognitive Level: Application
Nursing Process: NA
NCLEX: Psychosocial Integrity
Text Page: 56

16. Answer: 1
Rationale: Empathy plays a major therapeutic role in both the interpersonal model and the supportive therapy model.
Cognitive Level: Analysis
Nursing Process: NA
NCLEX: Psychosocial Integrity
Text Page: 57-58

17. Answer: 2
Rationale: The patient participating in interpersonal therapy has the role of participating in a relationship and sharing concerns with the therapist, who demonstrates uncritical and accepting behavior. The therapist demonstrates experience that the patient can use to formulate other relationships in all aspects of life, not

just in a family (Answer 4) and not just in a social situation (Answer 1). Nor will the patient be expected to be involved with group work because of interpersonal therapy. The only correct answer is 3.
Cognitive Level: Analysis
Nursing Process: Implementation
NCLEX: Psychosocial Integrity
Text Page: 53

18. Answer: 2
Rationale: Szasz believes that society must find a way to manage "undesirables," so it labels them as mentally ill. People who are so labeled usually are unable to conform to social norms, and they usually become incarcerated because of their refusal to conform. The other terms in 1, 3, and 4 are fictional.
Cognitive Level: Analysis
Nursing Process: NA
NCLEX: Psychosocial Integrity
Text Page: 54

19. Answer: 1
Rationale: Existential therapists help patients to focus on the importance of experiences in the present. It is a form of therapy that assumes a patient must be able to choose freely from what his or her life has to offer. The other answers are incorrect.
Cognitive Level: Analysis
Nursing Process: NA
NCLEX: Psychosocial Integrity
Text Page: 55

20. Answer: 1
Rationale: The medical model of psychiatric care refers to psychiatric care that is based on the traditional physician-patient relationship. It focuses on the diagnosis of a mental illness and subsequent treatment that is based on that diagnosis.
Cognitive Level: Application
Nursing Process: Implementation
NCLEX: Psychosocial Integrity
Text Page: 56

21. Answer: 4
Rationale: The medical model dominates modern psychiatric care. Other health professionals may be involved in interagency referrals, family assessment, and health teaching, but physicians are seen as the leaders of the team under this model.
Cognitive Level: Application
Nursing Process: Implementation
NCLEX: Psychosocial Integrity
Text Page: 56

22. Answer: 1
Rationale: The medical model proposes that all mental processes, even the most complex psychological processes, derive from operations of the brain. Several different types of brain disorders can lead to mental illness. Answers 2, 3, and 4 all indicate how the disorders are treated with only one methodology, which should indicate that they are probably not correct.
Cognitive Level: Analysis
Nursing Process: NA
NCLEX: Psychosocial Integrity
Text Page: 57

23. Answer: 1
Rationale: In the medical model of psychiatric care, the physician, as the healer, identifies the patient's illness and formulates a treatment plan.
Cognitive Level: Comprehension
Nursing Process: NA
NCLEX: Psychosocial Integrity
Text Page: 57

24. Answer: 4
Rationale: The DSM-IV TR is based on the medical model. All other responses are incorrect.
Cognitive Level: Knowledge
Nursing Process: NA
NCLEX: Psychosocial Integrity
Text Page: 54

25. Answer: 1
Rationale: The two components of a healthy state identified by Peplau are physiological demands and interpersonal conditions, or according to Sullivan, satisfaction and security. The only individual that meets the two criteria is indicated in Answer 1. The others are not indicative of both security and satisfaction.
Cognitive Level: Analysis
Nursing Process: NA
NCLEX: Psychosocial Integrity
Text Page: 53

CHAPTER 4

1. Answer: 3
Rationale: The Stuart Stress Adaptation Model is holistic, views nature as ordered on a social hierarchy, regards adaptation/maladaptation as distinct from health/illness, relates nursing activities to levels of prevention and the four stages of treatment, is based on standards of psychiatric nursing care and professional performance, and can be used across psychiatric settings throughout the care continuum.
Cognitive Level: Application
Nursing Process: NA
NCLEX: Psychosocial Integrity
Text Page: 61

2. Answer: 4
Rationale: The answer is the explanation the author gives.
Cognitive Level: Application
Nursing Process: NA
NCLEX: Psychosocial Integrity
Text Page: 61

3. Answer: 3
Rationale: Answer 2 will be performed eventually for the patient but the primary responsibility of the psychiatric nurse according the fifth assumption of Stuart's Stress Adaptation Model is to utilize the nursing process, standards of care, and professional performance, which, in this case, should start with a nursing assessment. Delegating responsibility to someone who will sit with the patient before knowing why the patient is still very emotionally distraught is not responsible nursing care, nor is getting a sedative order for the patient.
Cognitive Level: Application
Nursing Process: Assessment
NCLEX: Safe, Effective Care Environment: Management of Care
Text Page: 61

4. Answer: 1
Rationale: Alternative or deviant social behaviors are not necessarily indicative of illness.
Cognitive Level: Analysis
Nursing Process: Assessment
NCLEX: Psychosocial Integrity
Text Page: 62

5. Answer: 1
Rationale: These factors relate directly to autonomy, the condition that allows for definition and control over a domain.
Cognitive Level: Application
Nursing Process: Assessment
NCLEX: Psychosocial Integrity
Text Page: 62

6. Answer: 3
Rationale: Reality perception is the individual's ability to test assumptions about the world with empirical thought. Hallucinations and delusions indicate problems with reality perception.
Cognitive Level: Application
Nursing Process: Assessment
NCLEX: Psychosocial Integrity
Text Page: 62

7. Answer: 2
Rationale: Integration refers to a balance between what is expressed and what is repressed and a regulation of moods and emotions, and it includes the characteristics mentioned in the question.
Cognitive Level: Application
Nursing Process: Assessment
NCLEX: Psychosocial Integrity
Text Page: 62

8. Answer: 4
Rationale: The question asks for a reply relevant to the extent of mental illness. Replies 1 and 2 do not address the extent of mental illness and Reply 3 is false.
Cognitive Level: Application
Nursing Process: Implementation
NCLEX: Psychosocial Integrity
Text Page: 63

9. Answer: 4
Rationale: The study predicted that by the year 2020, unipolar major depression will become the second leading factor in disease burden.
Cognitive Level: Analysis
Nursing Process: Planning
NCLEX: Psychosocial Integrity
Text Page: 63

10. Answer: 2
Rationale: The only reply that addresses comparative treatment efficacy is Answer 2.
Cognitive Level: Application
Nursing Process: Implementation
NCLEX: Psychosocial Integrity
Text Page: 64

11. Answer: 1
Rationale: Under health care reform, making mental health coverage for the severely mentally ill commensurate with other health care coverage would actually yield a $2.2 billion net savings in the United States.
Cognitive Level: Application
Nursing Process: NA
NCLEX: Safe, Effective Care Environment: Management of Care
Text Page: 64

12. Answer: 1
Rationale: Predisposing factors include biological, psychological, and sociocultural components. Predisposing factors are those that place a person at risk for development of a stress-related disorder.
Cognitive Level: Application
Nursing Process: Implementation
NCLEX: Psychosocial Integrity
Text Page: 65

13. Answer: 3
Rationale: Precipitating stressors are stimuli that the individual perceives as challenging, threatening, or demanding. Dealing with them requires extra energy and produces a state of tension and stress.

Cognitive Level: Application
Nursing Process: Assessment
NCLEX: Psychosocial Integrity
Text Page: 64-65

14. Answer: 1
Rationale: The 42-year-old patient is dealing with two stressful life events that are socially undesirable. His cognitive appraisal of the stressors is that of loss and threat of loss. He gives no indication of psychological hardiness. The other people described are dealing with change they perceive as challenging but to which they are committed and over which they have some control. These factors indicate psychological hardiness.
Cognitive Level: Analysis
Nursing Process: NA
NCLEX: Psychosocial Integrity
Text Page: 67

15. Answer: 2
Rationale: Research suggests that daily hassles may be better predictors of psychological and physical health than major life events. The more frequent and intense the hassles people reported, the poorer was their overall mental and physical health.
Cognitive Level: Analysis
Nursing Process: NA
NCLEX: Health Promotion and Maintenance
Text Page: 67

16. Answer: 4
Rationale: Appraisal of a stressor is the processing and comprehension of the stressful situation that takes place on many levels including cognitive, affective, physiological, behavioral, and social.
Cognitive Level: Application
Nursing Process: Assessment
NCLEX: Psychosocial Integrity
Text Page: 67-68

17. Answer: 2
Rationale: Caplan described four phases of an individual's responses to stressful events.
Cognitive Level: Application
Nursing Process: Assessment
NCLEX: Psychosocial Integrity
Text Page: 67

18. Answer: 1
Rationale: Social response to stress and illness involves the search for meaning, which is a period of time in which people seek information about their problem. This is necessary for devising a coping strategy.
Cognitive Level: Application
Nursing Process: NA
NCLEX: Psychosocial Integrity
Text Page: 67

19. Answer: 1
Rationale: Social attributions in which the individual sees a problem as resulting from his or her own negligence may block active coping responses.
Cognitive Level: Application
Nursing Process: Assessment
NCLEX: Psychosocial Integrity
Text Page: 68

20. Answer: 2
Rationale: Coping resources include economic assets, abilities, skills, defensive techniques, social supports, and motivation. Coping mechanisms can be defined as any effort directed at stress management and include problem-focused, cognitive-focused, and emotion-focused mechanisms that can be constructive (assets) or destructive (liabilities).
Cognitive Level: Analysis
Nursing Process: NA
NCLEX: Psychosocial Integrity
Text Page: 68

21. Answer: 4
Rationale: Nursing diagnosis is concerned with the adaptive/maladaptive continuum of human responses; medical diagnosis is concerned with the health/illness continuum of health problems. Nurses assess risk factors and look for vulnerabilities; physicians assess disease states and look for causes. Nursing intervention consists of caregiving activities; medical intervention consists of curative treatments.
Cognitive Level: Analysis
Nursing Process: NA
NCLEX: Health Promotion and Maintenance
Text Page: 68-69

22. Answer: 2
Rationale: Responses to stress, whether actual or potential, are the subject of nursing diagnoses. Nursing diagnoses complement rather than replace medical diagnoses.
Cognitive Level: Application
Nursing Process: NA
NCLEX: Health Promotion and Maintenance
Text Page: 68-69

23. Answer: 4
Rationale: Patients with psychosis have these characteristics: regressive behavior, personality disintegration, significant reduction in the level of awareness, great difficulty in adequately functioning, and gross impairment in reality testing.
Cognitive Level: Application
Nursing Process: Implementation
NCLEX: Psychosocial Integrity
Text Page: 69

24. Answer: 3
Rationale: Nurses may use the nursing process to assess, analyze, plan, implement, and evaluate care for patients independent of physicians or other health care professionals. Nursing care will complement medical care.
Cognitive Level: Application
Nursing Process: Implementation
NCLEX: Safe, Effective Care Environment: Management of Care
Text Page: 71

25. Answer: 1
Rationale: The crisis stage occurs in the first days to weeks after a stressful event.
Cognitive Level: Application
Nursing Process: Assessment
NCLEX: Psychosocial Integrity
Text Page: 71

26. Answer: 1
Rationale: According to the Stuart Stress Adaptation Model, the nursing goal for the crisis stage is the stabilization of the patient.
Cognitive Level: Application
Nursing Process: Planning
NCLEX: Psychosocial Integrity
Text Page: 71

27. Answer: 1
Rationale: According to the Stuart Stress Adaptation Model, during the acute stage of treatment, the expected outcome of nursing care is symptom relief.
Cognitive Level: Application
Nursing Process: Outcome Identification
NCLEX: Psychosocial Integrity
Text Page: 71

28. Answer: 3
Rationale: According to the Stuart Stress Adaptation Model, mutual treatment planning, modeling, and teaching adaptive responses are appropriate nursing interventions for the acute stage of treatment.
Cognitive Level: Application
Nursing Process: Planning
NCLEX: Psychosocial Integrity
Text Page: 71

29. Answer: 3
Rationale: The desired outcome during the maintenance stage of treatment is improved patient functioning.
Cognitive Level: Application
Nursing Process: Outcome Identification
NCLEX: Psychosocial Integrity
Text Page: 71

30. Answer: 2
Rationale: Axis II of the DSM-IV will confirm or deny the presence of a diagnosed personality disorder.
Cognitive Level: Application
Nursing Process: Assessment
NCLEX: Psychosocial Integrity
Text Page: 70

31. Answer: 4
Rationale: Axis V reports the clinician's judgment of the individual's overall level of functioning.
Cognitive Level: Application
Nursing Process: Assessment
NCLEX: Psychosocial Integrity
Text Page: 70

32. Answer: 2
Rationale: Axis III allows the clinician to identify any physical disorder that is potentially relevant to the understanding or treatment of the individual.
Cognitive Level: Application
Nursing Process: Assessment
NCLEX: Psychosocial Integrity
Text Page: 70

CHAPTER 5

1. Answer: 2
Rationale: Although the 1999 report concluded that mental health treatment efficacy is well-documented and that many treatments are available for most mental health disorders, many questions for psychiatric nursing can be extrapolated, including the question about whether psychiatric nursing practice produces satisfied consumers.
Cognitive Level: Analysis
Nursing Process: Planning
NCLEX: Psychosocial Integrity
Text Page: 83

2. Answer: 3
Rationale: Little research has been done to examine psychiatric nursing practice patterns, evaluate the nature of the data supporting them, and demonstrate sound clinical decision making in a way that can be empirically supported. Psychiatric nursing currently relies on opinion-based processes and unproved theories.
Cognitive Level: Analysis
Nursing Process: NA
NCLEX: Safe, Effective Care Environment: Management of Care
Text Page: 76

3. Answer: 3
Rationale: Providing evidence-based practice requires searching the research literature, critically synthesizing

research findings, and applying relevant evidence to practice. The other activities are myths about what makes effective practitioners.
Cognitive Level: Analysis
Nursing Process: NA
NCLEX: Safe, Effective Care Environment: Management of Care
Text Page: 76

4. Answer: 3
Rationale: Evidence-based practice includes research findings, performance data, and consensus recommendations of recognized experts. Apart from situations requiring a regulatory basis, the best basis to substantiate clinical practice is the evidence of well-established research findings. Such evidence reflects verifiable, replicable facts and relationships that have been exposed to stringent scientific criteria.
Cognitive Level: Analysis
Nursing Process: NA
NCLEX: Safe, Effective Care Environment: Management of Care
Text Page: 76

5. Answer: 4
Rationale: In the hierarchy of research evidence, a meta-analysis of all relevant randomized, controlled trials will give the nurse the highest quality of information.
Cognitive Level: Analysis
Nursing Process: Planning
NCLEX: Safe, Effective Care Environment: Management of Care
Text Page: 77-78

6. Answer: 2
Rationale: Safety and effective care are two important characteristics in the development of practice guidelines. Answer 1 is a consideration but not a major characteristic. Answers 3 and 4 are not true.
Cognitive Level: Assessment
Nursing Process: NA
NCLEX: Safe, Effective Care Environment: Management of Care
Text Page: 78

7. Answer: 4
Rationale: Clinical pathways identify the key clinical processes and corresponding timelines to which a patient must adhere to achieve standard outcomes within a specified period of time. They require quality monitoring and interdisciplinary cooperation and they are less specific than clinical algorithms.
Cognitive Level: Comprehension
Nursing Process: NA
NCLEX: Safe, Effective Care Environment: Management of Care
Text Page: 80

8. Answer: 3
Rationale: Many algorithms are represented by flow charts that identify what clinical process might follow from a patient's clinical status and response to prior treatments and provide statements of what to do if treatment is not effective. Many nurses are familiar with flow charts because they are commonly used in nursing documentation.
Cognitive Level: Analysis
Nursing Process: NA
NCLEX: Safe, Effective Care Environment: Management of Care
Text Page: 80

9. Answer: 4
Rationale: Currently there is no research evidence to support the important contributions psychiatric nurses make to positive patient outcomes. Without such evidence, psychiatric nursing services can be deemed to be cost-ineffective and therefore unnecessary.
Cognitive Level: Analysis
Nursing Process: NA
NCLEX: Safe, Effective Care Environment: Management of Care
Text Page: 81

10. Answer: 3
Rationale: Each of the options listed above is important to evidence-based nursing practice, but only the use of rating scales directly relates to outcome measurement.
Cognitive Level: Analysis
Nursing Process: NA
NCLEX: Safe, Effective Care Environment: Management of Care
Text Page: 81-82

11. Answer: 2
Rationale: According to Stuart, accountability for patient care outcomes is a basic responsibility of professional nurses. Central to this accountability is the ability to examine nursing practice patterns, evaluate the nature of the data supporting them, and demonstrate sound clinical decision making in a way that can be empirically supported. Therefore the only correct answer is Answer 2. The client is willingly participating in a psychoeducational group to learn more about his disease process. This outcome can be measured and documented for inclusion as part of the performance data. Answer 1 indicates that the patient will make an attempt to abstain from illicit drugs and alcohol but is not an evidence-based outcome. In Answers 3 and 4, the client will go through the motions of securing employment and a place to live without rational, sound evidence of purpose or research indicating that this is part of a sound evidence-based plan.
Cognitive Level: Analysis

Nursing Process: Planning
NCLEX: Psychosocial Integrity
Text Page: 76

12. Answer: 4
Rationale: Textbooks become outdated, as do nursing journal articles. The DSM-IV is also like a textbook and is updated only periodically. The only correct answer is to find current relevant information by using electronic databases, which is the most current method for research indicated.
Cognitive Level: Application
Nursing Process: Planning
NCLEX: Psychosocial Integrity
Text Page: 77

13. Answer: 2
Rationale: Defining the clinical problem for this patient is the first step in evidence-based care. All other options can be useful to his future care, but with evidence-based care, it is most important to have a clear question to identify the clinical problems, identify the existing nursing interventions, and specify the expected outcome.
Cognitive Level: Analysis
Nursing Process: Planning
NCLEX: Psychosocial Integrity
Text Page: 77

14. Answer: 2
Rationale: In the evaluation phase of evidence-based care, the nurse asks whether the application of evidence leads to an improvement in care. This is done by examining clearly specified outcomes from the evidence-based plan. This also involves the use of outcome measurement and reevaluation. The best response here is Answer 2. Answer 1 looks at only medical evidence, while Answers 3 and 4 ask for subjective information from family and the patient and are anecdotal.
Cognitive Level: Application
Nursing Process: Evaluation
NCLEX: Psychosocial Integrity
Text Page: 78

15. Answer: 4
Rationale: The practice guidelines may vary widely but all are designed to provide detailed specification of methods and procedures to ensure effective treatment for each disorder.
Cognitive Level: Application
Nursing Process: Implementation
NCLEX: Safe, Effective Care Environment: Management of Care
Text Page: 78

16. Answer: 2
Rationale: The clinical pathway is used most often in inpatient settings and serves as a shortened version of the multidisciplinary plan of care of the patient.
Cognitive Level: Comprehension
Nursing Process: NA
NCLEX: Safe, Effective Care Environment: Management of Care
Text Page: 80

17. Answer: 2
Rationale: Clinical algorithms take practice guidelines to a greater level of specificity by providing step-by-step recommendations on issues such as treatment options, treatment sequencing, preferred dosage, and progress assessment.
Cognitive Level: Application
Nursing Process: Planning
NCLEX: Safe, Effective Care Environment: Management of Care
Text Page: 80

18. Answer: 2
Rationale: The categories of outcome indicators include clinical, functional, satisfaction, and financial. All other answers are incorrect.
Cognitive Level: Analysis
Nursing Process: NA
NCLEX: Health Promotion and Maintenance
Text Page: 81

19. Answer: 4
Rationale: A type of outcome measure is related not to the patient, but to the performance of the behavioral health care organization itself. One must consider the three dimensions when discussing these report cards: content, point of view, and intended audience. Answers 1, 2, and 3 are incorrect.
Cognitive Level: Comprehension
Nursing Process: NA
NCLEX: Safe, Effective Care Environment: Management of Care
Text Page: 82

20. Answer: 2
Rationale: In the evidence-based model for psychiatric nurses, the practitioners are being asked to describe what they do and how thy add value to the health care organization. Their responses should be couched with sensitivity for the issues of effectiveness, cost, and quality.
Cognitive Level: Analysis
Nursing Process Evaluation
NCLEX: Safe, Effective Care Environment: Management of Care
Text Page: 82

21. Answer: 3
Rationale: Practice guidelines can be developed in a variety of ways. The best mental health practice guidelines are based on a scientific review of the available clinical research literature to determine which treatments are safe and effective for particular psychiatric disorders. Answers 1, 2, and 4 are not correct.
Cognitive Level: Analysis
Nursing Process: Implementation
NCLEX: Safe, Effective Care Environment: Management of Care
Text Page: 78

22. Answer: 2
Rationale: Algorithms and protocols are the most specific set of treatment decisions based on the strongest evidence base. Answer 1 identifies all of the possible prevention and treatment options, while Answers 3 and 4 are broader than algorithms and protocols.
Cognitive Level: Comprehension
Nursing Process: NA
NCLEX: Health Promotion and Maintenance
Text Page: 79

23. Answer: 2
Rationale: The development of clinical pathways involves reviewing for efficiency and necessity the many activities that occur from the time the patient enters the health care facility through discharge and aftercare. These activities include preadmission work-ups, tests, consultations, treatments, activities, diet, and health teaching.
Cognitive Level: Application
Nursing Process: Assessment
NCLEX: Safe, Effective Care Environment: Management of Care
Text Page: 80

24. Answer: 2
Rationale: Psychiatric nurses should routinely use rating scales to assess their patients to determine their state at baseline (before beginning treatment), their progress during treatment, and the clinical progress they have made at the end of treatment. In this way nurses will be able to document the effectiveness of the care they provide.
Cognitive Level: Application
Nursing Process: Implementation
NCLEX: Safe, Effective Care Environment: Management of Care
Text Page: 81

25. Answer: 2
Rationale: A theory that arises out of practice is validated by research, which rebounds to direct practice and inform clinical care. The only correct answer is research. Answers 1, 3, and 4 are important to practice, but theory is validated by research.
Cognitive Level: Comprehension
Nursing Process: NA
NCLEX: Health Promotion and Maintenance
Text Page: 83

CHAPTER 6

1. Answer: 1
Rationale: Neurotransmitters are chemicals manufactured in the brain that are responsible for exciting or inhibiting brain cells in the production of an action.
Cognitive Level: Application
Nursing Process: Implementation
NCLEX: Psychosocial Integrity
Text Page: 88

2. Answer: 4
Rationale: Neurotransmitters are chemicals that assist communication between neurons and give rise to human activity, body functions, consciousness, intelligence, creativity, memory, dreams, and emotion.
Cognitive Level: Knowledge
Nursing Process: Implementation
NCLEX: Psychosocial Integrity
Text Page: 88, 93

3. Answer: 1
Rationale: The cerebellum is responsible for fine motor coordination, posture, balance, and integration of emotional processes.
Cognitive Level: Knowledge
Nursing Process: Implementation
NCLEX: Physiological Integrity: Physiological Adaptation
Text Page: 90

4. Answer: 4
Rationale: Serotonin, also called 5-HT, is derived from tryptophan, a dietary amino acid. It is located only in the brain, particularly in the raphe nuclei of the brainstem. It plays a role in regulation of mood.
Cognitive Level: Knowledge
Nursing Process: NA
NCLEX: Physiological Integrity: Physiological Adaptation
Text Page: 95

5. Answer: 2
Rationale: The hypothalamus is responsible for regulation of metabolism, temperature, and emotions.
Cognitive Level: Knowledge
Nursing Process: NA

NCLEX: Physiological Integrity: Physiological Adaptation
Text Page: 90

6. Answer: 1
Rationale: Dopamine is derived from tyrosine, a dietary amino acid. It is located mostly in the brainstem and is involved in control of complex movements, motivation, and cognition. It is involved in movement disorders such as Parkinson's disease and in many of the deficits seen in schizophrenia and other forms of psychosis.
Cognitive Level: Knowledge
Nursing Process: NA
NCLEX: Physiological Integrity: Physiological Adaptation
Text Page: 95

7. Answer: 2
Rationale: CT can image brain structures through a series of radiographs that are computer-constructed into "slices" of the brain that can be stacked by the computer, giving the image a three-dimensional appearance.
Cognitive Level: Comprehension
Nursing Process: Implementation
NCLEX: Physiological Integrity: Reduction of Risk Potential
Text Page: 98

8. Answer: 1
Rationale: When results of studies such as MRI are coupled with neuropsychological test results, the deficits in a person's performance, such as language or cognitive or sensory information processing, can be linked to the activity in the region of the brain responsible for those functions.
Cognitive Level: Knowledge
Nursing Process: Assessment
NCLEX: Physiological Integrity: Physiological Adaptation
Text Page: 97-98

9. Answer: 2
Rationale: Several hundred genetic tests are in clinical use for illnesses such as muscular dystrophies, cystic fibrosis, and sickle cell anemia.
Cognitive Level: Analysis
Nursing Process: Implementation
NCLEX: Physiological Integrity: Physiological Adaptation
Text Page: 101-102

10. Answer: 3
Rationale: Genetic counselors are trained to diagnose and explain disorders from a genetic perspective. They can review available options for testing and treatment and provide emotional support to individuals or families who have genetic disorders, are at risk for them, or need information about risks to their offspring.
Cognitive Level: Application
Nursing Process: Implementation
NCLEX: Psychosocial Integrity
Text Page: 102

11. Answer: 2
Rationale: Pharmacogenetics is a discipline that blends pharmacology with genomic capabilities and will eventually allow researchers to match DNA variants with individual responses to medical treatments. It will allow for custom drugs based on individual genetic profiles.
Cognitive Level: Knowledge
Nursing Process: NA
NCLEX: Physiological Integrity: Pharmacological and Parenteral Therapies
Text Page: 102

12. Answer: 1
Rationale: Before giving information or otherwise responding prematurely, it would be wise to discern the extent of the patient's knowledge and understanding of the condition as explained by the physician.
Cognitive Level: Application
Nursing Process: Assessment
NCLEX: Psychosocial Integrity
Text Page: 105

13. Answer: 4
Rationale: The limbic system is concerned with subjective emotional experiences and with changes in bodily functions associated with emotional states.
Cognitive Level: Analysis
Nursing Process: Assessment
NCLEX: Psychosocial Integrity
Text Page: 92, 96

14. Answer: 2
Rationale: PET scanning allows for the imaging of brain activity and function with the use of an injected radioactive substance that travels to the brain and shows up as a bright spot on the scan.
Cognitive Level: Application
Nursing Process: Implementation
NCLEX: Physiological Integrity: Reduction of Risk Potential
Text Page: 98

15. Answer: 3
Rationale: PET scanning allows for the imaging of brain activity and function with the use of an injected radioactive substance that travels to the brain and shows up as a bright spot on the scan. There is no electrical "jolt" involved. Answers 1 and 2 address an

assumption made by the nurse that the patient is referring to ECT, and answer4 is not factual.
Cognitive Level: Application
Nursing Process: Implementation
NCLEX: Physiological Integrity: Reduction of Risk Potential
Text Page: 98

16. Answer: 4
Rationale: MRIs visualize brain structure. They are not painful but require that the patient lie still.
Cognitive Level: Application
Nursing Process: Implementation
NCLEX: Physiological Integrity: Reduction of Risk Potential
Text Page: 98

17. Answer: 3
Rationale: Studies show that with depression, REM sleep is excessive, the deeper stages of sleep are decreased, and dreams may be unusually intense, leading to patient reports of fatigue, poor concentration, and irritability associated with sleep deprivation.
Cognitive Level: Synthesis
Nursing Process: Assessment
NCLEX: Psychosocial Integrity
Text Page: 99-100

18. Answer: 1
Rationale: It is known that natural killer cells, which are believed to play a role in tumor surveillance and the control of viral infections, seem to decrease with increasing levels of stress.
Cognitive Level: Application
Nursing Process: Implementation
NCLEX: Psychosocial Integrity
Text Page: 100-101

19. Answer: 3
Rationale: Only after a patient has been carefully screened can it be determined that the problems are amenable to psychiatric intervention.
Cognitive Level: Application
Nursing Process: Implementation
NCLEX: Psychosocial Integrity
Text Page: 104

20. Answer: 2
Rationale: Current evidence suggests that there is a significant genetic role in the cause of recurrent depression and bipolar disorder. A genetic counselor is well prepared to discuss the concerns of these individuals.
Cognitive Level: Application
Nursing Process: Implementation
NCLEX: Psychosocial Integrity
Text Page: 102

21. Answer: 1
Rationale: The frontal lobe is responsible primarily for intellectual functioning, including learning, abstracting, reasoning, and inhibition of impulses.
Cognitive Level: Analysis
Nursing Process: Assessment
NCLEX: Psychosocial Integrity
Text Page: 90

22. Answer: 4
Rationale: Gene therapy is still an experimental field. It holds potential for treating or even curing genetic and acquired diseases such as cancer or AIDS, but is not likely to be clinically applicable in psychiatry in the near future.
Cognitive Level: Application
Nursing Process: Implementation
NCLEX: Psychosocial Integrity
Text Page: 102

23. Answer: 1
Rationale: Changes in schedule that affect circadian rhythms, such as work shifts that alter usual sleep patterns, can result in fatigue that is not related to mental health status. Other factors that alter sleep include changes in light and darkness, and temperature changes. Answer 2 should not affect sleep, while Answers 3 and 4 should enhance sleep by reducing risk of nocturia (Answer 3) or indigestion (Answer 4).
Cognitive Level: Application
Nursing Process: Assessment
NCLEX: Physiological Integrity: Basic Care and Comfort
Text Page: 99-100

CHAPTER 7

1. Answer: 2
Rationale: The primary purpose would be to assess emotional factors that may have an effect on the patient's current condition. The patient has given clues to psychological distress. Holistic care requires the assessment of biological, psychological, and sociocultural health status.
Cognitive Level: Application
Nursing Process: Assessment
NCLEX: Psychosocial Integrity
Text Page: 108

2. Answer: 2
Rationale: Patients with whom the nurse has established rapport will feel understood by the examiner and will be more willing to cooperate with the examiner's questions.
Cognitive Level: Analysis
Nursing Process: Assessment

NCLEX: Psychosocial Integrity
Text Page: 109

3. Answer: 3
Rationale: Participant observation is a clinical approach that allows the nurse to critically observe a patient while structuring the examination in a way that allows for the broad exploration of many areas to screen for potential problems and for the in-depth exploration of obvious symptoms or maladaptive coping responses.
Cognitive Level: Application
Nursing Process: Implementation
NCLEX: Safe, Effective Care Environment: Management of Care
Text Page: 109

4. Answer: 3
Rationale: Many observations can be made during other aspects of the nursing assessment and specific questions can be blended into the general flow of the interview.
Cognitive Level: Application
Nursing Process: Implementation
NCLEX: Safe, Effective Care Environment: Management of Care
Text Page: 108

5. Answer: 1
Rationale: Dress, eye contact, personal hygiene, speech and use of language, personal space, and body language are a few aspects of the mental status examination that vary with culture and social status.
Cognitive Level: Application
Nursing Process: Assessment
NCLEX: Psychosocial Integrity
Text Page: 110

6. Answer: 2
Rationale: Confabulation means covering one's inability to remember by making up a story of something that might have happened.
Cognitive Level: Application
Nursing Process: Assessment
NCLEX: Psychosocial Integrity
Text Page: 113

7. Answer: 3
Rationale: Suicidal intent should be openly and directly investigated.
Cognitive Level: Application
Nursing Process: Implementation
NCLEX: Psychosocial Integrity
Text Page: 111

8. Answer: 1
Rationale: The mental status examination is designed to give a picture of the patient's current level of functioning.
Cognitive Level: Application
Nursing Process: NA
NCLEX: Psychosocial Integrity
Text Page: 108

9. Answer: 4
Rationale: Mood is the patient's self-report of his or her prevailing emotional/affective state. The nurse's empathic responses usually give clues to the patient's affect/mood.
Cognitive Level: Application
Nursing Process: Assessment
NCLEX: Psychosocial Integrity
Text Page: 111

10. Answer: 4
Rationale: Attentive listening, observation, and focused questions allow for the use of empathic statements and make a patient feel understood, and feeling understood fosters rapport.
Cognitive Level: Analysis
Nursing Process: Implementation
NCLEX: Safe, Effective Care Environment: Management of Care
Text Page: 109

11. Answer: 3
Rationale: Manic patients often dress in bright colors and mix a variety of patterns. Their attire may give them an eccentric or bizarre look.
Cognitive Level: Application
Nursing Process: Assessment
NCLEX: Psychosocial Integrity
Text Page: 110

12. Answer: 3
Rationale: Manic patients show excessive body movement, whereas many depressed patients show little body activity.
Cognitive Level: Analysis
Nursing Process: Assessment
NCLEX: Psychosocial Integrity
Text Page: 110

13. Answer: 3
Rationale: Reporting significant life events with little emotional response suggests a blunted or flattened affect.
Cognitive Level: Application
Nursing Process: Assessment
NCLEX: Psychosocial Integrity
Text Page: 111

14. Answer: 1
Rationale: Lability is identified when the patient's affect shifts rapidly, such as from happy to sad or angry to elated.
Cognitive Level: Application
Nursing Process: Assessment
NCLEX: Psychosocial Integrity
Text Page: 111

15. Answer: 2
Rationale: Because hallucinations are false sensory perceptions, the question posed in Answer 2 is the most pertinent.
Cognitive Level: Application
Nursing Process: Assessment
NCLEX: Psychosocial Integrity
Text Page: 111-112

16. Answer: 3
Rationale: Grandiose delusions are beliefs that one possesses greatness or special powers.
Cognitive Level: Application
Nursing Process: Assessment
NCLEX: Psychosocial Integrity
Text Page: 112

17. Answer: 4
Rationale: The question in Answer 4 tests judgment, but the other questions assess orientation to person, time, and place.
Cognitive Level: Analysis
Nursing Process: Assessment
NCLEX: Psychosocial Integrity
Text Page: 113

18. Answer: 3
Rationale: Interpersonal and intrapersonal intelligence form one's personal intelligence or "emotional quotient."
Cognitive Level: Application
Nursing Process: Assessment
NCLEX: Psychosocial Integrity
Text Page: 115

19. Answer: 2
Rationale: Recent memory is tested when the patient is asked to recall several words 15 minutes after hearing them for the first time.
Cognitive Level: Application
Nursing Process: Assessment
NCLEX: Psychosocial Integrity
Text Page: 113

20. Answer: 3
Rationale: These symptoms indicate the presence of a thought disorder seen more often in patients with schizophrenia than in those with panic or depression. Defensive coping is not a DSM-IV diagnosis.
Cognitive Level: Application
Nursing Process: Assessment
NCLEX: Psychosocial Integrity
Text Page: 113

21. Answer: 4
Rationale: Judgment involves making decisions that are constructive and adaptive. Answer 4 is the only question listed that tests this ability.
Cognitive Level: Application
Nursing Process: Assessment
NCLEX: Psychosocial Integrity
Text Page: 115-116

22. Answer: 2
Rationale: The Mini-Mental State Examination is a simplified scored form of the cognitive mental status examination. It consists of 11 questions and requires only 10 minutes to administer.
Cognitive Level: Application
Nursing Process: Assessment
NCLEX: Psychosocial Integrity
Text Page: 116

23. Answer: 3
Rationale: Interpreting proverbs gives clues to the patient's ability to move from concrete to abstract thinking by stating meaning in terms symbolic of human behavior or events.
Cognitive Level: Application
Nursing Process: Assessment
NCLEX: Psychosocial Integrity
Text Page: 115

24. Answer: 4
Rationale: Only Answer 4 contains observations about appearance.
Cognitive Level: Application
Nursing Process: Assessment
NCLEX: Psychosocial Integrity
Text Page: 109

25. Answer: 2
Rationale: Pressured speech is rapid, forcefully delivered speech that is often loud in volume and excessive in amount.
Cognitive Level: Application
Nursing Process: Assessment
NCLEX: Psychosocial Integrity
Text Page: 110

26. Answer: 1
Rationale: Thought insertion is the delusion that thoughts are placed into the mind by people or influences outside of the self.
Cognitive Level: Application
Nursing Process: Assessment
NCLEX: Psychosocial Integrity
Text Page: 112

27. Answer: 2
Rationale: Subtle emotions are transmitted during the mental status evaluation, but they may register only as gut feelings. Examples are subtle hostility that may make the nurse feel threatened or angry and sadness or hopelessness that may make the nurse feel sad.

Cognitive Level: Application
Nursing Process: Assessment
NCLEX: Psychosocial Integrity
Text Page: 110-111

28. Answer: 4
Rationale: Nursing observations must be documented in the medical record whether or not a behavioral rating scale is used.
Cognitive Level: Application
Nursing Process: Assessment
NCLEX: Psychosocial Integrity
Text Page: 118

CHAPTER 8

1. Answer: 4
Rationale: Awareness and knowledge must be accompanied by intervention skills if treatment is to be successful.
Cognitive Level: Analysis
Nursing Process: Implementation
NCLEX: Psychosocial Integrity
Text Page: 121

2. Answer: 3
Rationale: Six patient characteristics, influenced by social norms, cultural values, and spiritual beliefs, are known to act as risk factors, protective factors, or both. These are patient age, ethnicity, gender, education, income, and beliefs.
Cognitive Level: Application
Nursing Process: Assessment
NCLEX: Psychosocial Integrity
Text Page: 122

3. Answer: 4
Rationale: Simple actions, gestures, and attitudinal displays that are part of the nurse's culture may be offensive to a patient of a different culture. Understanding this indicates that the nurse will make an effort to display cultural sensitivity.
Cognitive Level: Application
Nursing Process: Planning
NCLEX: Psychosocial Integrity
Text Page: 121

4. Answer: 4
Rationale: By 2050, Hispanics will make up about 25% of the U.S. population, African Americans will make up about 14%, Asians and Pacific Islanders about 8%, and whites about 53%.
Cognitive Level: Analysis
Nursing Process: Planning
NCLEX: Psychosocial Integrity
Text Page: 123

5. Answer: 1
Rationale: Females are at greater risk for being diagnosed and treated for depression than males. The rate of depression among aging adults is lower than the rate in younger age groups.
Cognitive Level: Analysis
Nursing Process: Assessment
NCLEX: Psychosocial Integrity
Text Page: 122-123

6. Answer: 1
Rationale: Among the elderly, the prevalence of depression is reduced among those with high socioeconomic status and more education. Church attendance is also a positive and adaptive coping resource for many individuals. Recreational activities are not part of sociocultural assessment.
Cognitive Level: Analysis
Nursing Process: Planning
NCLEX: Psychosocial Integrity
Text Page: 123

7. Answer: 1
Rationale: Research suggests that members of minority groups delay seeking help until their problems are intense, chronic, and at a stage that is difficult to treat, and until community and family support systems have been exhausted. Delays in accessing care and early termination from care create a cyclical reliance on more costly health care services.
Cognitive Level: Application
Nursing Process: Assessment
NCLEX: Psychosocial Integrity
Text Page: 124

8. Answer: 3
Rationale: A person's belief system, worldview, religion, or spirituality can have a positive or negative effect on mental health. Belief systems play a vital role in determining whether a particular explanation and associated treatment plan will have meaning for the patient and others in the patient's social network. The statements in Answers 1 and 4 do not address the issue of the question asked by the patient, and the statement in Answer 2 is too narrow in scope.
Cognitive Level: Application
Nursing Process: Implementation
NCLEX: Psychosocial Integrity
Text Page: 126

9. Answer: 2
Rationale: Spirituality-based intervention programs, such as 12-step programs, which encourage the individual to surrender control to an external supreme being, are commonly used treatments for addictive disorders, including addiction to alcohol.
Cognitive Level: Application

Nursing Process: Implementation
NCLEX: Psychosocial Integrity
Text Page: 126

10. Answer: 2
Rationale: Although there appears to be distinctive male and female patterns of risk, when all psychiatric disorders are included, the prevalence of mental illness among males and females is roughly equal.
Cognitive Level: Application
Nursing Process: NA
NCLEX: Psychosocial Integrity
Text Page: 124

11. Answer: 3
Rationale: Stereotypes are depersonalized conceptions of individuals within a group.
Cognitive Level: Comprehension
Nursing Process: Assessment
NCLEX: Psychosocial Integrity
Text Page: 127

12. Answer: 3
Rationale: Incorporating the value of culture into all levels of care is desirable. Eliminating all staff bias is unlikely, hiring only minority health care providers is not desirable, and keeping access to care open for minority groups would be more relevant.
Cognitive Level: Application
Nursing Process: Implementation
NCLEX: Psychosocial Integrity
Text Page: 129-130

13. Answer: 3
Rationale: Answer 3 is the only statement about racial/ethnic psychobiological differences listed that is accurate.
Cognitive Level: Application
Nursing Process: Assessment
NCLEX: Psychosocial Integrity
Text Page: 130-131

14. Answer: 1
Rationale: In terms of treatment planning, the psychiatric nurse needs to be sensitive to sociocultural issues but also must transcend them. A central responsibility of the nurse is to understand what the illness means to the patient and the way in which the patient's beliefs can help to mediate the stressful events or make them easier to bear by redefining them as opportunities for personal growth.
Cognitive Level: Analysis
Nursing Process: Planning
NCLEX: Psychosocial Integrity
Text Page: 127

15. Answer: 3
Rationale: Risk factors interact constantly, so risk factors may assume greater or lesser significance for an individual over time. Cultural groups vary in terms of risk for specific mental health disorders, and sociocultural risk factors affect the nurse working with the patient during all phases of the nursing process.
Cognitive Level: Analysis
Nursing Process: Planning
NCLEX: Psychosocial Integrity
Text Page: 122

16. Answer: 2
Rationale: It has been found that as age increases, the prevalence of depression decreases. Older people have a greater capacity to adapt and tend to recover from depression more quickly than younger individuals; they are also less likely to have a recurrence.
Cognitive Level: Application
Nursing Process: Outcome Identification
NCLEX: Psychosocial Integrity
Text Page: 123

17. Answer: 3
Rationale: Disadvantagement factors, such as lack of basic resources and low education level, create profound problems in prevention, diagnosis, and treatment of psychiatric disorders.
Cognitive Level: Application
Nursing Process: Assessment
NCLEX: Psychosocial Integrity
Text Page: 127

18. Answer: 4
Rationale: The difference is gender-based. The lesser amount of stomach acid secreted by women means that benzodiazepines are better absorbed.
Cognitive Level: Application
Nursing Process: Assessment
NCLEX: Psychosocial Integrity
Text Page: 130-131

19. Answer: 4
Rationale: Males tend to have earlier onset of schizophrenia than females. The mean age of onset for males is 31; for females, 41. Age of onset is a critical factor in the prognosis for schizophrenia because early onset is associated with a longer course of illness and poorer prognosis. It is also known that women have a better response to both pharmacologic and psychosocial treatments.
Cognitive Level: Analysis
Nursing Process: Outcome Identification
NCLEX: Psychosocial Integrity
Text Page: 123

20. Answer: 3
Rationale: Lack of insurance, low access to primary physicians for referral, and language barriers that make it difficult to negotiate an unfamiliar system are factors

that promote a delay in seeking help. Minorities do not necessarily have better support systems.
Cognitive Level: Analysis
Nursing Process: Planning
NCLEX: Psychosocial Integrity
Text Page: 123

CHAPTER 9

1. Answer: 3
Rationale: Depression ranks as the second most common cause of disability measured in disability-adjusted life years in the United States, and four other psychiatric disorders are in the top 10 worldwide including alcohol use, bipolar disorder, schizophrenia, and obsessive-compulsive disorder.
Cognitive Level: Comprehension
Nursing Process: NA
NCLEX: Psychosocial Integrity
Text Page: 134

2. Answer: 1
Rationale: A large international study found that depression was the number one psychiatric cause of disability in the world. Four other psychiatric disorders also were among the top 10 including alcohol abuse, bipolar disorder, schizophrenia, and obsessive-compulsive disorder.
Cognitive Level: Analysis
Nursing Process: NA
NCLEX: Psychosocial Integrity
Text Page: 134

3. Answer: 1
Rationale: The interface between mental health care and the environment has become increasingly complex in recent years. It once consisted only of mental health providers and patients, but the interface now includes patients, providers, families, reimbursers and insurers; lawmakers and regulators, and the judiciary, and each of these components has its own agenda.
Cognitive Level: Analysis
Nursing Process: NA
NCLEX: Psychosocial Integrity
Text Page: 136

4. Answer: 4
Rationale: Behavioral health covers both mental illness and substance abuse disorders.
Cognitive Level: Analysis
Nursing Process: NA
NCLEX: Psychosocial Integrity
Text Page: 137

5. Answer: 1
Rationale: Recommendations under goal 1 are to (1) advance and implement a national campaign to reduce the stigma of seeking care and a national strategy for suicide prevention, and (2) address mental health with the same urgency as physical health. The other strategies listed help to achieve goals 2, 3, and 6, respectively, of the report of the New Freedom Commission on Mental Health.
Cognitive Level: Comprehension
Nursing Process: Implementation
NCLEX: Psychosocial Integrity
Text Page: 135

6. Answer: 4
Rationale: Gatekeeping is a process that limits direct access to specialists, hospitals, and expensive procedures. Patients select a primary care provider who manages everyday care and is a gatekeeper for referral to other health care providers.
Cognitive Level: Comprehension
Nursing Process: Implementation
NCLEX: Psychosocial Integrity
Text Page: 138

7. Answer: 4
Rationale: Preadmission certification ensures the proper treatment setting; utilization review evaluates the appropriateness and necessity of services; and case management focuses on desirable outcomes, appropriate lengths of stay, and efficient use of resources. Each of these helps control costs.
Cognitive Level: Application
Nursing Process: Implementation
NCLEX: Psychosocial Integrity
Text Page: 138-139

8. Answer: 3
Rationale: Capitation calls for the consumer to pay a fixed fee or a per-member-per-month premium. In return, the managed care company agrees to provide all medically necessary health care for all covered people.
Cognitive Level: Application
Nursing Process: Implementation
NCLEX: Psychosocial Integrity
Text Page: 138

9. Answer: 4
Rationale: Access is the degree to which services and information about care are easily obtained. The ideal comprehensive system would provide multiple points of entry for treatment, including direct access through self-referral.
Cognitive Level: Application
Nursing Process: Implementation
NCLEX: Psychosocial Integrity
Text Page: 139

10. Answer: 1
Rationale: Access is the degree to which services and information about care are easily obtained. When the

consumer-to-doctor ratio is high, access is often compromised.
Cognitive Level: Application
Nursing Process: NA
NCLEX: Psychosocial Integrity
Text Page: 139

11. Answer: 3
Rationale: Cost-effectiveness studies document the value of EAPs, particularly through their contributions to prevention in areas such as workplace education, skill development, and policy and environmental changes.
Cognitive Level: Application
Nursing Process: NA
NCLEX: Psychosocial Integrity
Text Page: 139-140

12. Answer: 3
Rationale: Substantial activity has taken place in state and federal legislatures to increase the mental health benefits offered by health insurance, but individuals with mental illness continue to fare significantly worse than the general population.
Cognitive Level: Analysis
Nursing Process: NA
NCLEX: Psychosocial Integrity
Text Page: 140

13. Answer: 4
Rationale: Although gains have been made in medical treatment for behavioral illness, little attention has been given to preventive, rehabilitative, and chronic care services. This is a topic worthy of nursing advocacy.
Cognitive Level: Application
Nursing Process: NA
NCLEX: Psychosocial Integrity
Text Page: 140

14. Answer: 3
Rationale: Clinical appropriateness is the degree to which the type, amount, and level of clinical services are delivered to promote the best clinical outcomes.
Cognitive Level: Application
Nursing Process: Assessment
NCLEX: Psychosocial Integrity
Text Page: 140

15. Answer: 3
Rationale: The goal of crisis treatment is stabilization, with the expected outcome being no harm to self or others.
Cognitive Level: Application
Nursing Process: Outcome Identification
NCLEX: Psychosocial Integrity
Text Page: 141

16. Answer: 2
Rationale: The goal of remission can probably be attained if the patient resumes medication therapy. The outcome of symptom relief will be attained during a short stay.
Cognitive Level: Analysis
Nursing Process: Outcome Identification
NCLEX: Psychosocial Integrity
Text Page: 141

17. Answer: 3
Rationale: A POS plan allows consumers to choose between delivery systems at the time they seek care. The other types of plans listed limit the clinicians and/or the agencies that can be utilized for health care services.
Cognitive Level: Comprehension
Nursing Process: NA
NCLEX: Psychosocial Integrity
Text Page: 138

18. Answer: 1
Rationale: Nurses who advocate for consumer empowerment for patients with mental health disorders will work to assist patients to do the following: achieve a sense of self responsibility, collaborate with health professionals to determine their treatment plans, be respected for the legitimacy of their points of view, and use resources from the entire community rather than just the formal mental health system.
Cognitive Level: Analysis
Nursing Process: Implementation
NCLEX: Psychosocial Integrity
Text Page: 141-142

19. Answer: 2
Rationale: The case manager has the greatest responsibility for allocating resources for a particular patient through the development of a comprehensive treatment plan; he or she then coordinates with all involved staff and agencies.
Cognitive Level: Analysis
Nursing Process: NA
NCLEX: Psychosocial Integrity
Text Page: 143

20. Answer: 4
Rationale: With cost-consciousness, greater emphasis is being placed on the continuum of care. The number of inpatient hospitalization days will continue to decrease, and nurses will be needed to staff alternate treatment sites.
Cognitive Level: Comprehension
Nursing Process: NA
NCLEX: Psychosocial Integrity
Text Page: 143

21. Answer: 2
Rationale: One recommendation from the report is to use health technology and telehealth to improve access and coordination of mental health care, especially for Americans in remote areas or in underserved populations.
Cognitive Level: Application
Nursing Process: Implementation
NCLEX: Psychosocial Integrity
Text Page: 135

22. Answer: 2
Rationale: The expected outcome for a patient during the acute stage of treatment is symptom relief. The expected outcome during crisis is that the patient does no harm to self or others. The expected outcome during maintenance is improved functioning. The expected outcome during health promotion is to attain an optimal quality of life.
Cognitive Level: Application
Nursing Process: Planning
NCLEX: Psychosocial Integrity
Text Page: 141

23. Answer: 1
Rationale: The expected goal for a patient in crisis is stabilization. The goal during the acute stage of treatment is remission. The goal during the maintenance stage of treatment is recovery. The goal during the health promotion phase is optimal level of wellness.
Cognitive Level: Application
Nursing Process: Planning
NCLEX: Psychosocial Integrity
Text Page: 141

24. Answer: 3
Rationale: A rehabilitation-oriented residential treatment program is a level of care provided during the maintenance stage of treatment in an integrated behavioral continuum of care. The expected outcome of care in this stage is improved functioning and the overall goal is recovery.
Cognitive Level: Application
Nursing Process: Outcome Identification
NCLEX: Psychosocial Integrity
Text Page: 141

CHAPTER 10

1. Answer: 2
Rationale: Although the staff acted ethically and observed the patient's right to give informed consent, the decision may have been coerced based on family pressure. Informed consent requires that the choice be freely made.
Cognitive Level: Application
Nursing Process: Assessment
NCLEX: Psychosocial Integrity
Text Page: 159

2. Answer: 4
Rationale: When requirements for making an informed decision are not met, the physician will need to confer with the patient.
Cognitive Level: Application
Nursing Process: Implementation
NCLEX: Psychosocial Integrity
Text Page: 159

3. Answer: 1
Rationale: It is a patient's right to be treated using the least restrictive setting and method.
Cognitive Level: Application
Nursing Process: Assessment
NCLEX: Psychosocial Integrity
Text Page: 160

4. Answer: 4
Rationale: Involuntary commitment means that the patient did not request hospitalization and may have opposed it or was indecisive and did not resist it. Further, most involuntary commitments are made on the grounds that the patient is dangerous to self or others, is mentally ill and in need of treatment, or is unable to provide for his or her own basic needs.
Cognitive Level: Application
Nursing Process: Assessment
NCLEX: Safe, Effective Care Environment: Management of Care
Text Page: 150

5. Answer: 4
Rationale: The Tarasoff decision gives mental health professionals a duty to warn prospective victims, but the extent and discharge of the duty vary from state to state. If unsure of how to proceed, the nurse should document the information and confer with the treatment team.
Cognitive Level: Application
Nursing Process: Implementation
NCLEX: Safe, Effective Care Environment: Management of Care
Text Page: 158

6. Answer: 4
Rationale: Patients who are admitted voluntarily lose none of their civil rights; they retain the right to make decisions to accept or reject specific treatments. The other items are matters that are unit policy rather than individual rights.
Cognitive Level: Application
Nursing Process: Planning

NCLEX: Safe, Effective Care Environment: Management of Care
Text Page: 150

7. Answer: 3
Rationale: Civil rights are not lost during a voluntary psychiatric hospital stay.
Cognitive Level: Application
Nursing Process: Implementation
NCLEX: Psychosocial Integrity
Text Page: 150

8. Answer: 3
Rationale: Under voluntary admission, any citizen of lawful age may apply in writing for admission to a public or private psychiatric hospital. The person agrees to receive treatment and abide by hospital rules. Voluntary admission is similar to medical hospitalization.
Cognitive Level: Application
Nursing Process: Assessment
NCLEX: Safe, Effective Care Environment: Management of Care
Text Page: 150

9. Answer: 2
Rationale: The criteria for involuntary commitment include the following: the patient is dangerous to self or others, the patient is mentally ill and in need of treatment, and the patient is unable to provide for his or her own basic needs.
Cognitive Level: Application
Nursing Process: Assessment
NCLEX: Safe, Effective Care Environment: Management of Care
Text Page: 150

10. Answer: 2
Rationale: Most state laws limit the length of emergency commitment to 48 to 72 hours; therefore diagnostic workups must be completed before the time limit. Completion within 36 hours allows time for converting emergency commitment to involuntary commitment if necessary.
Cognitive Level: Application
Nursing Process: Planning
NCLEX: Safe, Effective Care Environment: Management of Care
Text Page: 151

11. Answer: 1
Rationale: Consulting a lawyer is the right of all psychiatric patients. Release is determined by the type of commitment; choice of agency caregiver is not a basic patient right, nor is keeping all personal effects a basic right; and safety considerations override the right to personal property.
Cognitive Level: Analysis
Nursing Process: Implementation
NCLEX: Safe, Effective Care Environment: Management of Care
Text Page: 154

12. Answer: 4
Rationale: Elopement does not cancel court commitment.
Cognitive Level: Application
Nursing Process: Implementation
NCLEX: Safe, Effective Care Environment: Management of Care
Text Page: 152-153

13. Answer: 4
Rationale: Information about patients may not be shared with individuals outside the circle of confidentiality.
Cognitive Level: Analysis
Nursing Process: Implementation
NCLEX: Safe, Effective Care Environment: Management of Care
Text Page: 157

14. Answer: 2
Rationale: Psychiatric patients have the right to communicate with others outside of the hospital.
Cognitive Level: Analysis
Nursing Process: Implementation
NCLEX: Psychosocial Integrity
Text Page: 154

15. Answer: 1
Rationale: Competence or incompetence is determined in a court; it is not a medical decision.
Cognitive Level: Application
Nursing Process: Implementation
NCLEX: Safe, Effective Care Environment: Management of Care
Text Page: 155

16. Answer: 3
Rationale: Confidentiality requires that the nurse impart no information whatsoever, including acknowledging whether or not the person has been a patient at the facility.
Cognitive Level: Application
Nursing Process: Implementation
NCLEX: Safe, Effective Care Environment: Management of Care
Text Page: 157

17. Answer: 3
Rationale: Nurses are mandated reporters of suspected child abuse. To report or not is not discretionary.
Cognitive Level: Application
Nursing Process: Implementation

NCLEX: Safe, Effective Care Environment: Management of Care
Text Page: 157

18. Answer: 3
Rationale: A consent form for the specific treatment is required. Unless informed consent is given, the patient may sue the agency, the physician, and all who participated in the treatment.
Cognitive Level: Application
Nursing Process: Implementation
NCLEX: Safe, Effective Care Environment: Management of Care
Text Page: 159

19. Answer: 1
Rationale: Patients have the right to refuse treatment, even when treatment would be in their best interest.
Cognitive Level: Application
Nursing Process: Implementation
NCLEX: Safe, Effective Care Environment: Management of Care
Text Page: 160

20. Answer: 4
Rationale: Four elements are necessary to prove liability for malpractice: duty, negligent performance, harm to the patient, and proximate cause. If the patient sustained no harm, no tort liability exists.
Cognitive Level: Application
Nursing Process: NA
NCLEX: Safe, Effective Care Environment: Management of Care
Text Page: 164-165

21. Answer: 2
Rationale: GMBI individuals who have committed capital crimes are never freed. They are usually held in penal institutions or maximum-security forensic psychiatric hospitals.
Cognitive Level: Application
Nursing Process: Implementation
NCLEX: Safe, Effective Care Environment: Management of Care
Text Page: 165

22. Answer: 3
Rationale: Studies show that the vast majority of people with serious mental illness are not inherently violent and are no more dangerous than people in the general population. Further, violence is not associated with any specific psychiatric diagnosis.
Cognitive Level: Application
Nursing Process: Implementation
NCLEX: Safe, Effective Care Environment: Management of Care
Text Page: 151

23. Answer: 1
Rationale: The predictors of violence include prior violent behavior, noncompliance with medications, current substance abuse, and antisocial personality disorder.
Cognitive Level: Analysis
Nursing Process: Assessment
NCLEX: Safe, Effective Care Environment: Management of Care
Text Page: 151

24. Answer: 2
Rationale: If the patient is competent, the contracts she signs are legal and binding. Depression does not necessarily render one incapable of handling personal affairs.
Cognitive Level: Application
Nursing Process: NA
NCLEX: Safe, Effective Care Environment: Management of Care
Text Page: 154

25. Answer: 3
Rationale: Patients' rights include the right to consult with one's own private psychiatrist.
Cognitive Level: Application
Nursing Process: Implementation
NCLEX: Safe, Effective Care Environment: Management of Care
Text Page: 154

CHAPTER 11

1. Answer: 2
Rationale: The term *extended family* is used to describe a family in which the patient lives with others who are related by blood or marriage. A nuclear family consists of parents and their children. The terms *traditional* and *nontraditional* may be used to describe a family according to gender roles and employment status. *Household* is a less precise term referring to a residence consisting of an individual living alone or a group of people sharing a common dwelling and cooking facilities.
Cognitive Level: Application
Nursing Process: Implementation
NCLEX: Psychosocial Integrity
Text Page: 170

2. Answer: 3
Rationale: Characteristics of a functional family include that children assume age-appropriate responsibility and enjoy age-appropriate responsibility, the family can tolerate conflict without disintegration of family cohesion (Answer 1), distance is not used to solve problems (Answer 2), and overcloseness or fusion is avoided (Answer 4).

Cognitive Level: Application
Nursing Process: Assessment
NCLEX: Psychosocial Integrity
Text Page: 171

3. Answer: 4
Rationale: In a healthy family, the preservation of a positive emotional climate is more highly valued than doing what is "right." If the children are often grounded for infractions of rules, this may be an indicator of less-than-optimal family functioning, and this warrants further assessment by the nurse. The descriptions in Answers 1, 2, and 3 represent indicators of a functional family, including effective problem resolution, maintenance of emotional contact across generations, and the promotion of personal growth and creativity, respectively.
Cognitive Level: Application
Nursing Process: Assessment
NCLEX: Psychosocial Integrity
Text Page: 171

4. Answer: 2
Rationale: Culture within a family often determines the definition of family, the beliefs governing family relationships, the conflict and tensions present in the family and the responses (adaptive or maladaptive) to them, the norms of the family, how outside events are perceived and interpreted, and the type and frequency of family interventions that will be most effective. The educational level that family members achieve is less closely linked to culture than the other options presented.
Cognitive Level: Assessment
Nursing Process:
NCLEX: Psychosocial Integrity
Text Page: 171

5. Answer: 4
Rationale: A genogram typically includes three generations and includes the patient. Thus a great-grandparent may not necessarily be included in a genogram for an adult patient. The genogram includes first-degree relatives, such as parents, siblings (Answer 1), and children as well as second-degree relatives, such as aunts and uncles (Answer 3), nieces and nephews, grandparents, and grandchildren. All family members by marriage, partnership, or adoption, and step-family members also are included (Answer 2).
Cognitive Level: Application
Nursing Process: Assessment
NCLEX: Psychosocial Integrity
Text Page: 171-172

6. Answer: 3
Rationale: The family APGAR tool can be used to explore family roles and relationships. It includes an assessment of how resources, decisions, nurturing, emotional experiences, time, space, and money are shared within the family.
Cognitive Level: Application
Nursing Process: Assessment
NCLEX: Psychosocial Integrity
Text Page: 172-173

7. Answer: 1
Rationale: A competence paradigm promotes the use of natural support networks, focuses on growth-producing behaviors rather than treatment of problems (Answer 4) or negative outcomes (Answer 2), and uses a health-based developmental model rather than a disease-based medical model (Answer 3).
Cognitive Level: Application
Nursing Process: Implementation
NCLEX: Psychosocial Integrity
Text Page: 173

8. Answer: 1
Rationale: A pathology paradigm focuses on a disease-based medical model and a view of families as being pathological, pathogenic, or dysfunctional. The competence paradigm focuses on adaptive behaviors (Answer 2), care that is congruent with culture (Answer 3), and a cooperative partnership between patient and health care providers (Answer 4).
Cognitive Level: Application
Nursing Process: Evaluation
NCLEX: Psychosocial Integrity
Text Page: 173

9. Answer: 4
Rationale: Psychoeducational programs for families are designed primarily for education and support. Their aim is to improve the course of the family member's illness, reduce relapse rates, and improve patient and family functioning. As such, Answers 1, 2, and 3 represent more specific goals that are part of the overall purpose.
Cognitive Level: Application
Nursing Process: Implementation
NCLEX: Psychosocial Integrity
Text Page: 173

10. Answer: 3
Rationale: Programs designed to enhance personal and family effectiveness would most likely focus on topics such as behavior management, conflict resolution, communication skills, problem solving, stress management, assertiveness training, achieving a family balance, and meeting personal needs.
Cognitive Level: Application
Nursing Process: Planning
NCLEX: Psychosocial Integrity
Text Page: 174

11. Answer: 4
Rationale: Components of comprehensive programs for working with families should include a didactic component, a skill component, an emotional component, a family process component, and a social component. Debate is not part of the structure of these programs.
Cognitive Level: Knowledge
Nursing Process: NA
NCLEX: Psychosocial Integrity
Text Page: 174

12. Answer: 1
Rationale: Barriers to educating families for involvement in their loved one's treatment include professional bias against families based on exposure to family-system theories that suggest families cause or perpetuate the illness. The statements in Answers 2, 3, and 4 are true and do not represent a barrier to family education.
Cognitive Level: Application
Nursing Process: Assessment
NCLEX: Psychosocial Integrity
Text Page: 175

13. Answer: 3
Rationale: Family literature is available to help nurses understand family burden. The symbolic interactionism model explains family attitudes, beliefs, and behaviors toward the ill person in terms of the symbolic meaning that the experience of living with the ill person has for each family member.
Cognitive Level: Application
Nursing Process: Implementation
NCLEX: Psychosocial Integrity
Text Page: 175

14. Answer: 2
Rationale: Managed-care agencies give low priority to family services because they usually are not reimbursable services.
Cognitive Level: Analysis
Nursing Process: Implementation
NCLEX: Psychosocial Integrity
Text Page: 174-175

15. Answer: 1
Rationale: Symbolic interactionism suggests that the nurse learn to "walk in the shoes" of family members by asking questions that elicit a description of their situation. The question in Answer 1 is such a question. Answer 4 is partially correct because it seeks to elicit the family's view, but it is a closed-end question and is narrower in scope. Answers 2 and 3 are inappropriate because they are factual and do not increase understanding of the lived experience of family members.
Cognitive Level: Application
Nursing Process: Implementation
NCLEX: Psychosocial Integrity
Text Page: 175

16. Answer: 2
Rationale: Children of mentally ill parents face great difficulty. They are at high risk for problems with trust and intimacy, identity, self-esteem, and dependence on the approval of others.
Cognitive Level: Application
Nursing Process: Assessment
NCLEX: Psychosocial Integrity
Text Page: 177-178

17. Answer: 1
Rationale: The family of the patient being admitted often has needs and concerns that can be ameliorated by thoughtful, empathic nursing intervention.
Cognitive Level: Application
Nursing Process: Implementation
NCLEX: Psychosocial Integrity
Text Page: 177

18. Answer: 2
Rationale: A family member is often a valuable source of information. Answer 1 refers to an older, outdated approach to mental illness. Medication compliance is only one aspect of assessment (Answer 3), and Answer 4 is not necessarily a true statement.
Cognitive Level: Application
Nursing Process: Implementation
NCLEX: Psychosocial Integrity
Text Page: 176-177

19. Answer: 1
Rationale: Many families who are eligible for preventive services do not avail themselves of these services. As families become more aware of services, budgets will need to be increased.
Cognitive Level: Application
Nursing Process: Planning
NCLEX: Psychosocial Integrity
Text Page: 175

20. Answer: 3
Rationale: Hurt, anger, and resentment are common emotions among families with mentally ill members. The nurse should assess for this and give support as necessary.
Cognitive Level: Application
Nursing Process: Assessment
NCLEX: Psychosocial Integrity
Text Page: 178

21. Answer: 1
Rationale: Utilizing skills in family dynamics is critical in engaging in effective collaboration with the family. Knowledge of family dynamics can be used to assist the

patient and family to work together effectively to meet the goals of treatment and to empower them to achieve a more healthy family relationship.
Cognitive Level: Application
Nursing Process: Implementation
NCLEX: Psychosocial Integrity
Text Page: 170

22. Answer: 4
Rationale: Foci for collaboration with family are as follows: offering information on mental illness, improving family communication and problem solving, helping with service-system use, helping family members meet their own needs, and addressing special issues concerning the patient and concerning the family.
Cognitive Level: Application
Nursing Process: Implementation
NCLEX: Psychosocial Integrity
Text Page: 177-178

23. Answer: 2
Rationale: With chapters across the country, The National Alliance for the Mentally Ill (NAMI) offers support and education for mentally ill patients and their families. AMA is the American Medical Association. APNA is the American Psychiatric Nurses Association. A family therapist engages in therapy but is not a prime resource for ongoing support and education.
Cognitive Level: Application
Nursing Process: Implementation
NCLEX: Psychosocial Integrity
Text Page: 179

CHAPTER 12

1. Answer: 1
Rationale: Learning is more effective when patients participate in the learning experience. By including patients as active participants, the nurse helps restore their sense of control over their life and over their responsibility for their own actions.
Cognitive Level: Application
Nursing Process: Planning
NCLEX: Psychosocial Integrity
Text Page: 188-189

2. Answer: 3
Rationale: It is important to document both baseline content and process. In addition to the verbal content of the interview, the patient's nonverbal messages and the nurse's reactions to the patient give important clues to the patient's state.
Cognitive Level: Application
Nursing Process: Assessment
NCLEX: Psychosocial Integrity
Text Page: 186

3. Answer: 2
Rationale: In using information from secondary sources, nurses should not simply accept the assessment of another health care team member; instead, they should apply the information they obtain to their nursing framework for data collection and formulate their own impressions and diagnoses. This brings another perspective to the work of the health care team and promotes an unbiased receptivity to patients and their problems.
Cognitive Level: Application
Nursing Process: Assessment
NCLEX: Psychosocial Integrity
Text Page: 186

4. Answer: 1
Rationale: Patients should be regarded as a source of validation.
Cognitive Level: Application
Nursing Process: Assessment
NCLEX: Psychosocial Integrity
Text Page: 186

5. Answer: 1
Rationale: A medical diagnosis is the health problem or disease states of the patient. Nursing diagnoses identify patterns of response to actual or potential psychiatric illnesses and mental health problems. Nursing diagnoses proceed from inductive and deductive reasoning, logical decision making, knowledge of normal parameters, and sociocultural sensitivity.
Cognitive Level: Analysis
Nursing Process: NA
NCLEX: Psychosocial Integrity
Text Page: 186

6. Answer: 4
Rationale: Patient safety is always of paramount concern. After safety for the patient has been established, other goals of treatment can be effectively addressed.
Cognitive Level: Analysis
Nursing Process: Planning
NCLEX: Psychosocial Integrity
Text Page: 188

7. Answer: 2
Rationale: NOC stands for Nursing Outcomes Classification. The outcomes listed can serve as models for nurses. NIC stands for Nursing Interventions Classification; DSM-IV refers to the *Diagnostic and Statistical Manual of Mental Disorders*, Fourth Edition; the abbreviation NANDA stands for North American Nursing Diagnosis Association.
Cognitive Level: Application
Nursing Process: Outcome Identification
NCLEX: Psychosocial Integrity
Text Page: 188

8. Answer: 4
Rationale: Short-term goal statements should be specific, measurable, attainable, current, adequate, and mutually accepted. The outcomes identified in Answers 1 and 2 are not measurable. The outcome in Answer 4 is more specific and attainable than Answer 3, which is a statement rather than an action.
Cognitive Level: Application
Nursing Process: Outcome Identification
NCLEX: Psychosocial Integrity
Text Page: 188-189

9. Answer: 2
Rationale: The three domains that should be considered are cognitive, affective, and psychomotor. Cognitive relates to intellectual, affective is concerned with values, and psychomotor is concerned with the mastery of motor skills. Compliance with a medication regime requires one to know the dose and dosing intervals, value the effects of the medication, and have the ability to obtain the medication.
Cognitive Level: Analysis
Nursing Process: Outcome Identification
NCLEX: Psychosocial Integrity
Text Page: 189

10. Answer: 1
Rationale: This nursing diagnosis deals with patient safety, a primary concern for the psychiatric nurse caring for a patient exhibiting symptoms of mania.
Cognitive Level: Application
Nursing Process: Diagnosis
NCLEX: Psychosocial Integrity
Text Page: 187, 189

11. Answer: 1
Rationale: The nursing care plan includes interventions designed to achieve designated outcomes and which answer the question, "How/by what means can this be accomplished?" The rationale that is developed for the selection of specific interventions answers the "Why?"
Cognitive Level: Analysis
Nursing Process: Planning
NCLEX: Psychosocial Integrity
Text Page: 189

12. Answer: 3
Rationale: Building adequate incentives to change is critical to translating insight into action. The nurse should help the patient to see the consequences of his actions and to help him understand that old patterns do more harm than good. The patient will not learn new patterns until the motivation to acquire them is greater than the motivation to retain the old ones.
Cognitive Level: Application
Nursing Process: Implementation
NCLEX: Psychosocial Integrity
Text Page: 191-192

13. Answer: 4
Rationale: Nursing interventions that have been proved successful by research methods (evidence-based psychiatric nursing) should be the ones chosen for use by clinicians. Answer 3 is incorrect because not all interventions investigated have been proved effective.
Cognitive Level: Analysis
Nursing Process: Implementation
NCLEX: Psychosocial Integrity
Text Page: 191

14. Answer: 3
Rationale: Nursing behaviors relating to the implementation phase of the nursing process include considering available resources, implementing nursing activities, generating alternatives, and coordinating care with other team members.
Cognitive Level: Analysis
Nursing Process: Implementation
NCLEX: Psychosocial Integrity
Text Page: 185

15. Answer: 1
Rationale: Evaluation is a continuous, active process that begins early in the relationship and continues throughout. It is an activity that requires patient and family participation, because it is based on previously identified goals and level of satisfaction. It should be documented to demonstrate the value of nursing services to consumers.
Cognitive Level: Application
Nursing Process: Implementation
NCLEX: Psychosocial Integrity
Text Page: 191

16. Answer: 2
Rationale: The model and standard I are congruent.
Cognitive Level: Analysis
Nursing Process: Assessment
NCLEX: Psychosocial Integrity
Text Page: 186

17. Answer: 2
Rationale: Accountability means taking responsibility for one's own actions.
Cognitive Level: Analysis
Nursing Process: Implementation
NCLEX: Psychosocial Integrity
Text Page: 192

18. Answer: 2
Rationale: Autonomy has two interrelated components: (1) control over nursing tasks, which means having the opportunity for independent thought and

action, having use of time, skills, and ability, having authority and responsibility for implementing goals related to quality of care, and being able to initiate changes, and (2) participation in decision making regarding quality standards, one's job context, and setting of institutional policies.
Cognitive Level: Analysis
Nursing Process: NA
NCLEX: Psychosocial Integrity
Text Page: 192

19. Answer: 2
Rationale: Professional performance standards state the following: "The psychiatric-mental health nurse systematically evaluates the quality of care and effectiveness of psychiatric-mental health practice."
Cognitive Level: Analysis
Nursing Process: NA
NCLEX: Psychosocial Integrity
Text Page: 194

20. Answer: 1
Rationale: Administrative performance appraisal involves the review, management, and regulation of competent psychiatric nursing practice in which actual performance is compared with role expectations in a formal way. Clinical performance appraisal is guidance provided through a mentoring relationship with a more experienced, skilled, and educated nurse.
Cognitive Level: Application
Nursing Process: NA
NCLEX: Psychosocial Integrity
Text Page: 193-194

21. Answer: 4
Rationale: Clinical advancement programs allow the nurse to be promoted and economically rewarded for providing direct patient care. Such programs identify levels of professional development in nursing based on increased critical thinking and advanced application of nursing skills.
Cognitive Level: Analysis
Nursing Process: NA
NCLEX: Psychosocial Integrity
Text Page: 193

22. Answer: 3
Rationale: Despite its intensity, supervision is not therapy; purposes are different. Supervision aims to teach psychotherapeutic skills, whereas therapy seeks to alter a person's characteristic patterns of coping.
Cognitive Level: Analysis
Nursing Process: Implementation
NCLEX: Psychosocial Integrity
Text Page: 195

23. Answer: 1
Rationale: The standard about education reads as follows: "The psychiatric-mental health nurse acquires and maintains current knowledge in nursing practice." Nursing conditions include intellectual curiosity, desire for professional growth, and access to new information.
Cognitive Level: Application
Nursing Process: NA
NCLEX: Psychosocial Integrity
Text Page: 195

24. Answer: 2
Rationale: At the beginning level, a staff nurse who has no advanced degrees can be expected to use research findings in practice, with supervision.
Cognitive Level: Application
Nursing Process: Implementation
NCLEX: Psychosocial Integrity
Text Page: 200

25. Answer: 4
Rationale: The standard for resource use states that the psychiatric-mental health nurse should consider safety, effectiveness, and cost when planning and delivering patient care. Treatment decisions must be made in such a way as to maximize resources and maintain quality of care while engaging in patient advocacy.
Cognitive Level: Application
Nursing Process: Planning
NCLEX: Psychosocial Integrity
Text Page: 199

26. Answer: 3
Rationale: Collegiality means regarding other nurses as partners in caregiving who are valued and respected for their unique contributions regardless of educational, experiential, or specialty background. It suggests that nurses view themselves as members of a profession and that nurses trust, remain loyal to, and demonstrate commitment to other nurses.
Cognitive Level: Application
Nursing Process: Assessment
NCLEX: Psychosocial Integrity
Text Page: 196

CHAPTER 13

1. Answer: 3
Rationale: Primary prevention is lowering the incidence of a mental disorder or reducing the rate at which new cases of the disorder develop.
Cognitive Level: Application
Nursing Process: Implementation
NCLEX: Psychosocial Integrity
Text Page: 208

2. Answer: 2
Rationale: Epidemiological studies examine the incidence (number of new cases) and prevalence (number of current existing cases) of a disease or disorder in a defined population over a specified period of time. The nurse who is trying to plan for services would find this data very helpful. Answers 1, 3, and 4 refer to other methods of assessing community needs but they are not as well suited to gathering the data identified by this question.
Cognitive Level: Application
Nursing Process: Assessment
NCLEX: Psychosocial Integrity
Text Page: 209

3. Answer: 3
Rationale: The primary difference is the medical model's attempt to identify a single cause of a disease; the nursing model assumes that mental disorders result from the interplay of several risk and protective factors.
Cognitive Level: Application
Nursing Process: NA
NCLEX: Psychosocial Integrity
Text Page: 209-210

4. Answer: 2
Rationale: The health education strategy of primary prevention in mental health involves the strengthening of individuals and groups through building of competence or resilience. The other answers do not address this particular trait.
Cognitive Level: Application
Nursing Process: Planning
NCLEX: Psychosocial Integrity
Text Page: 211

5. Answer: 4
Rationale: Self-efficacy is a belief in one's personal capabilities and reflects the notion that a person has control over the events in his or her life and that his or her actions will be effective. People with a low sense of efficacy tend to avoid difficult tasks and have low aspirations and weak commitment to their goals.
Cognitive Level: Analysis
Nursing Process: Assessment
NCLEX: Psychosocial Integrity
Text Page: 211

6. Answer: 3
Rationale: The nurse's work in tertiary prevention involves rehabilitative efforts. Work satisfaction would be most clearly related to Answer 3.
Cognitive Level: Application
Nursing Process: Implementation
NCLEX: Psychosocial Integrity
Text Page: 211

7. Answer: 3
Rationale: The assessment phase of the nursing process is in use when the nurse identifies problem areas.
Cognitive Level: Application
Nursing Process: Assessment
NCLEX: Psychosocial Integrity
Text Page: 210

8. Answer: 4
Rationale: Low self-efficacy negatively affects an individual's thoughts, motivation, mood, and health. A person with low self-efficacy dwells on obstacles and personal deficiencies, and such a person is depression-prone. Successful interventions for groups with low self-efficacy can be planned and implemented.
Cognitive Level: Application
Nursing Process: Assessment
NCLEX: Psychosocial Integrity
Text Page: 211

9. Answer: 4
Rationale: Primary prevention is aimed at reducing the incidence of mental illness. Depression is a frequent outcome of low self-efficacy. Therefore a goal of intervention to raise self-efficacy is to reduce the incidence of depression in the group.
Cognitive Level: Analysis
Nursing Process: Outcome Identification
NCLEX: Psychosocial Integrity
Text Page: 211

10. Answer: 1
Rationale: Planning is the elaboration of strategies designed to achieve a specific goal.
Cognitive Level: Application
Nursing Process: Planning
NCLEX: Psychosocial Integrity
Text Page: 210

11. Answer: 4
Rationale: Factors that place a person at high risk include the presence of many stressors, fewer protective factors, and inadequate coping mechanisms. (Developmental tasks are considered universal.)
Cognitive Level: Analysis
Nursing Process: Assessment
NCLEX: Psychosocial Integrity
Text Page: 210

12. Answer: 2
Rationale: An indicated population is one made up of high-risk individuals identified as having biological markers that indicate a predisposition for the disorder.
Cognitive Level: Application
Nursing Process: Planning
NCLEX: Psychosocial Integrity
Text Page: 210

13. Answer: 2
Rationale: Being a minority, living in poverty, being elderly, and having no social support are sociocultural risk factors.
Cognitive Level: Analysis
Nursing Process: Assessment
NCLEX: Psychosocial Integrity
Text Page: 210

14. Answer: 3
Rationale: Knowledge of normal growth and development is necessary for assessing a person's functioning and for choosing appropriate preventive nursing interventions.
Cognitive Level: Application
Nursing Process: Implementation
NCLEX: Psychosocial Integrity
Text Page: 210

15. Answer: 2
Rationale: Assessment is the first phase of the nursing process.
Cognitive Level: Analysis
Nursing Process: Planning
NCLEX: Psychosocial Integrity
Text Page: 210

16. Answer: 2
Rationale: Health education for patients with mental health disorders can include interventions to increase the coping skills of the individual or group, such as problem solving, communication skills, tolerance of stress and frustration, motivation, hope, anger management, and self-esteem. Answers 1, 3, and 4 do not relate to an increase in coping skills related to anger management.
Cognitive Level: Application
Nursing Process: Implementation
NCLEX: Psychosocial Integrity
Text Page: 212

17. Answer: 2
Rationale: Health education used as a primary prevention strategy involves the strengthening of individuals and groups through competence building. Competence building improves self-efficacy.
Cognitive Level: Comprehension
Nursing Process: Implementation
NCLEX: Psychosocial Integrity
Text Page: 211

18. Answer: 1
Rationale: Groups that tend to be important to adolescents include those that discuss peer relationships, sexuality, or potential problems such as drug abuse or promiscuity. Groups devoted to normal growth and development and childrearing are groups of most importance to parents. Career selection does not relate directly to health education, but it may indirectly affect the stressors in one's life.
Cognitive Level: Analysis
Nursing Process: Implementation
NCLEX: Psychosocial Integrity
Text Page: 212

19. Answer: 3
Rationale: Health education and competency building are synonymous as primary prevention strategies.
Cognitive Level: Application
Nursing Process: Implementation
NCLEX: Psychosocial Integrity
Text Page: 211

20. Answer: 1
Rationale: Providing social support includes cushioning the effects of potential stressors. Improving links between the individual and the community, strengthening natural caregiving networks, using informal support groups, and providing nursing support all are ways to increase social support for an individual.
Cognitive Level: Application
Nursing Process: Implementation
NCLEX: Psychosocial Integrity
Text Page: 214-215

21. Answer: 4
Rationale: Answer 4 clarifies the characteristics of self-help groups about which the individual had misconceptions.
Cognitive Level: Application
Nursing Process: Implementation
NCLEX: Psychosocial Integrity
Text Page: 215-216

22. Answer: 2
Rationale: Self-help groups are supportive and educative rather than therapeutic. Members lead the group and implement principles of self-governance (Answer 2). They are focused on a single life-disrupting event (Answer 3). Membership is voluntary and nonprofit in orientation (Answer 4).
Cognitive Level: Application
Nursing Process: Implementation
NCLEX: Psychosocial Integrity
Text Page: 216

CHAPTER 14

1. Answer: 2
Rationale: A situational crisis occurs when a life event upsets an individual's psychological equilibrium. Loss of a job can give rise to a situational crisis.

Cognitive Level: Application
Nursing Process: Assessment
NCLEX: Psychosocial Integrity
Text Page: 223

2. Answer: 1
Rationale: A situational crisis occurs when an accidental, uncommon, or unexpected event upsets psychological equilibrium.
Cognitive Level: Application
Nursing Process: Assessment
NCLEX: Psychosocial Integrity
Text Page: 223

3. Answer: 2
Rationale: Maturational crises are developmental events requiring role change.
Cognitive Level: Application
Nursing Process: Assessment
NCLEX: Psychosocial Integrity
Text Page: 223

4. Answer: 1
Rationale: A situational crisis occurs when an accidental, uncommon, or unexpected event upsets psychological equilibrium.
Cognitive Level: Application
Nursing Process: Assessment
NCLEX: Psychosocial Integrity
Text Page: 223

5. Answer: 2
Rationale: Crisis intervention therapy is usually limited to 6 weeks' duration.
Cognitive Level: Application
Nursing Process: Implementation
NCLEX: Safe, Effective Care Environment: Management of Care
Text Page: 225

6. Answer: 1
Rationale: The patient is probably experiencing a maturational crisis related to the role changes required by the birth of the baby. Crisis intervention is appropriate.
Cognitive Level: Application
Nursing Process: Assessment
NCLEX: Psychosocial Integrity
Text Page: 223

7. Answer: 4
Rationale: A return to the precrisis level of functioning is the expected outcome for crisis intervention.
Cognitive Level: Application
Nursing Process: Outcome Identification
NCLEX: Psychosocial Integrity
Text Page: 225

8. Answer: 2
Rationale: Self-esteem is threatened when role mastery is not attained. Role mastery is achieved when the person attains work, sexual, and family role successes.
Cognitive Level: Application
Nursing Process: Assessment
NCLEX: Psychosocial Integrity
Text Page: 225

9. Answer: 1
Rationale: Balancing factors are important in the development and resolution of a crisis and include the precipitating stressor, the patient perception of the stressor, the nature and strength of a patient's support systems and coping resources, and previous strengths and coping mechanisms. Family, friends, clergy, and coworkers are considered part of the patient's support system.
Cognitive Level: Application
Nursing Process: Assessment
NCLEX: Psychosocial Integrity
Text Page: 225

10. Answer: 3
Rationale: Biological function is achieved when a person is safe and life is not threatened.
Cognitive Level: Application
Nursing Process: Implementation
NCLEX: Safe, Effective Care Environment: Management of Care
Text Page: 225

11. Answer: 1
Rationale: The patient's perception is a key factor. What may be trivial to one may seem overwhelming to another, and vice versa. If the patient does not perceive the event as problematic, a crisis may be averted.
Cognitive Level: Application
Nursing Process: Assessment
NCLEX: Psychosocial Integrity
Text Page: 226

12. Answer: 2
Rationale The generic approach is designed to reach high-risk individuals and large groups as quickly as possible.
Cognitive Level: Application
Nursing Process: Planning
NCLEX: Psychosocial Integrity
Text Page: 227

13. Answer: 1
Rationale: Catharsis is the release of feelings that takes place as the patient talks about the event. The nurse solicits the patient's feelings about the situation by asking open-ended, explorative questions and focusing on feelings.

Cognitive Level: Application
Nursing Process: Implementation
NCLEX: Psychosocial Integrity
Text Page: 228

14. Answer: 2
Rationale: Environmental manipulation includes interventions that directly change the patient's physical or interpersonal situation. These interventions provide situational support or remove stress.
Cognitive Level: Application
Nursing Process: Implementation
NCLEX: Psychosocial Integrity
Text Page: 227

15. Answer: 3
Rationale: This type of crisis intervention can be effective with all types of crises. It is particularly useful in combined situational and maturational crises.
Cognitive Level: Application
Nursing Process: Implementation
NCLEX: Psychosocial Integrity
Text Page: 227

16. Answer: 3
Rationale: Because of time constraints, nurses performing crisis intervention use techniques that are active, focused, and explorative to carry out the interventions. Interventions must be aimed at achieving quick resolution. Nurses must be creative, flexible, and competent in the use of many techniques.
Cognitive Level: Application
Nursing Process: Implementation
NCLEX: Psychosocial Integrity
Text Page: 228

17. Answer: 1
Rationale: Clarification is used when a nurse helps the patient identify the relationship among events, behavior, and feelings. For example, clarification can mean helping a patient see that it was after he was passed over for a promotion that he thought he was too sick to go to work.
Cognitive Level: Application
Nursing Process: Implementation
NCLEX: Psychosocial Integrity
Text Page: 228

18. Answer: 2
Rationale: Support of defenses encourages the use of adaptive defenses and discourages maladaptive and unhealthy coping strategies.
Cognitive Level: Application
Nursing Process: Implementation
NCLEX: Psychosocial Integrity
Text Page: 228

19. Answer: 3
Rationale: Raising self-esteem helps a patient regain feelings of self-worth by communicating confidence that the patient has strengths and can find solutions to problems.
Cognitive Level: Application
Nursing Process: Implementation
NCLEX: Psychosocial Integrity
Text Page: 228

20. Answer: 3
Rationale: The patient is using denial, admits to anxiety, and has self-doubts. These would be appropriate targets for intervention.
Cognitive Level: Application
Nursing Process: Assessment
NCLEX: Psychosocial Integrity
Text Page: 228

21. Answer: 1
Rationale: Whenever a patient alludes to the possibility of suicide the nurse should actively explore the topic.
Cognitive Level: Application
Nursing Process: Assessment
NCLEX: Psychosocial Integrity
Text Page: 226

22. Answer: 4
Rationale: Safety contracting is an accepted, effective method of deterring suicide.
Cognitive Level: Application
Nursing Process: Implementation
NCLEX: Safe, Effective Care Environment: Management of Care
Text Page: 228

23. Answer: 2
Rationale: The last phase of crisis intervention is evaluation, when the nurse and patient evaluate whether the intervention resulted in a positive resolution of the crisis. One area is to explore whether the patient has returned to the precrisis level of functioning.
Cognitive Level: Application
Nursing Process: Evaluation
NCLEX: Psychosocial Integrity
Text Page: 229

24. Answer: 3
Rationale: Praying represents a coping mechanism previously and successfully used by the patient.
Cognitive Level: Analysis
Nursing Process: Assessment
NCLEX: Psychosocial Integrity
Text Page: 226

25. Answer: 3
Rationale: The only correct answer here is Answer 3. Mobile crisis teams provide front-line interdisciplinary

crisis intervention to individuals, families, and communities. Crisis intervention usually is not available only during non-daytime hours (Answer 1), nor is it usually available in primary care physicians' offices (Answer 2), nor do caregivers usually discriminate or treat certain groups of individuals only if they are located in such facilities (Answer 4).
Cognitive Level: Analysis
Nursing Process: NA
NCLEX: Psychosocial Integrity
Text Page: 232

CHAPTER 15

1. Answer: 3
Rationale: Psychiatric rehabilitation is the process of helping the person return to the highest possible level of functioning.
Cognitive Level: Application
Nursing Process: Implementation
NCLEX: Safe, Effective Care Environment: Management of Care
Text Page: 239

2. Answer: 4
Rationale: Rehabilitative psychiatric nursing takes place in the context of a multidisciplinary treatment team. Other team members may include psychiatrists, psychologists, social workers, occupational therapists, rehabilitation counselors, case managers, consumer team members, family advocates, employment specialists, and job coaches.
Cognitive Level: Analysis
Nursing Process: NA
NCLEX: Safe, Effective Care Environment: Management of Care
Text Page: 240

3. Answer: 3
Rationale: In traditional medical rehabilitation, the focus is on disease, illness, and symptoms. Psychiatric rehabilitation focuses on wellness and health, not symptoms.
Cognitive Level: Application
Nursing Process: Implementation
NCLEX: Health Promotion and Maintenance
Text Page: 240

4. Answer: 1
Rationale: The patient-helper relationship in psychiatric rehabilitation is an adult-to-adult relationship that is more egalitarian and promotes choices and empowerment, whereas the traditional medical model uses an expert-to-patient relationship.
Cognitive Level: Application
Nursing Process: Implementation
NCLEX: Psychosocial Integrity
Text Page: 240

5. Answer: 2
Rationale: Although deficits are assessed, implementation focuses on the reinforcement of identified strengths.
Cognitive Level: Application
Nursing Process: Implementation
NCLEX: Psychosocial Integrity
Text Page: 240

6. Answer: 3
Rationale: Secondary symptoms of mental illness are caused by a person's response to the illness or its treatment (e.g., loneliness and social isolation).
Cognitive Level: Application
Nursing Process: Evaluation
NCLEX: Psychosocial Integrity
Text Page: 242

7. Answer: 1
Rationale: The Vellenga study identified several themes that are related to secondary symptoms: stigmatization, alienation, loss of relationships and vocational opportunities, distress caused by the effects of the illness, acceptance of self as having a mental illness, and the need for acceptance by others.
Cognitive Level: Application
Nursing Process: Implementation
NCLEX: Psychosocial Integrity
Text Page: 242

8. Answer: 4
Rationale: The nurse's response should be aimed at dispelling the myth that mentally ill patients are dangerous and continue to be dangerous after discharge.
Cognitive Level: Application
Nursing Process: Implementation
NCLEX: Psychosocial Integrity
Text Page: 243

9. Answer: 2
Rationale: Answer 1 indicates that the family will need to make changes to meet the needs of the patient. This is not necessarily true. Instead, the nurse should assess the family's understanding of the patient's problem and the plan of care. Answer 3 indicates that the family will be responsible for meeting all of the patient's needs, but this is not indicated. Instead, the family structure should be assessed, including developmental stage, roles, responsibilities, norms, and values. In Answer 4, help with ADLs has not been indicated for this patient. Therefore the only correct answer is Answer 2.
Cognitive Level: Application
Nursing Process: Assessment

NCLEX: Safe, Effective Care Environment: Management of Care
Text Page: 244

10. Answer: 2
Rationale: Daily hassles are concerns, worries, and events that disrupt daily life and well being. The hassles of most frequent concern are money; loneliness; boredom; crime; past, present, and future accomplishments; communication problems; and physical health.
Cognitive Level: Application
Nursing Process: Assessment
NCLEX: Psychosocial Integrity
Text Page: 249

11. Answer: 1
Rationale: The only conclusion that can be drawn based on the assessment data is that he currently has low readiness to function in the community.
Cognitive Level: Analysis
Nursing Process: Assessment
NCLEX: Health Promotion and Maintenance
Text Page: 244

12. Answer: 4
Rationale: For families of patients with schizophrenia, the problems most often described were poor grooming and personal care, suspiciousness, and talking to self.
Cognitive Level: Application
Nursing Process: Assessment
NCLEX: Safe, Effective Care Environment: Management of Care
Text Page: 244

13. Answer: 2
Rationale: Usual assessment findings are increased family stress and conflict, a tendency of members to blame each other for the illness, difficulty understanding or accepting the illness, tension during family gatherings, and disproportionate family time, energy, or money expended on the ill member.
Cognitive Level: Application
Nursing Process: Assessment
NCLEX: Safe, Effective Care Environment: Management of Care
Text Page: 245

14. Answer: 3
Rationale: Norbeck and associates identified four categories of support needs as emotional support, feedback support exemplified by affirmation, cognitive or informational support, and instrumental support exemplified by resources and respite.
Cognitive Level: Application
Nursing Process: Assessment
NCLEX: Safe, Effective Care Environment: Management of Care
Text Page: 246

15. Answer: 4
Rationale: Families often express grief, anger, powerlessness, and the need for social support. Powerlessness, however, is the only one of these aspects of subjective burden for which there is a NANDA nursing diagnosis.
Cognitive Level: Analysis
Nursing Process: Diagnosis
NCLEX: Psychosocial Integrity
Text Page: 245

16. Answer: 3
Rationale: Patients, too, can contribute to and provide support for their families by helping with household tasks, showing concern for others, thanking the family for their help, sharing positive personal characteristics such as sense of humor, caring for themselves by following the treatment plan, and giving others peace of mind by communicating how they are feeling.
Cognitive Level: Application
Nursing Process: Implementation
NCLEX: Psychosocial Integrity
Text Page: 247

17. Answer: 3
Rationale: The best knowledge is that which is gained firsthand by observing how the agency responds to a patient in need of services. It would be unethical to pretend to be someone who is in need of services.
Cognitive Level: Application
Nursing Process: Implementation
NCLEX: Safe, Effective Care Environment: Management of Care
Text Page: 246

18. Answer: 4
Rationale: Consumer-run psychosocial programs offer various levels of service, from drop-in socialization centers to a full range of rehabilitative services. The patient will be able to become involved in meaningful social and vocational activities.
Cognitive Level: Application
Nursing Process: Implementation
NCLEX: Safe, Effective Care Environment: Management of Care
Text Page: 249

19. Answer: 4
Rationale: Training in community living averts hospitalization. It allows for the assessment of patient skills and the establishment of realistic collaborative goals. Staff contact is reduced as patient function improves.
Cognitive Level: Application
Nursing Process: Implementation

NCLEX: Safe, Effective Care Environment: Management of Care
Text Page: 249

20. Answer: 3
Rationale: These interventions are the basis of practice in psychiatric nursing rehabilitation.
Cognitive Level: Application
Nursing Process: Implementation
NCLEX: Health Promotion and Maintenance
Text Page: 246-247

21. Answer: 1
Rationale: Effective programs for families of people with serious mental illnesses include empowerment and education.
Cognitive Level: Analysis
Nursing Process: NA
NCLEX: Safe, Effective Care Environment: Management of Care
Text Page: 256

22. Answer: 2
Rationale: Education that is offered in a supportive environment can increase self-esteem, improve job qualifications, and encourage some consumers to pursue higher education.
Cognitive Level: Analysis
Nursing Process: Planning
NCLEX: Psychosocial Integrity
Text Page: 253

23. Answer: 1
Rationale: The only correct answer is number 1. There are several common trouble spots in family life that can be anticipated. Learning ways to handle these troublesome areas empowers the family by giving them a sense of control over their lives. Some of these trouble spots include mechanics of everyday life, including the need for privacy and control over personal space, keeping a regular schedule, television usage, money management, grooming, alcohol and drug use, and a need for relatives to remember to take care of themselves.
Cognitive Level: Application
Nursing Process: Implementation
NCLEX: Psychosocial Integrity
Text Page: 253

24. Answer: 3
Rationale: Family education has become a primary nursing intervention when providing rehabilitative services to relatives of people with severe mental illness. Nurses have established workshops for family members that have been well received and have helped families cope with the challenges presented by the mental illness. Programming for these workshops can include information and skill-building exercises. The experiences of the more seasoned family members can be particularly helpful because they can share their successes and failures in using various coping strategies and provide needed social support.
Cognitive Level: Application
Nursing Process: Implementation
NCLEX: Psychosocial Integrity
Text Page: 253-254

25. Answer: 3
Rationale: Program evaluation is conducted to inform administrators about the relevance and cost effectiveness of the services they offer. Program evaluation is evolving as program funders and the public demand greater accountability from service providers.
Cognitive Level: Application
Nursing Process: NA
NCLEX: Safe, Effective Care Environment: Management of Care
Text Page: 255

CHAPTER 16

1. Answer: 4
Rationale: Anxiety is a subjective human experience. The nurse can infer that a patient is anxious based on selected behaviors but must validate this with the patient.
Cognitive Level: Comprehension
Nursing Process: Assessment
NCLEX: Psychosocial Integrity
Text Page: 260

2. Answer: 4
Rationale: Moderate anxiety is characterized by a focus on only immediate concerns and by the demonstration of a narrowed perceptual field as the person sees, hears, and grasps less. The person blocks out selected areas but can attend to more if directed to do so.
Cognitive Level: Application
Nursing Process: Assessment
NCLEX: Psychosocial Integrity
Text Page: 261

3. Answer: 2
Rationale: Panic level anxiety is associated with awe, dread, and terror. The person is disorganized, is unable to relate to others, and experiences distorted perceptions and loss of rational thought. He or she is unable to do things even with direction.
Cognitive Level: Application
Nursing Process: Assessment
NCLEX: Psychosocial Integrity
Text Page: 261

4. Answer: 1
Rationale: Safety is of highest priority because the patient in panic is at high risk for self-injury related to increased non–goal-directed motor activity, distorted perceptions, and disordered thoughts.
Cognitive Level: Analysis
Nursing Process: Planning
NCLEX: Psychosocial Integrity
Text Page: 278

5. Answer: 2
Rationale: Lorazepam (Ativan) is a benzodiazepine used to treat anxiety. It may be given as a prn medication.
Cognitive Level: Application
Nursing Process: Implementation
NCLEX: Psychosocial Integrity
Text Page: 277

6. Answer: 2
Rationale: Behaviorist theory proposes that anxiety is a product of frustration caused by anything that interferes with attaining a desired goal.
Cognitive Level: Application
Nursing Process: Planning
NCLEX: Psychosocial Integrity
Text Page: 264

7. Answer: 1
Rationale: Restlessness is a behavioral symptom of mild anxiety, while edginess is an affective symptom, and inability to concentrate is a cognitive symptom.
Cognitive Level: Application
Nursing Process: Assessment
NCLEX: Psychosocial Integrity
Text Page: 261

8. Answer: 2
Rationale: Task-oriented reactions are thoughtful, deliberate attempts to solve problems, resolve conflicts, and gratify needs. They are consciously directed and action oriented and can include attack, withdrawal, and compromise.
Cognitive Level: Application
Nursing Process: Assessment
NCLEX: Psychosocial Integrity
Text Page: 268

9. Answer: 1
Rationale: Ego defense mechanisms operate unconsciously and usually involve some degree of self-deception and reality distortion.
Cognitive Level: Application
Nursing Process: Assessment
NCLEX: Psychosocial Integrity
Text Page: 268-269

10. Answer: 2
Rationale: Displacement is defined as the shifting of an emotion from its original source to a person or object less threatening.
Cognitive Level: Analysis
Nursing Process: Assessment
NCLEX: Psychosocial Integrity
Text Page: 269

11. Answer: 2
Rationale: Repression is the involuntary exclusion of a painful or conflictual thought, impulse, or memory from awareness.
Cognitive Level: Application
Nursing Process: Assessment
NCLEX: Psychosocial Integrity
Text Page: 269

12. Answer: 3
Rationale: Rationalization is the offering of a socially acceptable or apparently logical reason as a justification for an unacceptable impulse, feeling, behavior, or motive.
Cognitive Level: Analysis
Nursing Process: Assessment
NCLEX: Psychosocial Integrity
Text Page: 269

13. Answer: 1
Rationale: Projection is the attributing of one's thoughts or impulses to another person.
Cognitive Level: Application
Nursing Process: Assessment
NCLEX: Psychosocial Integrity
Text Page: 269

14. Answer: 3
Rationale: Reaction formation is the development of behavior patterns or conscious attitudes that are the opposite of what one really feels or would like to do.
Cognitive Level: Analysis
Nursing Process: Assessment
NCLEX: Psychosocial Integrity
Text Page: 269

15. Answer: 1
Rationale: The woman has a persistent fear of open places. The extreme physical and emotional reaction is consistent with panic-level anxiety experienced when the feared situation is imminent.
Cognitive Level: Analysis
Nursing Process: Assessment
NCLEX: Psychosocial Integrity
Text Page: 271

16. Answer: 1
Rationale: Approximately 40% to 60% of patients with OCD respond favorably to selective serotonin reuptake

inhibitor therapy. Drugs such as clomipramine, fluvoxamine, paroxetine, fluoxetine, and sertraline are often prescribed.
Cognitive Level: Application
Nursing Process: Planning
NCLEX: Psychosocial Integrity
Text Page: 276

17. Answer: 3
Rationale: Severe anxiety is characterized by a reduced perceptual field as evidenced by inability to follow directions. All behavior is aimed at relieving anxiety as evidenced by the rituals he performs.
Cognitive Level: Application
Nursing Process: Assessment
NCLEX: Psychosocial Integrity
Text Page: 261

18. Answer: 4
Rationale: This remark acknowledges the patient's feelings but addresses his need to know important areas of the unit.
Cognitive Level: Application
Nursing Process: Implementation
NCLEX: Psychosocial Integrity
Text Page: 278

19. Answer: 1
Rationale: Obsessive-compulsive patients may be so consumed by rituals that they are not able to stop long enough to eat, go to the bathroom, or sleep. Sleeping 6 hours a night in comparison with sleeping only 1 hour indicates improvement.
Cognitive Level: Application
Nursing Process: Evaluation
NCLEX: Psychosocial Integrity
Text Page: 274

20. Answer: 1
Rationale: The autonomic nervous system, which comprises parasympathetic and sympathetic systems, is responsible for the individual's physiological responses to anxiety. The parasympathetic system conserves body responses, and the sympathetic system activates body responses. Sympathetic reactions predominate in anxiety.
Cognitive Level: Application
Nursing Process: Implementation
NCLEX: Psychosocial Integrity
Text Page: 261

21. Answer: 3
Rationale: Posttraumatic stress disorder (PTSD) follows exposure to a traumatic event. Symptoms include a tendency to relive the experience, a feeling of emotional "numbness," inability to relate, and persistent symptoms of arousal.
Cognitive Level: Analysis
Nursing Process: Assessment
NCLEX: Psychosocial Integrity
Text Page: 271

22. Answer: 2
Rationale: Anxiety is communicated interpersonally. Just as patients can become more anxious when the nurse is anxious, so too can nurses experience anxiety that has been transmitted by the patient.
Cognitive Level: Application
Nursing Process: Implementation
NCLEX: Psychosocial Integrity
Text Page: 280

23. Answer: 4
Rationale: Double approach-avoidance conflicts result in what is often called ambivalence.
Cognitive Level: Analysis
Nursing Process: Assessment
NCLEX: Psychosocial Integrity
Text Page: 265

24. Answer: 3
Rationale: A depressed individual usually makes negative appraisals that are pervasive and global, is absolute about negative evaluations, believes mistakes or defects are beyond redemption, and has a global view that nothing will turn out right.
Cognitive Level: Application
Nursing Process: Assessment
NCLEX: Psychosocial Integrity
Text Page: 273

25. Answer: 3
Rationale: Helping the patient connect anxiety and the use of the symptom is an initial therapeutic step. The nurse acknowledges the patient's feeling, attempts to label it, helps the patient describe feelings, and associates them with the use of a specific behavioral pattern.
Cognitive Level: Analysis
Nursing Process: Implementation
NCLEX: Psychosocial Integrity
Text Page: 280

26. Answer: 1
Rationale: Sometimes patients jump to erroneous conclusions. Questioning the evidence used by the patient to support a particular belief can be helpful. The source of Quentin's data was his own thinking, rather than information supplied by superiors. The nurse could help Quentin see that his superiors would consider his prior work record rather than make a precipitous decision to fire him.
Cognitive Level: Application
Nursing Process: Implementation

NCLEX: Psychosocial Integrity
Text Page: 280

CHAPTER 17

1. Answer: 2
Rationale: Somatization disorder is often characterized by multiple vague complaints that encourage others to take care of the individual and enable the individual to avoid demands of adult responsibility. The patients described in the other options have either a physiological basis for the complaint (Answers 1 and 3) or a disturbed body image (Answer 4).
Cognitive Level: Application
Nursing Process: Assessment
NCLEX: Psychosocial Integrity
Text Page: 287

2. Answer: 3
Rationale: Conversion disorder is a type of somatoform disorder in which symptoms of some physical illness appear without any underlying organic cause. The organic symptom reduces the patient's anxiety and usually gives a clue to the conflict.
Cognitive Level: Application
Nursing Process: Assessment
NCLEX: Psychosocial Integrity
Text Page: 287

3. Answer: 3
Rationale: Spending time with a patient focusing on strengths and positive attributes builds self-esteem and self-confidence. This intervention also reduces secondary gains.
Cognitive Level: Application
Nursing Process: Planning
NCLEX: Psychosocial Integrity
Text Page: 287-288, 297

4. Answer: 3
Rationale: The therapy selected will be one that can be used over the long term. Relaxation training, which helps the patient control tension and anxiety and thereby reduce pain, can be an effective long-term strategy. Benzodiazepines and opioids are both habit-forming, and they are not useful for the long term. Response prevention rarely is used to treat chronic pain.
Cognitive Level: Analysis
Nursing Process: Planning
NCLEX: Psychosocial Integrity
Text Page: 298

5. Answer: 4
Rationale: The exhaustion phase of the general adaptation syndrome often is associated with loss. Ms. C. has lost her husband and her ability to live at home.
Cognitive Level: Analysis
Nursing Process: Assessment
NCLEX: Psychosocial Integrity
Text Page: 285-286

6. Answer: 1
Rationale: Coping resources are characteristics of the person, group, or environment that help people adapt to stress. A social support system is considered a coping resource; the other distracters for this question would be considered stressors.
Cognitive Level: Analysis
Nursing Process: Assessment
NCLEX: Psychosocial Integrity
Text Page: 292

7. Answer: 2
Rationale: If the patient has said that she feels pressured, this suggests that the NCLEX to learn to say "no" to some requests made by her family, friends, and employer. Answer 2 is the only role-playing situation listed that addresses this problem.
Cognitive Level: Analysis
Nursing Process: Implementation
NCLEX: Psychosocial Integrity
Text Page: 292

8. Answer: 4
Rationale: The patient uses compensation in an attempt to prove that he is healthy and in control of his body.
Cognitive Level: Analysis
Nursing Process: Assessment
NCLEX: Psychosocial Integrity
Text Page: 292

9. Answer: 4
Rationale: Preoccupation with an imagined defect in appearance suggests body dysmorphic disorder.
Cognitive Level: Analysis
Nursing Process: Assessment
NCLEX: Psychosocial Integrity
Text Page: 295

10. Answer: 2
Rationale: Disturbed body image is a nursing diagnosis that is useful in most instances when body dysmorphic disorder is present. There are no data to support activity intolerance or ineffective sexuality pattern, and more data would be necessary to support ineffective role performance.
Cognitive Level: Analysis
Nursing Process: Diagnosis
NCLEX: Psychosocial Integrity
Text Page: 294

11. Answer: 4
Rationale: The patient has distorted thinking about the size of her nose, and she has highly negative and self-critical thoughts. Cognitive-behavioral therapy can address and change these automatic responses.
Cognitive Level: Application
Nursing Process: Planning
NCLEX: Psychosocial Integrity
Text Page: 296

12. Answer: 1
Rationale: Psychophysiological illness should never be dismissed as "all in one's head." This approach will cause the patient to withdraw from the nurse and prevent the formation of a therapeutic relationship.
Cognitive Level: Application
Nursing Process: Implementation
NCLEX: Psychosocial Integrity
Text Page: 296-297

13. Answer: 1
Rationale: Hypochondriasis involves preoccupation with fears of having a serious disease on the basis of the person's misinterpretation of bodily symptoms.
Cognitive Level: Analysis
Nursing Process: Assessment
NCLEX: Psychosocial Integrity
Text Page: 288

14. Answer: 3
Rationale: Questioning the evidence is a cognitive restructuring technique that can be effective in changing distorted thinking. Patients with hypochondriasis often ignore any possibilities except those that support their distorted thinking. Learning that headaches, visual disturbances, weakness, and vomiting can have causes other than brain tumors can be helpful.
Cognitive Level: Application
Nursing Process: Implementation
NCLEX: Psychosocial Integrity
Text Page: 296

15. Answer: 1
Rationale: "Doctor shopping" occurs when a patient makes an effort to find a physician who will find an organic basis for the symptoms he or she is exhibiting. The patient demonstrating this behavior rejects any suggestion that there may be a psychological component associated with the physical symptom.
Cognitive Level: Analysis
Nursing Process: Assessment
NCLEX: Psychosocial Integrity
Text Page: 286

16. Answer: 2
Rationale: During the stage of resistance, the body adapts to stress, functions at a lower-than-optimal level, and requires a greater-than-usual expenditure of energy for survival.
Cognitive Level: Application
Nursing Process: Assessment
NCLEX: Psychosocial Integrity
Text Page: 285

17. Answer: 3
Rationale: Psychophysiological disorders have stress-related physical symptoms associated with organic pathology. Treatment of symptoms and mitigation of psychological factors are indicated.
Cognitive Level: Application
Nursing Process: Assessment
NCLEX: Psychosocial Integrity
Text Page: 286

18. Answer: 4
Rationale: This approach acknowledges the reality of the patient's symptoms and suggests the possibility of stress as a contributing factor.
Cognitive Level: Application
Nursing Process: Implementation
NCLEX: Psychosocial Integrity
Text Page: 286

19. Answer: 2
Rationale: Dependency is the need for others to care for the patient. Clinicians have observed that may patients with somatization disorder display dependency. Having physical symptoms allows a patient to meet dependency needs in a socially acceptable way.
Cognitive Level: Application
Nursing Process: Planning
NCLEX: Psychosocial Integrity
Text Page: 287

20. Answer: 3
Rationale: An empathetic response may pave the way for discussion of the effect and meaning of illness for Mr. T.
Cognitive Level: Application
Nursing Process: Implementation
NCLEX: Psychosocial Integrity
Text Page: 296

21. Answer: 4
Rationale: Because the patient with a somatoform disorder is using physical symptoms to express feelings, the goal of verbalizing feelings is appropriate.
Cognitive Level: Application
Nursing Process: Planning
NCLEX: Psychosocial Integrity
Text Page: 294

22. Answer: 4
Rationale: The process of insight-oriented therapy for patients with psychophysiological disorders requires

that the patient's underlying feelings be recognized and supportively confronted.
Cognitive Level: Application
Nursing Process: Implementation
NCLEX: Psychosocial Integrity
Text Page: 297

23. Answer: 3
Rationale: Chlordiazepoxide (Librium) is a benzodiazepine. Tolerance to benzodiazepines develops quickly and leaves the patient needing larger doses of the drug to obtain the desired effect. Because tolerance and dependence on benzodiazepines occur, their use should be of short term.
Cognitive Level: Analysis
Nursing Process: Diagnosis
NCLEX: Psychosocial Integrity
Text Page: 299

24. Answer: 2
Rationale: Conversion symptoms serve the purpose of relieving the patient's anxiety, which is engendered by a conflict. When the symptom must be given up before the conflict is resolved and the patient has no alternative strategy for coping with the repressed anxiety, another symptom may replace the first.
Cognitive Level: Analysis
Nursing Process: Assessment
NCLEX: Psychosocial Integrity
Text Page: 296-297

25. Answer: 4
Rationale: One of the most important ways of promoting adaptive psychophysiological responses involves changing health habits. People who adopt positive health practices and good health measures can prevent biopsychosocial illnesses.
Cognitive Level: Application
Nursing Process: Planning
NCLEX: Psychosocial Integrity
Text Page: 298

CHAPTER 18

1. Answer: 2
Rationale: Self-esteem is most threatened during adolescence, when concepts of self are being modified and new self-decisions are being made.
Cognitive Level: Application
Nursing Process: Assessment
NCLEX: Psychosocial Integrity
Text Page: 306

2. Answer: 2
Rationale: Self-esteem disturbance is defined as having a negative self-evaluation or negative feelings about self or self-capabilities, which may be directly or indirectly expressed.
Cognitive Level: Application
Nursing Process: Diagnosis
NCLEX: Psychosocial Integrity
Text Page: 308

3. Answer: 4
Rationale: Identity diffusion is manifested by behaviors that include disruptions in relationships and problems with intimacy.
Cognitive Level: Application
Nursing Process: Assessment
NCLEX: Psychosocial Integrity
Text Page: 309-310

4. Answer: 3
Rationale: Depersonalization is characterized by feelings of detachment, isolation, alienation, unreality, confusion, and a dreamlike view of the world.
Cognitive Level: Application
Nursing Process: Assessment
NCLEX: Psychosocial Integrity
Text Page: 310-311

5. Answer: 3
Rationale: Each patient described faces threats to security, self-control, and wholeness. However, Gloria's perception of the change is the most negative and potentially jeopardizes her relationships with her peers, thus having a negative effect on her self-esteem.
Cognitive Level: Analysis
Nursing Process: Assessment
NCLEX: Psychosocial Integrity
Text Page: 314

6. Answer: 1
Rationale: Acceptance involves giving support without making demands. Simply sitting with a patient shows acceptance.
Cognitive Level: Application
Nursing Process: Implementation
NCLEX: Psychosocial Integrity
Text Page: 320

7. Answer: 1
Rationale: The first step in expanding self-awareness may be to confirm the identity of a patient with limited ego resources.
Cognitive Level: Application
Nursing Process: Implementation
NCLEX: Psychosocial Integrity
Text Page: 308

8. Answer: 2
Rationale: Simple, concrete directions are appropriate interventions for a patient with self-concept disturbance

evidenced by distorted thinking, passivity, loss of initiative, and inability to make decisions.
Cognitive Level: Application
Nursing Process: Implementation
NCLEX: Psychosocial Integrity
Text Page: 320

9. Answer: 4
Rationale: When patients have difficulty describing feelings, the nurse can use the technique of verbalizing how he or she might have felt in the same situation.
Cognitive Level: Application
Nursing Process: Implementation
NCLEX: Psychosocial Integrity
Text Page: 321-322

10. Answer: 2
Rationale: Letting the patient know that he or she is responsible for his or her own behavior reduces the projection of patient problems onto the environment and fosters empowerment.
Cognitive Level: Application
Nursing Process: Implementation
NCLEX: Psychosocial Integrity
Text Page: 322

11. Answer: 2
Rationale: Empathic communication helps the patient accept his or her own feelings and thoughts. This acceptance is the basis for self-exploration.
Cognitive Level: Analysis
Nursing Process: Planning
NCLEX: Psychosocial Integrity
Text Page: 321

12. Answer: 4
Rationale: Abby shows self-awareness and commitment to change, whereas the remarks of the others express only self-awareness.
Cognitive Level: Analysis
Nursing Process: Evaluation
NCLEX: Psychosocial Integrity
Text Page: 322

13. Answer: 1
Rationale: Self-ideal is one's perception of how one should behave on the basis of personal standards.
Cognitive Level: Application
Nursing Process: Assessment
NCLEX: Psychosocial Integrity
Text Page: 305

14. Answer: 2
Rationale: The self-concept development of a young child is most influenced by the parents. Initially the child views himself or herself as an extension of the parents and is highly sensitive to their perceptions of him or her.
Cognitive Level: Application
Nursing Process: Implementation
NCLEX: Psychosocial Integrity
Text Page: 303-304

15. Answer: 1
Rationale: This remark shows understanding of what the patient has said, and it would encourage the patient to continue talking. Answer 2 is probing, Answer 3 changes the focus, and Answer 4 gives premature advice.
Cognitive Level: Application
Nursing Process: Implementation
NCLEX: Psychosocial Integrity
Text Page: 305

16. Answer: 3
Rationale: This answer gives the correct sequence for addressing the problem of helping the patient alter self-concept. Self-awareness and self-exploration allow self-evaluation. Self-evaluation makes formulation of a plan possible, and support helps the patient achieve goals.
Cognitive Level: Analysis
Nursing Process: Planning
NCLEX: Psychosocial Integrity
Text Page: 320-326

17. Answer: 3
Rationale: Self-actualization is at the highest level of Maslow's hierarchy of needs and is highly desirable. Attaining self-actualization indicates that the alteration in self-concept has been resolved.
Cognitive Level: Application
Nursing Process: Planning
NCLEX: Psychosocial Integrity
Text Page: 327

18. Answer: 1
Rationale: Some degree of ego strength, such as the capacity for reality testing, self-control, or a degree of ego integration, is needed as a foundation for later nursing care.
Cognitive Level: Application
Nursing Process: Planning
NCLEX: Psychosocial Integrity
Text Page: 321

19. Answer: 1
Rationale: Sympathy reinforces self-pity, and self-pity stands in the way of the patient's realizing that the power to change lies within himself or herself, which is the desired outcome of patient self-exploration.
Cognitive Level: Application
Nursing Process: Planning
NCLEX: Psychosocial Integrity
Text Page: 322-323

20. Answer: 4
Rationale: Expressions of low self-esteem can be direct or indirect. The statement in Answer 4 is an indirect statement that is categorized as illusions and unrealistic goals. Other indirect expressions are exaggerated sense of self, boredom, and polarizing view of life. The statements in the other answers represent direct expressions of low self-esteem, including self-criticism (Answer 1), physical manifestations (Answer 2), and disturbed relationships (Answer 3).
Cognitive Level: Application
Nursing Process: Assessment
NCLEX: Psychosocial Integrity
Text Page: 308

21. Answer: 2
Rationale: Encouraging the patient to examine feelings and behavior related to a stressor is part of nursing interventions at level 1 expanded self-awareness. Answer 1 represents level 2 self-exploration. Answer 3 represents level 4 realistic planning, and Answer 4 represents level 3 self-evaluation.
Cognitive Level: Application
Nursing Process: Implementation
NCLEX: Psychosocial Integrity
Text Page: 320

22. Answer: 3
Rationale: Encouraging the patient to examine feelings and behavior related to a stressor is part of nursing interventions at level 2 self-exploration. Answer 1 represents level 4 realistic planning, while Answer 2 represents level 3 self-evaluation. Answer 4 represents level 1 expanded self-awareness.
Cognitive Level: Application
Nursing Process: Implementation
NCLEX: Psychosocial Integrity
Text Page: 321

23. Answer: 2
Rationale: Clarifying that the patient's beliefs affect her feelings and behaviors helps the patient to define the problem clearly and is part of level 3 self-evaluation. Answer 1 helps the nurse to work with whatever ego strength the patient has and represents level 1 expanded self-awareness. Answer 3 helps the patient to accept her own thoughts and feelings and represents level 2 self-exploration. Answer 4 helps the patient to identify alternative solutions and represents level 4 realistic planning.
Cognitive Level: Application
Nursing Process: Implementation
NCLEX: Psychosocial Integrity
Text Page: 324

24. Answer: 2
Rationale: Helping the patient to understand that she can change only herself and not others is part of level 4 realistic planning. Answer 1 helps the patient to accept her own thoughts and feelings and represents level 2 self-exploration. Answer 3 helps the nurse to work with whatever ego strength the patient has and represents level 1 expanded self-awareness. Answer 4 helps the patient to define the problem clearly and is part of level 3 self-evaluation.
Cognitive Level: Application
Nursing Process: Implementation
NCLEX: Psychosocial Integrity
Text Page: 325

25. Answer: 1
Rationale: Commitment to action is the fifth level of nursing intervention. At this time, the nurse helps the patient to commit to the goal and relates to the patient how the nurse sees the patient, correcting a poor self-image. Answers 2, 3, and 4 represent interventions at levels 3, 4, and 1, respectively.
Cognitive Level: Application
Nursing Process: Implementation
NCLEX: Psychosocial Integrity
Text Page: 326

CHAPTER 19

1. Answer: 4
Rationale: Suppression of emotions for a prolonged period is less adaptive than showing emotional responsiveness to loss.
Cognitive Level: Analysis
Nursing Process: Assessment
NCLEX: Safe, Effective Care Environment: Management of Care
Text Page: 331

2. Answer: 3
Rationale: Loss of one's job can precipitate a grief reaction. Mr. J. is showing emotional responsiveness to his loss as evidenced by initial disbelief, anger, and pain.
Cognitive Level: Analysis
Nursing Process: Assessment
NCLEX: Psychosocial Integrity
Text Page: 331

3. Answer: 2
Rationale: Mourning begins with introjection of the lost object. Denial, suppression, and dissociation are seen in delayed grief reactions.
Cognitive Level: Application
Nursing Process: Assessment

NCLEX: Psychosocial Integrity
Text Page: 345-346

4. Answer: 1
Rationale: Inability to cry or express emotions and speaking of the deceased in the present tense suggest the use of denial.
Cognitive Level: Application
Nursing Process: Assessment
NCLEX: Psychosocial Integrity
Text Page: 331

5. Answer: 3
Rationale: This reply is empathetic and allows the nurse to begin teaching the husband the value of expressing feelings related to loss.
Cognitive Level: Application
Nursing Process: Implementation
NCLEX: Psychosocial Integrity
Text Page: 343

6. Answer: 3
Rationale: It is appropriate to help the daughter understand the grieving process, including the fact that normal grieving can take a year or more.
Cognitive Level: Application
Nursing Process: Implementation
NCLEX: Psychosocial Integrity
Text Page: 331

7. Answer: 4
Rationale: Seasonal affective disorder is a fall and winter disorder thought to be associated with shortened hours of daylight and abnormal melatonin metabolism.
Cognitive Level: Analysis
Nursing Process: Assessment
NCLEX: Psychosocial Integrity
Text Page: 334

8. Answer: 4
Rationale: The key element is change. In depression, patients and family see the depression as a change from their usual selves. In mania, others note major changes in usual patterns and responses while patients may indicate they are more creative or active.
Cognitive Level: Application
Nursing Process: Assessment
NCLEX: Psychosocial Integrity
Text Page: 334

9. Answer: 2
Rationale: Severely depressed patients may have suicidal ideation but lack the cognitive ability to plan an attempt and the energy to implement a plan. As depression lifts, the patient may be better able to plan a suicide attempt and may have sufficient energy to carry out a plan. Self-report of feeling less depressed does not mean the risk for self-injury is diminished. Vigilance continues to be necessary.
Cognitive Level: Application
Nursing Process: Planning
NCLEX: Psychosocial Integrity
Text Page: 350

10. Answer: 3
Rationale: Rapport is best established through shared time and supportive companionship, even if the patient talks little. The nurse's presence indicates his or her belief that the patient has worth.
Cognitive Level: Application
Nursing Process: Implementation
NCLEX: Psychosocial Integrity
Text Page: 351

11. Answer: 3
Rationale: Depressed patients need reassurance that their current pain and despair are not permanent. Nurses can convey a sense of hope that treatment will produce change, albeit slowly.
Cognitive Level: Application
Nursing Process: Implementation
NCLEX: Psychosocial Integrity
Text Page: 354

12. Answer: 2
Rationale: Depressed patients often say they feel too full to eat. Fullness may be related to slow stomach emptying. Seeing large portions and thinking one is expected to eat a large amount can be overwhelming. Serving six small, calorie-dense meals often helps the patient increase caloric intake while reducing the patient's negative response to food.
Cognitive Level: Application
Nursing Process: Planning
NCLEX: Psychosocial Integrity
Text Page: 351

13. Answer: 3
Rationale: Cognitive therapy focuses on changing distortions and negative thinking patterns that affect the patient's feelings and behaviors.
Cognitive Level: Application
Nursing Process: Implementation
NCLEX: Psychosocial Integrity
Text Page: 354

14. Answer: 3
Rationale: The expected outcome for a depressed patient is that he or she will be emotionally responsive and return to a pre-illness level of functioning.
Cognitive Level: Application
Nursing Process: Outcome Identification

NCLEX: Psychosocial Integrity
Text Page: 348

15. Answer: 2
Rationale: When depression leads to inadequate hygiene, nurses must matter-of-factly assist the patient to bathe and dress, explaining that the nurse is helping because the patient is unable to do it independently.
Cognitive Level: Application
Nursing Process: Implementation
NCLEX: Psychosocial Integrity
Text Page: 350

16. Answer: 1
Rationale: Patients should be made aware that antidepressant medications work slowly, requiring 2 to 6 weeks for amelioration of symptoms. Patients without this knowledge may discontinue taking the medication, thinking it is not working.
Cognitive Level: Application
Nursing Process: Planning
NCLEX: Safe, Effective Care Environment: Management of Care
Text Page: 351

17. Answer: 2
Rationale: Acute manic states are also life threatening. These patients show poor judgment, excessive risk taking, and an inability to evaluate realistic danger and the consequences of their actions. Extreme hyperactivity can lead to exhaustion and death.
Cognitive Level: Application
Nursing Process: Implementation
NCLEX: Safe, Effective Care Environment: Management of Care
Text Page: 350

18. Answer: 3
Rationale: Hypomania is a state just below mania at which psychomotor activity and other symptoms are less pronounced than those observed when a patient is in the manic state.
Cognitive Level: Application
Nursing Process: Assessment
NCLEX: Psychosocial Integrity
Text Page: 333

19. Answer: 1
Rationale: Manic states are characterized by expansive, abnormally elevated, or irritable moods, impaired social or occupational functioning, increased motor activity, decreased sleep, grandiosity, and rapid, pressured speech.
Cognitive Level: Analysis
Nursing Process: Assessment
NCLEX: Psychosocial Integrity
Text Page: 333

20. Answer: 2
Rationale: Manic patients require reduced environmental stimuli; thus a single room is preferable to a double room. Manic patients often require increased nursing supervision and limit setting to counteract impulsivity, so placing the patient near the nurse's station is preferable to placing him near the entrance, where elopement is easier.
Cognitive Level: Application
Nursing Process: Planning
NCLEX: Safe, Effective Care Environment: Management of Care
Text Page: 351

21. Answer: 3
Rationale: A less stimulating environment would be therapeutic for Mr. A. Because verbal interventions have not been successful in providing the necessary structure, another approach to limit setting should be tried. When sufficient staff members are assembled, one nurse should set limits by saying, "Mr. A., we are here to walk to your room with you." The presence of other staff members ensures that the limit setting can be safely implemented.
Cognitive Level: Application
Nursing Process: Implementation
NCLEX: Psychosocial Integrity
Text Page: 350

22. Answer: 4
Rationale: Bipolar patients are maintained on medication indefinitely to prevent recurrences. The earlier and the more thoroughly the patient understands this need, the more likely it is that he or she will comply with the long-term treatment plan.
Cognitive Level: Application
Nursing Process: Implementation
NCLEX: Psychosocial Integrity
Text Page: 352

23. Answer: 1
Rationale: Inadequate nutrition, dehydration, weight loss, and sleep deprivation are frequent physiological consequences of manic episodes. It is easy for staff members to focus on the arresting affective, cognitive, and behavioral aspects while ignoring basic physical needs of patients.
Cognitive Level: Application
Nursing Process: Planning
NCLEX: Psychosocial Integrity
Text Page: 336, 354, 356

24. Answer: 2
Rationale: Remaining in the dining room does not ensure adequate intake. The patient may argue rather than eat. Providing calorie-dense foods that can be eaten or drunk "on the run" is a better strategy.

Recording food and fluid intake and daily weights is appropriate for evaluation purposes.
Cognitive Level: Analysis
Nursing Process: Planning
NCLEX: Psychosocial Integrity
Text Page: 351

25. Answer: 3
Rationale: Manic patients often have unattainable goals and grandiose self-appraisals. Identifying realistic goals and self-appraisals is indicative of appropriate emotional responsiveness.
Cognitive Level: Evaluation
Nursing Process: Evaluation
NCLEX: Psychosocial Integrity
Text Page: 356

26. Answer: 1
Rationale: ECT remains a viable treatment for depressed patients who do not respond to antidepressants. Light therapy is more useful for seasonal affective disorder than for severe depression. Neuroleptics and benzodiazepines are not therapies of choice for depression.
Cognitive Level: Analysis
Nursing Process: Planning
NCLEX: Safe, Effective Care Environment: Management of Care
Text Page: 352

CHAPTER 20

1. Answer: 2
Rationale: Direct self-destructive behavior includes any form of suicidal threats, attempts, gestures, and completed suicide. Indirect self-destructive behavior is any behavior that is detrimental to the person's physical well-being and that potentially may result in death.
Cognitive Level: Analysis
Nursing Process: Assessment
NCLEX: Psychosocial Integrity
Text Page: 364

2. Answer: 2
Rationale: To think about or attempt self-destruction, the individual must have low self-regard.
Cognitive Level: Analysis
Nursing Process: Diagnosis
NCLEX: Psychosocial Integrity
Text Page: 365

3. Answer: 1
Rationale: The most prominent behavior associated with noncompliance is refusal to admit the seriousness of the illness. This denial interferes with acceptance of treatment.
Cognitive Level: Application
Nursing Process: Planning
NCLEX: Psychosocial Integrity
Text Page: 366

4. Answer: 1
Rationale: Noncompliant people struggle for control. Serious illness is seen as a betrayal by the body. Patients wish to reassert control and prove mastery over their bodies.
Cognitive Level: Analysis
Nursing Process: Implementation
NCLEX: Health Promotion and Maintenance
Text Page: 366

5. Answer: 2
Rationale: The lethality of self-injury is usually low, and patients who self-injure seek relief of tension. Suicide attempts are directed by the wish to die. Care-planning strategies will differ based on underlying patient motivation.
Cognitive Level: Analysis
Nursing Process: Planning
NCLEX: Psychosocial Integrity
Text Page: 367

6. Answer: 2
Rationale: The three aspects of personality most closely associated with increased risk for suicide are hostility, impulsivity, and depression. These traits cross diagnostic groups.
Cognitive Level: Application
Nursing Process: Implementation
NCLEX: Psychosocial Integrity
Text Page: 371

7. Answer: 4
Rationale: The psychiatric diagnoses most closely associated with suicide risk are mood disorders, substance abuse, and schizophrenia.
Cognitive Level: Analysis
Nursing Process: Assessment
NCLEX: Psychosocial Integrity
Text Page: 371

8. Answer: 1
Rationale: Suicide threats are warnings—indirect or direct, verbal or nonverbal—that the person plans to attempt suicide.
Cognitive Level: Application
Nursing Process: Assessment
NCLEX: Psychosocial Integrity
Text Page: 367

9. Answer: 2
Rationale: Answer 2 is directly related to the diagnosis. The other outcomes are desirable but are more appropriate for other diagnoses.

Cognitive Level: Application
Nursing Process: Outcome Identification
NCLEX: Safe, Effective Care Environment: Management of Care
Text Page: 375-376

10. Answer: 3
Rationale: This reply shows empathy, an important quality in developing a relationship. The reply also begins assessment of risk. It is important to determine whether the patient has a plan, the lethality of the method chosen, and whether the patient has the means to implement the plan.
Cognitive Level: Application
Nursing Process: Implementation
NCLEX: Psychosocial Integrity
Text Page: 367

11. Answer: 4
Rationale: Most suicidal patients have some ambivalence. With this strategy, the nurse is appealing to the healthy part of the patient's self that wants to survive and is better able to cope with life.
Cognitive Level: Application
Nursing Process: Implementation
NCLEX: Safe, Effective Care Environment: Management of Care
Text Page: 367

12. Answer: 2
Rationale: The highest suicide rate for any group in this country is among people over age 65, especially white men over 85. Although this group constitutes 12.6% of the total U.S. population, it accounts for about 18.1% of suicide deaths. White males over the age of 50 represent the greatest number of these deaths.
Cognitive Level: Analysis
Nursing Process: Assessment
NCLEX: Psychosocial Integrity
Text Page: 365

13. Answer: 1
Rationale: One-to-one supervision communicates concern to the patient as it offers help in controlling impulses to harm the self.
Cognitive Level: Application
Nursing Process: Implementation
NCLEX: Safe, Effective Care Environment: Management of Care
Text Page: 378

14. Answer: 2
Rationale: Patient involvement in evaluation of progress can provide reinforcement and incentive to work toward a goal.
Cognitive Level: Application
Nursing Process: Evaluation
NCLEX: Safe, Effective Care Environment: Management of Care
Text Page: 381

15. Answer: 3
Rationale: A final issue related to suicidal behavior is the effect of a completed suicide on the clinical staff. Psychiatric nurses will inevitably experience a patient suicide at some time in their careers. When a patient commits suicide, staff response can split the interdisciplinary treatment team. Thus interventions must be aimed not only at helping the individual clinician heal but also at preserving the integrity of the treatment team.
Cognitive Level: Application
Nursing Process: Planning
NCLEX: Psychosocial Integrity
Text Page: 381

16. Answer: 2
Rationale: The treatment plan must first address the goal of protecting the patient from harm. The development of insight and the substitution of healthy coping mechanisms come later.
Cognitive Level: Application
Nursing Process: Implementation
NCLEX: Safe, Effective Care Environment: Management of Care
Text Page: 381

17. Answer: 4
Rationale: This explanation is honest and suggests caring as well as collaboration between the nurse and patient. The other choices are impersonal and do little to convey caring.
Cognitive Level: Application
Nursing Process: Implementation
NCLEX: Safe, Effective Care Environment: Management of Care
Text Page: 378

18. Answer: 1
Rationale: The subject of suicide is not taboo. It should be approached matter-of-factly. If the patient is having suicidal thoughts, he or she is often relieved to be able to talk about them openly.
Cognitive Level: Application
Nursing Process: Implementation
NCLEX: Psychosocial Integrity
Text Page: 368

19. Answer: 1
Rationale: Family history of suicide is a significant risk factor for self-destructive behavior. In addition, monozygotic twins have a high concordance rate for suicide.
Cognitive Level: Application
Nursing Process: Assessment

NCLEX: Psychosocial Integrity
Text Page: 370

20. Answer: 1
Rationale: Self-destructive people have low self-esteem. The nurse may intervene by treating the patient as someone deserving of attention and concern. Positive attributes of the patient should be recognized with genuine praise.
Cognitive Level: Application
Nursing Process: Planning
NCLEX: Psychosocial Integrity
Text Page: 379

21. Answer: 4
Rationale: While under constant supervision the patient is never left alone, even momentarily. Unit restriction requires that the patient remain on the unit at all times.
Cognitive Level: Application
Nursing Process: Implementation
NCLEX: Safe, Effective Care Environment: Management of Care
Text Page: 378

22. Answer: 2
Rationale: Nursing care of suicidal patients should initially be directed toward protection, increasing patient self-esteem, and helping patients to become aware of their feelings, to label them, and to express them appropriately.
Cognitive Level: Application
Nursing Process: Implementation
NCLEX: Psychosocial Integrity
Text Page: 379

23. Answer: 2
Rationale: This question will give the nurse information as to whether a plan exists, the lethality of the method chosen, and the accessibility of the method.
Cognitive Level: Application
Nursing Process: Implementation
NCLEX: Psychosocial Integrity
Text Page: 367

24. Answer: 3
Rationale: Jumping from a high place into swift water when one cannot swim is a highly lethal method. Enacting the plan at night when there is little traffic means there is little provision for rescue. She has a car and can drive, and therefore she has access to the means she has chosen.
Cognitive Level: Analysis
Nursing Process: Assessment
NCLEX: Psychosocial Integrity
Text Page: 367

25. Answer: 4
Rationale: One-to-one supervision is appropriate for suicidal patients who refuse to sign no-harm contracts. In addition, she speaks of "another time," and the plan that was implemented was highly lethal with little provision for being discovered.
Cognitive Level: Analysis
Nursing Process: Planning
NCLEX: Safe, Effective Care Environment: Management of Care
Text Page: 378

CHAPTER 21

1. Answer: 4
Rationale: The information processing of individuals with schizophrenia may be altered by brain deficits affecting memory and attention that then affect retention, ability to focus, and ability to make decisions.
Cognitive Level: Application
Nursing Process: Planning
NCLEX: Psychosocial Integrity
Text Page: 387-388

2. Answer: 2
Rationale: When cognitive functioning is disrupted, self-care deficit may be severe. The nurse may need to dress the patient. Each step of the process of dressing should be undertaken singly, and a simple explanation as to what is expected should be given.
Cognitive Level: Application
Nursing Process: Implementation
NCLEX: Psychosocial Integrity
Text Page: 392

3. Answer: 4
Rationale: Patients with disrupted cognitive functioning have difficulty focusing on an activity in a sustained, concentrated fashion. They may need direction. Because multi-stage commands are often not understood, simple direction should be given one step at a time.
Cognitive Level: Application
Nursing Process: Implementation
NCLEX: Psychosocial Integrity
Text Page: 392, 405

4. Answer: 1
Rationale: When asked, the nurse should point out that he or she is not experiencing the same stimuli but should accept the reality of the hallucinations for the patient. Being able to communicate with the nurse at the time the hallucinations are occurring is helpful to the patient. Interactive discussion of hallucinations is a vital element in the development of reality-testing skills.
Cognitive Level: Application
Nursing Process: Implementation

NCLEX: Psychosocial Integrity
Text Page: 410

5. Answer: 4
Rationale: The two most consistent neurobiological research findings in schizophrenia are imaging studies that show reduced brain volume and abnormal function, and neurochemical studies that show alterations of neurotransmitter systems affecting the prefrontal cortex and the limbic system.
Cognitive Level: Application
Nursing Process: Implementation
NCLEX: Physiological Integrity: Physiological Adaptation
Text Page: 396-397

6. Answer: 4
Rationale: Developing trust is fundamental to developing a nurse-patient relationship. The nurse must demonstrate consistent and genuine caring. Schedule brief (5- to 10-minute), frequent contacts initially. Increase time gradually based on patient agreement.
Cognitive Level: Application
Nursing Process: Implementation
NCLEX: Psychosocial Integrity
Text Page: 402

7. Answer: 3
Rationale: Developing trust is fundamental to working with a delusional patient. There is much assessment data to gather before questioning the facts and their meaning and discussing the consequences of the delusion.
Cognitive Level: Application
Nursing Process: Implementation
NCLEX: Psychosocial Integrity
Text Page: 407-408

8. Answer: 2
Rationale: Engaging the patient in physical activity will help distract the patient and keep her from focusing solely on the delusion. The patient can focus on the delusion while looking as though she is reading or listening to music. The latter two activities are better addressed somewhat later in the course of treatment.
Cognitive Level: Application
Nursing Process: Implementation
NCLEX: Psychosocial Integrity
Text Page: 407-408

9. Answer: 3
Rationale: When the patient or family is aware of the symptoms of an impending relapse, they can use symptom-management strategies to prevent the relapse.
Cognitive Level: Application
Nursing Process: Implementation
NCLEX: Psychosocial Integrity
Text Page: 413

10. Answer: 2
Rationale: Caffeine intake greater than 250 mg daily or smoking 10 to 20 cigarettes daily dramatically reduces the effectiveness of antipsychotic and antianxiety drugs and lithium. The need to limit the use of these substances is an important teaching point.
Cognitive Level: Analysis
Nursing Process: Planning
NCLEX: Physiological Integrity: Pharmacological and Parenteral Therapies
Text Page: 415

11. Answer: 4
Rationale: Interacting with at least one person is desirable to reduce complete withdrawal and isolation. Such interaction provides the basis for formation of trust and the development of a nurse-patient relationship.
Cognitive Level: Application
Nursing Process: Planning
NCLEX: Psychosocial Integrity
Text Page: 402

12. Answer: 1
Rationale: Individuals with paranoid schizophrenia are usually distrustful of others and socially withdrawn. They often have delusions of persecution and auditory hallucinations that further serve to isolate them from others.
Cognitive Level: Analysis
Nursing Process: Diagnosis
NCLEX: Psychosocial Integrity
Text Page: 402-403

13. Answer: 4
Rationale: Problems in cognitive functioning include impaired short-term and long-term memory, poor concentration, distractibility and poor concentration, loose associations, tangentiality, incoherence, illogical speech, concrete thinking, indecisiveness, impaired judgment, and delusions.
Cognitive Level: Application
Nursing Process: Assessment
NCLEX: Psychosocial Integrity
Text Page: 390

14. Answer: 1
Rationale: The person with schizophrenia has brain malfunction resulting in poor memory and attention. The information should be repeated as often as necessary in a kindly, matter-of-fact manner.
Cognitive Level: Application
Nursing Process: Implementation
NCLEX: Psychosocial Integrity
Text Page: 390

15. Answer: 4
Rationale: Patients with schizophrenia are considered to have neurobiological problems. "Soft signs" are

neurological deficits consistent with brain dysfunction of the frontal or parietal lobes. Soft signs include astereognosis, agraphesthesia, dysdiadochokinesia, impaired fine motor skills, increased eye blinking, abnormal smooth pursuit eye movements, and muscle twitches. By contrast, hard signs include loss of function, weakness, diminished reflexes, and paralysis.
Cognitive Level: Application
Nursing Process: Assessment
NCLEX: Psychosocial Integrity
Text Page: 394-395

16. Answer: 3
Rationale: Impulsive activity, talking to people who are not present, and covering the ears are behaviors that may indicate the patient is responding to auditory hallucinations.
Cognitive Level: Analysis
Nursing Process: Assessment
NCLEX: Psychosocial Integrity
Text Page: 409

17. Answer: 1
Rationale: Positive symptoms of schizophrenia represent an excess or distortion of normal function. Delusions and hallucinations are considered psychotic disorders of thinking. The other symptoms listed are noted in schizophrenia, but they are not considered thought disorders.
Cognitive Level: Analysis
Nursing Process: Assessment
NCLEX: Psychosocial Integrity
Text Page: 392

18. Answer: 3
Rationale: An appropriate outcome for a delusional patient is that the patient will interpret reality correctly.
Cognitive Level: Analysis
Nursing Process: Outcome Identification
NCLEX: Psychosocial Integrity
Text Page: 403

19. Answer: 3
Rationale: It is appropriate for the nurse to help the patient place the delusion in a time frame and to identify triggers that may be related to stress or anxiety.
Cognitive Level: Application
Nursing Process: Implementation
NCLEX: Psychosocial Integrity
Text Page: 407-408

20. Answer: 1
Rationale: This question is not appropriate. It is nurse-centered rather than patient-centered. If the patient is talking with the nurse about auditory hallucinations, it is likely that some degree of trust exists. The other information will help the nurse identify ongoing interventions.
Cognitive Level: Application
Nursing Process: Assessment
NCLEX: Psychosocial Integrity
Text Page: 410

21. Answer: 4
Rationale: The patient and family should be made aware of symptom triggers to which the patient is particularly reactive. Triggers may precipitate relapse. Teaching the family to modify this behavior is ideal; but if it is impossible, the patient can be taught to contact a mental health provider.
Cognitive Level: Analysis
Nursing Process: Assessment
NCLEX: Psychosocial Integrity
Text Page: 393, 416

22. Answer: 3
Rationale: Psychotic patients often are preoccupied with internal stimuli and find it difficult to comprehend the words and actions of others. They may misinterpret both words and actions. To gain cooperation, use simple, explicit, concrete explanations and directions.
Cognitive Level: Application
Nursing Process: Implementation
NCLEX: Psychosocial Integrity
Text Page: 407

23. Answer: 1
Rationale: Ms. C. evidences self-care deficit in the areas of bathing/hygiene, dressing/grooming, feeding, and toileting.
Cognitive Level: Analysis
Nursing Process: Diagnosis
NCLEX: Psychosocial Integrity
Text Page: 402-403

24. Answer: 3
Rationale: Believing that others can hear one's unexpressed thoughts is called thought broadcasting.
Cognitive Level: Application
Nursing Process: Assessment
NCLEX: Psychosocial Integrity
Text Page: 392

25. Answer: 3
Rationale: Loose associations reflect a disturbance in thinking in which speech shifts from topic to topic in a random, seemingly unrelated manner. When severe, it results in incoherence.
Cognitive Level: Application
Nursing Process: Assessment
NCLEX: Psychosocial Integrity
Text Page: 391

26. Answer: 4
Rationale: Early identification of signs of impending relapse provides time for intervention with

symptom-management techniques and support systems. Symptom self-management promotes personal empowerment.
Cognitive Level: Application
Nursing Process: Planning
NCLEX: Psychosocial Integrity
Text Page: 405

27. Answer: 2
Rationale: Clozapine, olanzapine, and risperidone are atypical antipsychotics that provide a better response with fewer side effects than the older typical antipsychotic medications. Olanzapine probably will be the drug of choice, because recent research indicates it may have some treatment advantages over risperidone and because it is a safer alternative than clozapine.
Cognitive Level: Application
Nursing Process: Planning
NCLEX: Physiological Integrity: Pharmacological and Parenteral Therapies
Text Page: 410

CHAPTER 22

1. Answer: 4
Rationale: Interdependent relationships allow reliance on others as well as independence. Each lets the other be dependent or independent without needing to control the person's behavior.
Cognitive Level: Application
Nursing Process: Assessment
NCLEX: Psychosocial Integrity
Text Page: 424

2. Answer: 3
Rationale: The three features of personality disorders are: (1) the individual has acquired few strategies for relating, and his or her approaches are inflexible and maladaptive, (2) the individual's needs, perceptions, and behavior tend to foster vicious circles that continue unhelpful patterns and provoke negative reactions from others, and (3) the individual's adaptation is characterized by tenuous stability, fragility, and lack of resilience when faced with stress.
Cognitive Level: Application
Nursing Process: Planning
NCLEX: Psychosocial Integrity
Text Page: 424

3. Answer: 1
Rationale: Antisocial individuals are exploitative and manipulative. They prefer to control others to avoid being controlled.
Cognitive Level: Analysis
Nursing Process: Assessment
NCLEX: Psychosocial Integrity
Text Page: 427

4. Answer: 2
Rationale: Impaired social interaction describes a state in which the person participates in insufficient, excessive, or ineffective social exchange. The last of these three is seen with the patient with antisocial personality disorder.
Cognitive Level: Application
Nursing Process: Analysis
NCLEX: Psychosocial Integrity
Text Page: 428

5. Answer: 3
Rationale: Narcissistic individuals are egocentric people who have fragile self-esteem that drives them to seek admiration and appreciation. As part of this, they display a sense of entitlement, believing they have rights to special treatment.
Cognitive Level: Application
Nursing Process: Assessment
NCLEX: Psychosocial Integrity
Text Page: 429

6. Answer: 1
Rationale: The staff always must seek to convey acceptance of the patient because this is a building block for a therapeutic relationship. Inappropriate behaviors such as manipulation should be identified, their negative consequences to the patient should be discussed, and more adaptive behaviors should be substituted.
Cognitive Level: Application
Nursing Process: Implementation
NCLEX: Psychosocial Integrity
Text Page: 439

7. Answer: 2
Rationale: Patients with antisocial personality disorder usually do not accept responsibility for their actions, and they are unable to problem-solve constructively.
Cognitive Level: Analysis
Nursing Process: Assessment
NCLEX: Psychosocial Integrity
Text Page: 432

8. Answer: 2
Rationale: Projection places responsibility for antisocial behavior outside oneself.
Cognitive Level: Application
Nursing Process: Assessment
NCLEX: Psychosocial Integrity
Text Page: 432

9. Answer: 3
Rationale: Splitting is the inability to integrate good and bad aspects of an object, resulting in treating the

object as all good or all bad. Projective identification is the practice of projecting certain aspects of the self onto another, who then responds to the negative or positive projections in a manner consistent with the projections. When a patient idealizes the nurse, the nurse has a tendency to lose objectivity and move toward over-involvement, overprotection, and indulgence. In this instance, two staff members are protective and indulgent, while others are more realistic.
Cognitive Level: Analysis
Nursing Process: Assessment
NCLEX: Psychosocial Integrity
Text Page: 432

10. Answer: 1
Rationale: Splitting is the inability to integrate the good and bad aspects of an object. The boyfriend is either perfect or the worst person in the world.
Cognitive Level: Application
Nursing Process: Assessment
NCLEX: Psychosocial Integrity
Text Page: 432

11. Answer: 2
Rationale: Narcissism is extreme self-centeredness requiring constant praise, admiration, and appreciation. When this is not forthcoming from others, rage often results.
Cognitive Level: Application
Nursing Process: Assessment
NCLEX: Psychosocial Integrity
Text Page: 432

12. Answer: 3
Rationale: Individuals with antisocial personality disorder are personable and persuasive, often able to convince judges of their good intentions. They are seldom able to maintain the good intentions they profess and revert to antisocial behaviors.
Cognitive Level: Analysis
Nursing Process: Assessment
NCLEX: Psychosocial Integrity
Text Page: 427

13. Answer: 3
Rationale: Features of borderline personality disorder include instability, impulsivity, hypersensitivity, self-destructive behavior, profound mood shifts, and unstable and intense interpersonal relationships.
Cognitive Level: Application
Nursing Process: Planning
NCLEX: Psychosocial Integrity
Text Page: 427

14. Answer: 3
Rationale: When a patient idealizes the nurse, the nurse tends to lose objectivity and move toward over-involvement, overprotection, and indulgence.
Cognitive Level: Application
Nursing Process: Implementation
NCLEX: Psychosocial Integrity
Text Page: 432-433

15. Answer: 1
Rationale: Milieu work is most effective if it focuses on realistic expectations, the process of decision making, and the process of developing interactional behaviors in the here and now.
Cognitive Level: Comprehension
Nursing Process: Implementation
NCLEX: Psychosocial Integrity
Text Page: 438

16. Answer: 3
Rationale: The features described most closely correspond with histrionic personality disorder, a cluster B disorder.
Cognitive Level: Analysis
Nursing Process: Assessment
NCLEX: Psychosocial Integrity
Text Page: 427

17. Answer: 1
Rationale: Devaluation and rejection are based on narcissistic injury. Based on the tendency to see people as all good or all bad, devaluation and rejection of the all-bad object are logical to the person.
Cognitive Level: Comprehension
Nursing Process: Assessment
NCLEX: Psychosocial Integrity
Text Page: 432

18. Answer: 4
Rationale: The behavior described is an example of manipulation. The goal of such behavior is to create conflict in the hope that while family and staff are "fighting among themselves," no one will focus on or place pressure on the patient to change maladaptive social responses.
Cognitive Level: Analysis
Nursing Process: Assessment
NCLEX: Psychosocial Integrity
Text Page: 438

19. Answer: 1
Rationale: Countertransference, a therapist's strong reaction to the patient, should be suspected when the nurse expresses excessively strong positive feelings or excessively strong negative feelings. In this nurse's statement, we see that the countertransference has shifted from positive to negative.
Cognitive Level: Analysis
Nursing Process: Implementation
NCLEX: Psychosocial Integrity
Text Page: 439

20. Answer: 3
Rationale: Although an obvious attempt to manipulate, the patient's proposal provides an opportunity to focus on the patient's feelings about treatment. Answer 3 allows exploration. The other options do not permit exploration.
Cognitive Level: Application
Nursing Process: Implementation
NCLEX: Psychosocial Integrity
Text Page: 439

21. Answer: 4
Rationale: Impulsivity is manifested by an inability to plan, unreliability, unpredictability, failure to learn from experience, and poor judgment. An impulsive person acts to immediately gratify needs without considering the consequences of the action.
Cognitive Level: Application
Nursing Process: Assessment
NCLEX: Psychosocial Integrity
Text Page: 430

22. Answer: 1
Rationale: Setting and maintaining limits is essential to helping the patient improve function. Staff members must collaborate in enforcing clear limits. Frequent meetings that allow the sharing of information are necessary if staff members are to avoid allowing the patient play one against another.
Cognitive Level: Application
Nursing Process: Implementation
NCLEX: Psychosocial Integrity
Text Page: 438-439

23. Answer: 3
Rationale: While each of the options might be part of a plan to care for a patient who is seeking to modify impulsive behavior, the strategy that will help explore the causes and consequences of impulsive behavior is keeping a diary as described above.
Cognitive Level: Application
Nursing Process: Implementation
NCLEX: Psychosocial Integrity
Text Page: 439

24. Answer: 1
Rationale: Behavioral change is slow and difficult, especially for one who sees no advantage to change. Nurses become frustrated with a lack of progress. Focusing on strengths changes the nurse's perspective from negative to positive. Focusing on patient strengths also is important lest patients receive constant negative messages from staff members.
Cognitive Level: Application
Nursing Process: Implementation
NCLEX: Psychosocial Integrity
Text Page: 439

25. Answer: 2
Rationale: A matter-of-fact approach does not reinforce self-mutilating behavior.
Cognitive Level: Application
Nursing Process: Implementation
NCLEX: Psychosocial Integrity
Text Page: 440

26. Answer: 3
Rationale: The establishment of a therapeutic nurse-patient relationship is fundamental to successful treatment. The interventions listed will foster an atmosphere of trust and open expression of thoughts and feelings.
Cognitive Level: Analysis
Nursing Process: Planning
NCLEX: Psychosocial Integrity
Text Page: 437-438

27. Answer: 4
Rationale: Impaired social interaction is a possibility for any patient with a personality disorder. Antisocial patients rarely experience anxiety. Self-mutilation is most common to patients with borderline personality disorder. Formal thought disorder is rarely seen among patients with personality disorders.
Cognitive Level: Analysis
Nursing Process: Diagnosis
NCLEX: Psychosocial Integrity
Text Page: 433

CHAPTER 23

1. Answer: 1
Rationale: Mr. B.'s history suggests a physiological basis for his cognitive disturbance. Vital signs will tell the nurse more about his physical condition.
Cognitive Level: Analysis
Nursing Process: Assessment
NCLEX: Physiological Integrity: Physiological Adaptation
Text Page: 447

2. Answer: 2
Rationale: Defining characteristics of sensory-perceptual alteration are present. For impaired environmental interpretational syndrome to be diagnosed, the confusional state must have been present for 3 to 6 months.
Cognitive Level: Analysis
Nursing Process: Diagnosis
NCLEX: Physiological Integrity: Physiological Adaptation
Text Page: 447-448

3. Answer: 2
Rationale: Reality orientation is generally helpful to patients with cognitive impairment. A patient who is

misinterpreting reality should be reoriented by a nurse who uses a calm manner and soothing voice. Reorientation is the least restrictive way of addressing his behaviors. Restraints or holding him down would increase his agitation; leaving him alone with his girlfriend ignores the hospital's responsibility for his safety.
Cognitive Level: Analysis
Nursing Process: Implementation
NCLEX: Safe, Effective Care Environment: Management of Care
Text Page: 463-464

4. Answer: 4
Rationale: Only Answer 4 is likely to result in substantial intake.
Cognitive Level: Analysis
Nursing Process: Implementation
NCLEX: Physiological Integrity: Basic Care and Comfort
Text Page: 463-464

5. Answer: 1
Rationale: Delirium is the behavioral response to widespread disturbances in cerebral metabolism and usually represents a sudden decline from the previous level of functioning. It usually is considered a medical emergency.
Cognitive Level: Application
Nursing Process: Assessment
NCLEX: Psychosocial Integrity
Text Page: 447-448

6. Answer: 3
Rationale: An empathic response is always helpful, as is gentle, diplomatic reorientation. Abrupt confrontation with reality will increase anxiety, but implicitly agreeing that her husband will come home is fostering false hope.
Cognitive Level: Application
Nursing Process: Implementation
NCLEX: Psychosocial Integrity
Text Page: 466

7. Answer: 3
Rationale: When cognitive ability diminishes in the evening, the pattern is called sundown syndrome. Diminished cognitive ability may result in patient disorientation and agitation.
Cognitive Level: Analysis
Nursing Process: Assessment
NCLEX: Psychosocial Integrity
Text Page: 452

8. Answer: 2
Rationale: Sundown syndrome may be associated with having fewer orienting environmental stimuli, such as planned activities, meals, and contact with others. Frequent interactions with staff members will increase stimuli and provide opportunities for reorientation.
Cognitive Level: Application
Nursing Process: Implementation
NCLEX: Psychosocial Integrity
Text Page: 452

9. Answer: 3
Rationale: The maladaptive cognitive responses of the patient with Alzheimer's disease are associated with the presence of neuritic plaques, neurofibrillary tangles, and cortical atrophy.
Cognitive Level: Analysis
Nursing Process: Diagnosis
NCLEX: Psychosocial Integrity
Text Page: 461

10. Answer: 2
Rationale: This statement is true. Progress is being made in identifying genetic markers that indicate a potential for developing Alzheimer's disease, but tests currently are not available.
Cognitive Level: Application
Nursing Process: Implementation
NCLEX: Psychosocial Integrity
Text Page: 455

11. Answer: 1
Rationale: Delirium is considered a reversible disorder when the cause has been discovered and treated. Most patients who are otherwise healthy can return to their former living arrangements.
Cognitive Level: Application
Nursing Process: Implementation
NCLEX: Psychosocial Integrity
Text Page: 448

12. Answer: 4
Rationale: Slower metabolism and excretion of drugs predisposes the elderly to toxic reactions marked by maladaptive cognitive responses. This is particularly true with anticholinergics and benzodiazepines.
Cognitive Level: Analysis
Nursing Process: Planning
NCLEX: Psychosocial Integrity
Text Page: 456-457

13. Answer: 4
Rationale: In these situations nurses, should identify themselves each time they enter the room and give the patient simple explanations and directives. A patient with cognitive impairment cannot be expected to remember the nurse from visit to visit and will respond better to easily comprehended information. The nurse also should be prepared to repeat directions as often as necessary.
Cognitive Level: Application

Nursing Process: Implementation
NCLEX: Psychosocial Integrity
Text Page: 463-464

14. Answer: 1
Rationale: Restraints may be ordered to keep IV lines open as well as to protect the delirious patient from self-injury or from injuring others. Restraints should not be used until other less-restrictive approaches have been tried, because they often increase, rather than decrease, agitation. A person in restraint always should be under the continuous, direct supervision of a staff member.
Cognitive Level: Analysis
Nursing Process: Planning
NCLEX: Safe, Effective Care Environment: Management of Care
Text Page: 463-464

15. Answer: 2
Rationale: Agnosia is difficulty recognizing well-known objects.
Cognitive Level: Application
Nursing Process: Assessment
NCLEX: Psychosocial Integrity
Text Page: 452

16. Answer: 2
Rationale: Confabulation is the process of making up a response to a question when one cannot remember the answer. It is a face-saving strategy that helps the individual deny memory loss.
Cognitive Level: Application
Nursing Process: Assessment
NCLEX: Psychosocial Integrity
Text Page: 451

17. Answer: 4
Rationale: This measure will best protect patient dignity and preserve functional status at this time.
Cognitive Level: Application
Nursing Process: Planning
NCLEX: Physiological Integrity: Basic Care and Comfort
Text Page: 469

18. Answer: 4
Rationale: Acetylcholinesterase inhibitors such as donepezil and tacrine are increasingly being prescribed to treat Alzheimer's disease. These drugs allow greater concentration of acetylcholine in the brain, thereby improving cognitive function.
Cognitive Level: Analysis
Nursing Process: Planning
NCLEX: Physiological Integrity: Pharmacological and Parenteral Therapies
Text Page: 465

19. Answer: 2
Rationale: A medium-intensity light will reduce shadows and reduce the agitation that comes with misinterpreted stimuli. A weaker-intensity light, such as the typical night light, may produce shadows.
Cognitive Level: Application
Nursing Process: Implementation
NCLEX: Physiological Integrity: Basic Care and Comfort
Text Page: 466

20. Answer: 3
Rationale: Achieving optimum cognitive functioning relates directly to the problem of disturbed thought processes. The other options make appropriate short-term goals.
Cognitive Level: Analysis
Nursing Process: Planning
NCLEX: Psychosocial Integrity
Text Page: 461

21. Answer: 2
Rationale: The behaviors noted are neither adaptive nor totally maladaptive.
Cognitive Level: Synthesis
Nursing Process: Assessment
NCLEX: Psychosocial Integrity
Text Page: 460

22. Answer: 3
Rationale: The area of perception includes misinterpretations, illusions, and hallucinations. Because the patient believes that another nurse is her niece, this can be construed to be a misinterpretation of reality, and as such would be a misperception.
Cognitive Level: Application
Nursing Process: Implementation
NCLEX: Psychosocial Integrity
Text Page: 447

23. Answer: 2
Rationale: Nonaggressive psychomotor behavior includes behaviors characterized by an increase in gross motor movement that does not have a negative effect on others but draws attention because of its repetitive nature. Examples include restlessness, wandering, and pacing.
Cognitive Level: Application
Nursing Process: Assessment
NCLEX: Psychosocial Integrity
Text Page: 452

24. Answer: 1
Rationale: In the adolescent population, dementia is most likely to be associated with juvenile-type Huntington's disease, Wilson's disease, subacute sclerosing panencephalitis, AIDS, substance abuse (especially

inhalants), and head trauma. The other listed disorders are more likely to affect the elderly.
Cognitive Level: Analysis
Nursing Process: Assessment
NCLEX: Physiological Integrity: Physiological Adaptation
Text Page: 458

25. Answer: 4
Rationale: In the prediagnostic phase, families need information that helps them to understand their situation. A single-session consultation is conducted at the time of diagnosis. Support groups and counseling are useful during the role-change phase. Options to reduce caregiver stress are helpful during the chronic caregiving phase.
Cognitive Level: Application
Nursing Process: Implementation
NCLEX: Psychosocial Integrity
Text Page: 468

CHAPTER 24

1. Answer: 4
Rationale: The signs and symptoms listed are consistent with alcohol withdrawal delirium. It usually has its onset 3 to 5 days after the last drink and lasts 2 to 3 days. It is considered a medical emergency.
Cognitive Level: Analysis
Nursing Process: Assessment
NCLEX: Psychosocial Integrity
Text Page: 480-481, 491

2. Answer: 4
Rationale: Maintaining physiologic stability is of highest priority. Withdrawal delirium is often accompanied by loss of fluid and electrolytes through vomiting, diarrhea, and diaphoresis.
Cognitive Level: Analysis
Nursing Process: Planning
NCLEX: Health Promotion and Maintenance
Text Page: 496

3. Answer: 2
Rationale: Admitting to being an alcoholic and staying alcohol-free for a day at a time is basic to the AA program. Members are mutually supported in the effort at abstinence. Being alcohol-free for 24 hours is a manageable goal, whereas many find that contemplating longer periods of sobriety is beyond their abilities.
Cognitive Level: Application
Nursing Process: Implementation
NCLEX: Psychosocial Integrity
Text Page: 506

4. Answer: 3
Rationale: Dysfunctional families often try to protect the patient, avoid confrontation, and blame themselves. These are called enabling behaviors. Making the patient responsible for the consequences of his drinking is difficult and usually requires professional support and/or involvement in Al-Anon.
Cognitive Level: Application
Nursing Process: Implementation
NCLEX: Psychosocial Integrity
Text Page: 505

5. Answer: 1
Rationale: Substances that may potentially contain alcohol must be avoided. The use of antacids would be safe.
Cognitive Level: Application
Nursing Process: Implementation
NCLEX: Safe, Effective Care Environment: Management of Care
Text Page: 499

6. Answer: 4
Rationale: Impairment should be documented by more than one person. The impaired nurse then must be relieved of duty. Further intervention can be planned and implemented at a later time.
Cognitive Level: Application
Nursing Process: Implementation
NCLEX: Safe, Effective Care Environment: Management of Care
Text Page: 510

7. Answer: 4
Rationale: Most health care agencies have employee assistance programs. Counseling for substance abuse is better provided by professionals in a neutral setting than by peers or administrators in the clinical area.
Cognitive Level: Application
Nursing Process: Implementation
NCLEX: Psychosocial Integrity
Text Page: 508

8. Answer: 1
Rationale: Direct offers of support are appropriate just as they are if a colleague is dealing with any other health problem. Avoiding mention is like trying to hide an elephant in the living room. Surreptitious observation and checking are demeaning.
Cognitive Level: Application
Nursing Process: Implementation
NCLEX: Psychosocial Integrity
Text Page: 511

9. Answer: 1
Rationale: PCP ingestion often produces an acutely psychotic state in which the patient is markedly agitated. Violence toward self or others is common. Because the

drug produces anesthesia, the patient may be unaware of pain.
Cognitive Level: Application
Nursing Process: Planning
NCLEX: Safe, Effective Care Environment: Management of Care
Text Page: 499

10. Answer: 2
Rationale: The safety of the patient and others is an important concern. Patients who have ingested PCP often display unprovoked violence and agitation. It is important that the benzodiazepine be administered as soon as the patient is taken to the seclusion room. The seclusion room provides an environment of minimal stimulation, essential to calming the patient.
Cognitive Level: Application
Nursing Process: Implementation
NCLEX: Safe, Effective Care Environment: Management of Care
Text Page: 499

11. Answer: 2
Rationale: Heroin, a CNS depressant, causes sedation. Opiate withdrawal produces flu-like symptoms rather than acute psychosis.
Cognitive Level: Application
Nursing Process: Implementation
NCLEX: Safe, Effective Care Environment: Management of Care
Text Page: 480-481, 485

12. Answer: 1
Rationale: Opiate withdrawal produces flu-like symptoms.
Cognitive Level: Application
Nursing Process: Assessment
NCLEX: Safe, Effective Care Environment: Management of Care
Text Page: 480-481

13. Answer: 1
Rationale: Tolerance to opiates develops when used repeatedly (i.e., a larger amount of the drug is needed to produce the desired effect). If the patient uses heroin or another opiate individually or in conjunction with other drugs, tolerance may be present. In addition, cross-tolerance develops among CNS depressants, meaning that as tolerance to one drug develops, tolerance develops to all other drugs in the group as well.
Cognitive Level: Analysis
Nursing Process: Assessment
NCLEX: Psychosocial Integrity
Text Page: 474

14. Answer: 1
Rationale: Opiate overdose results in lowered blood pressure, a rise in pulse, and respiratory depression.
Cognitive Level: Application
Nursing Process: Assessment
NCLEX: Safe, Effective Care Environment: Management of Care
Text Page: 480-481

15. Answer: 2
Rationale: Naltrexone is an opiate antagonist. It will reverse CNS depression caused by opiates. Nalmefene is a newer opiate antagonist that may be ordered in lieu of naltrexone.
Cognitive Level: Application
Nursing Process: Planning
NCLEX: Safe, Effective Care Environment: Management of Care
Text Page: 499-500

16. Answer: 1
Rationale: Screening tests increase the accuracy of assessment. Exploring alcohol use before a surgical procedure is important, because excessive use may result in the patient experiencing withdrawal symptoms or other alcohol-related problems postoperatively.
Cognitive Level: Application
Nursing Process: Assessment
NCLEX: Safe, Effective Care Environment: Management of Care
Text Page: 477-478

17. Answer: 3
Rationale: Total abstinence is ideal but may not be a realistic long-term goal. It is rare for an addicted person to suddenly stop substance use forever. Most try at least once to use substances in a controlled way. Thus a long-term goal of abstinence or reduced use may help the individual cope with relapses and returns to treatment.
Cognitive Level: Analysis
Nursing Process: Outcome Identification
NCLEX: Health Promotion and Maintenance
Text Page: 494

18. Answer: 1
Rationale: Acknowledging the problem is an appropriate short-term goal. Answer 2 may or may not be of initial value, while Answers 3 and 4 are intermediate to long-term goals.
Cognitive Level: Analysis
Nursing Process: Outcome Identification
NCLEX: Psychosocial Integrity
Text Page: 493-495

19. Answer: 3
Rationale: Initial short-term goals related to abstinence should focus on self. Relationships, job, education, and other issues should be deferred unless they are roadblocks to recovery.

Cognitive Level: Application
Nursing Process: Outcome Identification
NCLEX: Psychosocial Integrity
Text Page: 494-495

20. Answer: 2
Rationale: Physiological stabilization is basic to the success of other goals. When abstinence and a support system to promote abstinence have been developed, attention can be turned to learning about dependence and recovery and developing alternative coping skills.
Cognitive Level: Analysis
Nursing Process: Outcome Identification
NCLEX: Safe, Effective Care Environment: Management of Care
Text Page: 494-495

21. Answer: 2
Rationale: Endorphins or enkephalins are neurotransmitters that bond with opiate receptors in the brain. Release of endorphins occurs with strenuous exercise and medication, and results in a feeling of well-being and reduced cravings.
Cognitive Level: Application
Nursing Process: Implementation
NCLEX: Health Promotion and Maintenance
Text Page: 491

22. Answer: 1
Rationale: Believing one can control drug use despite addiction is based in the coping mechanism of denial. Denial, rationalization, and minimization are coping mechanisms often used by patients who abuse drugs or alcohol.
Cognitive Level: Application
Nursing Process: Assessment
NCLEX: Psychosocial Integrity
Text Page: 492

23. Answer: 2
Rationale: The relevant guidelines are: the longer the half-life of the drug, the longer the withdrawal symptoms will last and the less intense the withdrawal symptoms will be.
Cognitive Level: Application
Nursing Process: Planning
NCLEX: Safe, Effective Care Environment: Management of Care
Text Page: 491

24. Answer: 3
Rationale: Withdrawal from alcohol, barbiturates, and benzodiazepines is similar. The goal is to prevent severe withdrawal symptoms by giving a drug with a similar action that is tapered down and eventually discontinued.
Cognitive Level: Application
Nursing Process: Planning
NCLEX: Safe, Effective Care Environment: Management of Care
Text Page: 480-481

25. Answer: 4
Rationale: A nontolerant individual would be comatose with a BAL of 0.40 g/dl. The fact that the patient can still walk and talk strongly suggests that the patient's body has developed tolerance to alcohol.
Cognitive Level: Analysis
Nursing Process: Assessment
NCLEX: Safe, Effective Care Environment: Management of Care
Text Page: 474

26. Answer: 1
Rationale: Cognitive-behavioral approaches are aimed at improving self-control and social skills to reduce substance use. Self-control strategies include goal-setting, self-monitoring, analysis of drinking antecedents, and learning of alternative coping skills. Social-skills training focuses on learning skills for forming and maintaining interpersonal relationships, assertiveness, and drink refusal.
Cognitive Level: Application
Nursing Process: Implementation
NCLEX: Psychosocial Integrity
Text Page: 504

27. Answer: 1
Rationale: Abstinence and relapse should be viewed as a process rather than distinct events. Recovery is not an all-or-nothing proposition. Success can be measured by improvements, while relapse can be viewed as an error from which to learn—a temporary setback on the road to recovery.
Cognitive Level: Application
Nursing Process: Implementation
NCLEX: Health Promotion and Maintenance
Text Page: 495, 504-505

28. Answer: 3
Rationale: Ineffective coping is a nursing diagnosis that could be used for a patient who abuses any of the mood-altering drugs. Other nursing diagnoses that have wide application to patients who abuse mood-altering drugs are: disturbed sensory perception, disturbed thought processes, and disturbed family processes.
Cognitive Level: Analysis
Nursing Process: Diagnosis
NCLEX: Psychosocial Integrity
Text Page: 495

CHAPTER 25

1. Answer: 3
Rationale: Self-examination before beginning therapeutic work is wise. If the nurse suspects that he or she has an eating disorder, he or she may not be able to provide care for patients who cannot regulate their eating responses.
Cognitive Level: Application
Nursing Process: Implementation
NCLEX: Psychosocial Integrity
Text Page: 527

2. Answer: 4
Rationale: On the continuum of eating regulation responses, a healthy person has balanced eating patterns with appropriate caloric intake and a healthy body weight. Progressing along the continuum from adaptive to maladaptive responses would be occasional overeating or skipping of meals (Answer 3), overeating or fasting under stress (Answer 1), severe dieting or frequent binging/fasting/night eating (Answer 2), and finally anorexia, bulimia, binge-eating disorder, or night eating syndrome.
Cognitive Level: Analysis
Nursing Process: Assessment
NCLEX: Psychosocial Integrity
Text Page: 518

3. Answer: 1
Rationale: The education plan should be built around the concept that self-demand feeding in children promotes adaptive eating regulation responses. This is often difficult to accept for parents who have acquired maladaptive eating regulation responses or who believe various myths about feeding.
Cognitive Level: Application
Nursing Process: Planning
NCLEX: Psychosocial Integrity
Text Page: 524

4. Answer: 2
Rationale: This information relates directly to motivation for change. Answers 3 and 4 evaluate patient insight. Answer 1 relates to environmental support for change.
Cognitive Level: Application
Nursing Process: Assessment
NCLEX: Psychosocial Integrity
Text Page: 525

5. Answer: 4
Rationale: The outcome is a more comprehensive statement than short-term goals that contribute to eventual outcome attainment. The other options should be considered short-term goals.
Cognitive Level: Analysis
Nursing Process: Outcome Identification
NCLEX: Psychosocial Integrity
Text Page: 528

6. Answer: 1
Rationale: Anorectic patients use denial about the appropriateness of body weight, their nutritional intake, their insistence of normalcy, and their need for help.
Cognitive Level: Application
Nursing Process: Assessment
NCLEX: Psychosocial Integrity
Text Page: 525

7. Answer: 2
Rationale: For an anorexic patient, the major issue is about control of the person's life and fears. Whether the fear is of maturity, independence, failure, sexuality, or parental demands, anorectics believe the solution to the problem lies in controlling their food intake and their bodies. With increasing family concern, anorectics also control the focus of significant others.
Cognitive Level: Application
Nursing Process: Planning
NCLEX: Psychosocial Integrity
Text Page: 525

8. Answer: 2
Rationale: The assessment data are most consistent with the medical diagnosis of anorexia nervosa, a disorder in which intense fear of gaining weight leads to a body weight 15% below normal for height and amenorrhea.
Cognitive Level: Analysis
Nursing Process: Assessment
NCLEX: Psychosocial Integrity
Text Page: 527

9. Answer: 1
Rationale: Hospitalization would be appropriate because reinstatement of physiologic stability is a high priority and may not be possible on an outpatient basis because of the patient's reluctance to accept treatment. Vital signs are below normal, skin turgor indicates dehydration, there has been weight loss of more than 30% of the patient's body weight over the past 3 months, and further assessment of fluid and electrolyte balance is necessary.
Cognitive Level: Analysis
Nursing Process: Assessment
NCLEX: Psychosocial Integrity
Text Page: 522

10. Answer: 3
Rationale: The patient is malnourished and is experiencing dehydration, as evidenced by the low BP, poor skin turgor, and high urine specific gravity. For this reason, highest priority should be placed on restoring

circulating volume, followed by increasing caloric intake. When the primary physiological needs are being met (according to Maslow), secondary needs such as body image can be addressed, and powerlessness can be explored if it applies.
Cognitive Level: Analysis
Nursing Process: Diagnosis
NCLEX: Psychosocial Integrity
Text Page: 529

11. Answer: 1
Rationale: A nurse-patient contract obtains commitment to the treatment process. By signing a contract, the patient will understand the treatment she will be receiving and will be able to make informed decisions about treatment and honoring the contract.
Cognitive Level: Application
Nursing Process: Implementation
NCLEX: Psychosocial Integrity
Text Page: 529

12. Answer: 3
Rationale: Anorectic patients are underweight; the patient with bulimia has experienced less weight loss. Both may be malnourished. Anorectics deny hunger. Bulimics experience hunger. Anorectics have body-image distortion; bulimics are more likely to experience body-image dissatisfaction.
Cognitive Level: Analysis
Nursing Process: Assessment
NCLEX: Psychosocial Integrity
Text Page: 528

13. Answer: 1
Rationale: Nursing interventions that help to achieve this goal involve the use of protocols that specify the number of meals and their timing, and that the diet is balanced. Exercise for the purpose of compensating for additional caloric intake is discouraged. Contracts should be enforced 100% of the time. The frequency of weighing is also determined as part of a treatment protocol and is not used as a reward for eating.
Cognitive Level: Application
Nursing Process: Outcome Identification
NCLEX: Psychosocial Integrity
Text Page: 529-530

14. Answer: 2
Rationale: The first goal is that the patient is able to eat meals that are served. From there, the patient may assume some control over scheduling of meals and food selection. Finally, the patient can shop for food and prepare it under supervision.
Cognitive Level: Application
Nursing Process: Outcome Identification
NCLEX: Psychosocial Integrity
Text Page: 539

15. Answer: 3
Rationale: It is often difficult to secure patient cooperation with treatment. A contract helps engage the patient in the therapeutic alliance and obtains commitment to the treatment process.
Cognitive Level: Application
Nursing Process: Implementation
NCLEX: Psychosocial Integrity
Text Page: 538

16. Answer: 3
Rationale: Eating disorders clearly involve cognitive distortions and faulty thinking about body shape, body weight, and food. Research has shown that cognitive-behavioral therapy is superior to other types of psychotherapy.
Cognitive Level: Application
Nursing Process: Planning
NCLEX: Psychosocial Integrity
Text Page: 530-531

17. Answer: 2
Rationale: Bingeing is a maladaptive eating response to feelings of isolation and loneliness and is not a cure for those feelings. The other statements do not represent cognitive distortions.
Cognitive Level: Analysis
Nursing Process: Assessment
NCLEX: Psychosocial Integrity
Text Page: 530-531

18. Answer: 1
Rationale: Antidepressant medications have been shown to have a therapeutic benefit for many patients with bulimia and binge-eating disorder. Because the side-effect profile is least troublesome for SSRI antidepressants, this is the type of medication the nurse can expect to be used.
Cognitive Level: Application
Nursing Process: Planning
NCLEX: Psychosocial Integrity
Text Page: 533, 535

19. Answer: 2
Rationale: Constructive strategies for coping with anxiety include the use of progressive relaxation, imagery, and meditation. Each is designed to replace feelings of anxiety with feelings of relaxation and well-being.
Cognitive Level: Application
Nursing Process: Planning
NCLEX: Psychosocial Integrity
Text Page: 531

20. Answer: 3
Rationale: Answers 1, 2, and 4 represent questions that should be answered as part of the evaluation of care for a patient with an eating disorder. Answer 3 is not

within the evaluation parameters because there is no absolute evidence that neurotransmitter imbalances are a cause of eating disorders.
Cognitive Level: Application
Nursing Process: Evaluation
NCLEX: Psychosocial Integrity
Text Page: 543

21. Answer: 2
Rationale: A person with bulimia typically is of average weight or is slightly overweight and has a history of unsuccessful dieting. The individuals in Answers 1 and 3 have excessive weight, and the individual in Answer 4 uses dance and calorie counting, rather than bingeing and purging, to maintain weight.
Cognitive Level: Analysis
Nursing Process: Assessment
NCLEX: Psychosocial Integrity
Text Page: 520

22. Answer: 2
Rationale: Comorbid major depression or dysthymia has been reported in 50% to 75% of people with anorexia and bulimia, and obsessive-compulsive disorder may be found in as many as 25% of patients with anorexia nervosa. Anxiety disorders and substance abuse also occur, but their incidence is lower than depression. Individuals who have binge-eating disorder, not anorexia nervosa, are more likely to have a personality disorder. Schizophrenia is not reported to be associated with anorexia nervosa.
Cognitive Level: Application
Nursing Process: Assessment
NCLEX: Psychosocial Integrity
Text Page: 522

23. Answer: 3
Rationale: Parents need to be aware of the difference between physical hunger and psychological hunger. The meal patterns in Answer 1 are excessive and could lead to overweight in some children. Indicating an interest in learning about healthy eating patterns (Answer 2) is a good first step but is not an outcome. Using food as a reward (Answer 4) is not healthy and is not an appropriate outcome.
Cognitive Level: Analysis
Nursing Process: Evaluation
NCLEX: Psychosocial Integrity
Text Page: 524

24. Answer: 4
Rationale: Individuals with anorexia nervosa without bingeing or purging tend to deny the experience of hunger, are introverted, rarely use laxatives or diuretics, and tend to be sexually inactive.
Cognitive Level: Application
Nursing Process: Assessment
NCLEX: Psychosocial Integrity
Text Page: 528

25. Answer: 2
Rationale: Individuals with bulimia nervosa without bingeing or purging tend to abuse laxatives and/or diuretics and tend to be extroverted and sexually active, and experience hunger.
Cognitive Level: Application
Nursing Process: Assessment
NCLEX: Psychosocial Integrity
Text Page: 528

26. Answer: 1
Rationale: In magnification, the patient overestimates the significance of undesirable events. Stimuli are embellished with meaning not supported by objective analogies, such as the statement in Answer 1. The remaining answers list other types of cognitive distortions that often accompany maladaptive eating responses.
Cognitive Level: Application
Nursing Process: Assessment
NCLEX: Psychosocial Integrity
Text Page: 531

27. Answer: 3
Rationale: Personalization is an egocentric interpretation of impersonal events or overinterpretation of events related to the self, such as the statement in Answer 3. The remaining answers list other types of cognitive distortions that often accompany maladaptive eating responses.
Cognitive Level: Application
Nursing Process: Assessment
NCLEX: Psychosocial Integrity
Text Page: 531

CHAPTER 26

1. Answer: 2
Rationale: Giving a direct answer is appropriate because the patient is seeking information. Answer 1 may cause her to needlessly blame herself. Answer 3 denies her right to be distressed. Answer 4 is challenging.
Cognitive Level: Application
Nursing Process: Implementation
NCLEX: Psychosocial Integrity
Text Page: 542

2. Answer: 1
Rationale: A transsexual is a person who is anatomically a male or female but who expresses strong conviction that he or she has the mind and feelings of the opposite sex.
Cognitive Level: Application

Nursing Process: Assessment
NCLEX: Psychosocial Integrity
Text Page: 542

3. Answer: 4
Rationale: Cognitive dissonance arises when two opposing beliefs exist at the same time.
Cognitive Level: Application
Nursing Process: Assessment
NCLEX: Psychosocial Integrity
Text Page: 540

4. Answer: 3
Rationale: In the stage of anxiety, the nurse may exhibit behaviors that hinder the discussion of sexual issues such as talking too much, failing to listen, and being preoccupied with facts rather than feelings.
Cognitive Level: Application
Nursing Process: Assessment
NCLEX: Psychosocial Integrity
Text Page: 540

5. Answer: 2
Rationale: The sexual expression of patients with psychiatric illness may be inappropriate and, at times, intrusive. The patient may not be able to understand or control sexual thoughts or impulses. Nursing intervention should protect the patient from the consequences of his own poor judgment whenever possible and should be achieved in a neutral, nonjudgmental manner.
Cognitive Level: Application
Nursing Process: Implementation
NCLEX: Psychosocial Integrity
Text Page: 545

6. Answer: 4
Rationale: This question is more sensitive than the other answers and is worded so as to make the patient more comfortable in answering.
Cognitive Level: Application
Nursing Process: Assessment
NCLEX: Psychosocial Integrity
Text Page: 541

7. Answer: 4
Rationale: Termination is a time for evaluating progress and bidding farewell. Patients who view their nurses in a positive fashion are often reluctant to terminate and seek to continue the relationship on a social basis after discharge. Helping the patient clarify the therapeutic aspect of the nursing role is appropriate.
Cognitive Level: Application
Nursing Process: Implementation
NCLEX: Psychosocial Integrity
Text Page: 552-553

8. Answer: 3
Rationale: When patients behave seductively toward nurses, it is appropriate to set limits firmly and matter-of-factly.
Cognitive Level: Application
Nursing Process: Implementation
NCLEX: Psychosocial Integrity
Text Page: 552-553

9. Answer: 2
Rationale: Masters and Johnson believe that attitudes and ignorance are responsible for most sexual dysfunction. Their therapeutic model emphasizes education about sexual function, alleviation of performance anxiety, and an increase in warm, comfortable feelings between partners. There is no attempt to employ the uncovering used in psychoanalytic treatment.
Cognitive Level: Application
Nursing Process: Planning
NCLEX: Psychosocial Integrity
Text Page: 558

10. Answer: 1
Rationale: Evaluation factors include patient sense of well-being, functioning ability, and satisfaction with treatment.
Cognitive Level: Application
Nursing Process: Evaluation
NCLEX: Psychosocial Integrity
Text Page: 558

11. Answer: 1
Rationale: Vaginismus is defined as recurrent or persistent involuntary spasm of the musculature of the outer third of the vagina that interferes with coitus.
Cognitive Level: Application
Nursing Process: Assessment
NCLEX: Psychosocial Integrity
Text Page: 550

12. Answer: 2
Rationale: Sexual dysfunction is a state in which an individual expresses concern about his or her sexuality. This diagnosis would be equally applicable to either of the patients described above.
Cognitive Level: Analysis
Nursing Process: Diagnosis
NCLEX: Psychosocial Integrity
Text Page: 547-548

13. Answer: 3
Rationale: Understanding that one should say "no" is much simpler than saying "no" when under pressure. A sex education program must give students tools with which to make appropriate decisions and the behavioral skills necessary to implement the decisions.

Role playing assertive ways of saying "no" is the only behaviorally focused intervention listed.
Cognitive Level: Application
Nursing Process: Planning
NCLEX: Psychosocial Integrity
Text Page: 552

14. Answer: 3
Rationale: Sexually, men and women in good health can function effectively throughout the life span. The other answers are sexual myths that the nurse should address.
Cognitive Level: Analysis
Nursing Process: Evaluation
NCLEX: Psychosocial Integrity
Text Page: 546-547

15. Answer: 4
Rationale: Sexual attraction and fantasy are part of the human experience. Nurses are not immune. Nurses, however, must recognize and deal appropriately with the feelings or risk interference with the quality of care. The feelings should not be denied, nor should they be tested or shared with the patient. It is the nurse's responsibility to preserve professional boundaries. Consultation is a constructive way of dealing with the situation.
Cognitive Level: Analysis
Nursing Process: Implementation
NCLEX: Psychosocial Integrity
Text Page: 552

16. Answer: 3
Rationale: Exploration of fears and feelings should be the initial intervention after the patient's statement of concern. Each of the other interventions might be appropriate at a later time.
Cognitive Level: Application
Nursing Process: Implementation
NCLEX: Psychosocial Integrity
Text Page: 544-545

17. Answer: 1
Rationale: A nursing history should include questions about sexual health. The side effects of several groups of drugs include impotence or delayed ejaculation in men and diminished responsiveness in women.
Cognitive Level: Knowledge
Nursing Process: Assessment
NCLEX: Psychosocial Integrity
Text Page: 545-546

18. Answer: 3
Rationale: Antihypertensive medications, antihistamines, anticholinergics, chemotherapeutic agents, and anti-seizure drugs can cause reduced sexual desire and/or orgasmic disorders in both men and women. The other drug classes listed are not known for these types of effects.
Cognitive Level: Application
Nursing Process: Assessment
NCLEX: Psychosocial Integrity
Text Page: 545

19. Answer: 4
Rationale: Validating terminology is a vital first step. After the nurse understands the patient's complaint, further assessment can take place.
Cognitive Level: Application
Nursing Process: Assessment
NCLEX: Psychosocial Integrity
Text Page: 541

20. Answer: 4
Rationale: An expected outcome is a broad statement relating to resolution of maladaptive sexual response. Answer 4 meets this description. Answers 1, 2, and 3 are more circumscribed and are considered short-term goals.
Cognitive Level: Application
Nursing Process: Outcome Identification
NCLEX: Psychosocial Integrity
Text Page: 548-549

21. Answer: 2
Rationale: Hypersexuality may be the first symptom of a manic episode. In depression, sexuality responses tend to be decreased. There are no specific patterns of altered sexuality associated with personality disorders or obsessive-compulsive disorder.
Cognitive Level: Application
Nursing Process: Assessment
NCLEX: Psychosocial Integrity
Text Page: 545

22. Answer: 1
Rationale: Many people who have transient variations in sexual response do not have a medically diagnosed health problem. Those with more severe or persistent problems are classified as having one of the disorders outlined in Answers 2, 3, and 4.
Cognitive Level: Application
Nursing Process: Assessment
NCLEX: Psychosocial Integrity
Text Page: 548

23. Answer: 2
Rationale: Sildenafil is taken in pill form 1 hour before sex and requires sexual stimulation to be effective. It has been effective for many men suffering from erectile dysfunction, although any relationship issues also must be addressed for satisfactory treatment of this dysfunction.
Cognitive Level: Application

Nursing Process: Implementation
NCLEX: Physiological Integrity: Pharmacological and Parenteral Therapies
Text Page: 558

24. Answer: 3
Rationale: Patients who believe they are transsexual and request surgical reassignment must: have two therapists agree that the surgery is indicated, be of legal age, and live in the preferred gender identity role for at least 1 year. Follow-up care also is generally recommended, but Answer 4 is a false statement.
Cognitive Level: Application
Nursing Process: Implementation
NCLEX: Psychosocial Integrity
Text Page: 556

25. Answer: 4
Rationale: Revictimization is a social problem that many survivors of sexual abuse encounter in that they also become victims of sexual violence at least once in an adult relationship. Answers 1, 2, and 3 identify behavioral problems after sexual abuse.
Cognitive Level: Application
Nursing Process: Assessment
NCLEX: Psychosocial Integrity
Text Page: 556

CHAPTER 27

1. Answer: 1
Rationale: This question requires identification of the therapeutic nursing intervention that would reduce the patient's risk for developing drug interactions. There are drug interactions that can occur with other medications, alcohol, nutrients, and herbs. Of the four answers given, Answer 1 will help the nurse ensure adequate nutrition and hydration. The specific implementation or nursing intervention requires the nurse to apply knowledge of risk factors for the development of drug interactions. These include the following: drug coadministration, high doses, geriatric status, debilitation or dehydration, concurrent illness, compromised organ-system functioning, inadequate patient education, history of medication nonadherence or noncompliance, and failure to include the patient in treatment planning.
Cognitive Level: Application
Nursing Process: Implementation
NCLEX: Physiological Integrity: Pharmacological and Parenteral Therapies
Text Page: 569

2. Answer: 2
Rationale: This question requires the application of knowledge about selective serotonin reuptake inhibitors (SSRIs) to a specific plan for medication education. When teaching patients who are taking tricyclic antidepressants (TCAs), one must emphasize that patients should dangle their legs over the bed and change positions slowly to prevent postural hypotension. It is also advisable for patients to increase fluids, exercise, and roughage intake to prevent the anticholinergic effects of antidepressants. Foods that contain tyramine (e.g., Chianti, nuts, cheese) are prohibited when patients are taking monoamine oxidase inhibitors (MAOIs).

The primary synaptic activity for SSRIs is to inhibit the reuptake of 5HT. The possible clinical effects of 5 HT include the following: GI disturbances and sexual dysfunction. Fluoxetine hydrochloride (Prozac), an SSRI that is usually administered in the morning to reduce the potential of a side-effect profile that is 2+ for insomnia/agitation, also demonstrates a 3+ for GI disturbances. To reduce nausea, the patient should be advised to take the medicine with meals.
Cognitive Level: Application
Nursing Process: Planning
NCLEX: Psychosocial Integrity
Text Pages: 579-583

3. Answer: 1
Rationale: This question requires analytical decision making to identify hypertensive crises and data for the evaluation process. Knowing when the last dose of the monoamine oxidase inhibitor (MAOI) was taken helps determine immediate treatment. Although the ingestion of alcohol is pertinent to determining what tyramine-containing foods the patient may have had, it is not as crucial as knowing when the last dose of MAOI was consumed. Although natural foods may produce similar bioactivity and other antidepressants should not be taken along with an MAOI, these answers do not reflect medication assessment and evaluation.

The patient is experiencing the clinical manifestation of hypertensive crisis. The classic symptoms of this condition are severe occipital headache, dilated pupils, hypertension, and palpitations or arrhythmias. This syndrome can be caused when the patient who is taking an MAOI ingests food containing tyramine, an amino acid released from foods that undergo hydrolysis (e.g., fermentation, aging, pickling, smoking, spoilage). This inhibits the monoamine oxidase and allows tyramine to reach the adrenergic nerve endings and cause the release of excess norepinephrine, which causes hypertensive crisis. To confirm the physical syndrome, first determine whether the patient is taking an MAOI. Knowing when the last dose was ingested provides a window for the duration of hypertension and therapeutic nursing interventions.
Cognitive Level: Analysis
Nursing Process: Evaluation
NCLEX: Safe Physiological Integrity: Pharmacological and Parenteral Therapies
Text Page: 583

4. Answer: 4
Rationale: Blurred vision, an anticholinergic side effect of antidepressant and antipsychotic medications, will usually resolve within 1 to 2 weeks. The most therapeutic intervention is the one that assesses the patient's recall of medication teaching. Moreover, it offers a strategy to assist the patient to cope during work time. Other interventions for blurred vision include the use of large print and cautioning the patient against operating potentially hazardous equipment.

The nurse must apply knowledge of the anticholinergic side effects of antidepressants and antipsychotics to select the appropriate nursing intervention for the patient's problem. Although ECT may be offered when patients are unable to take medication, it is premature to suggest ECT or other medications, and these suggestions reflect a knowledge deficit. It is considered best to encourage patients to maintain activities of daily living and work, if possible.
Cognitive Level: Application
Nursing Process: Implementation
NCLEX: Psychosocial Integrity
Text Page: 582

5. Answer: 1
Rationale: Most patients who respond initially to antidepressant therapy require at least 1 year of therapy and may take medication on a lifetime basis. This is similar to patients who take antihypertensives or insulin. The patient's statement alerts the nurse to set clear therapy goals that extend beyond medication assessment. Prozac takes 2 to 4 weeks to reach a steady state and is maintained in the body for several weeks after it is discontinued, but the nurse's suggestion of tapering off the medication is a wise intervention for this patient, who seems impulsive about medication adherence.

A patient with a knowledge deficit and nonadherence potential requires communication that recalls prior teaching and that builds on the knowledge he or she already has. Reminding the patient of the time it takes to become depressed provides anticipatory guidance about the possibility of needing medication on a lifetime basis. Sarcastic humor is usually a poor response that demeans the patient and may reflect the nurse's impatience and a judgmental attitude toward the patient, and a laissez-faire response does not reflect a caring attitude. Withdrawal usually is not a problem for medications with a long half-life.
Cognitive Level: Analysis
Nursing Process: Implementation
NCLEX: Psychosocial Integrity
Text Page: 567, 598

6. Answer: 3
Rationale: By blocking dopamine, antipsychotic medications produce extrapyramidal side effects. Akathisia is internal or external restless fidgeting or pacing. Patients with akathisia demonstrate motoric restlessness and complain of feeling their muscles quiver. When this condition has advanced, the patient will say that he or she is not able to sit still or lie down quietly. The nurse will want to observe whether the patient's legs are shaking. If the patient's feet are not shaking, the nurse will observe that his or her arms will start to shake. The therapeutic treatment is the administration of anticholinergic agents such as benztropine (Cogentin), trihexyphenidyl (Artane), or procyclidine (Kemadrin).

Diphenhydramine (Benadryl), an antihistamine, also may be administered. The other three medication selections are antipsychotic agents: Zyprexa, an atypical antipsychotic; Moban, an antipsychotic (dihydroindolone); and Mellaril (phenothiazine), a typical antipsychotic.
Cognitive Level: Application
Nursing Process: Evaluation
NCLEX: Physiological Integrity: Pharmacological and Parenteral Therapies
Text Page: 592

7. Answer: 2
Rationale: No consent form is required for this 24-hour urine and serum collection. Blood may be drawn at any time during the collection (if using Vacutainer, one red, red-gray, or gold top tube is needed). In the morning, the first voiding is discarded, then the collection is timed and urine is collected for 24 hours. All urine is stored in a clean, 3-L plastic container that is refrigerated when not in use and then delivered to the lab. Teaching the patient the procedure for a 24-hour creatinine clearance as part of a prelithium workup (urinalysis, BUN, TSH, T3 and T4, FBS, and a complete physical examination with history and workup for family history of renal disease, diabetes mellitus, hypertension, diuretic use, and analgesic abuse) is required.
Cognitive Level: Application
Nursing Process: Implementation
NCLEX: Safe, Effective Care Environment: Management of Care
Text Page: 585

8. Answer: 1
Rationale: Amitriptyline (Elavil) is a tricyclic antidepressant (TCA) medication (tertiary amine). The TCAs are very toxic when ingested at levels of 1000 mg to 3000 mg, and overdosage and suicide attempts with this medication are extremely dangerous and often require emergency medical attention.

Because an overdose often requires only a 1-week supply of medication, it is the nurse's responsibility to suggest that the prescription be dispensed in weekly doses. In the above situation, the patient has a history of self-directed lethality, and prudence is the best approach. By asking the patient to help the nurse determine the easiest method of dispensing medication, the

nurse allows the patient control and offers respect and mutuality.
Cognitive Level: Analysis
Nursing Process: Implementation
NCLEX: Safe, Effective Care Environment: Management of Care
Text Page: 578, 597

9. Answer: 2
Rationale: Tardive dyskinesia usually occurs with long-term conventional antipsychotic agent treatment and is evidenced by stereotypical involuntary movements (e.g., tongue protrusion, lip smacking, chewing, blinking, grimacing, choreiform movements of the limbs and trunk, and foot tapping). Although there is no treatment for tardive dyskinesia, preventive measures such as frequent use of the AIMS and supervised drug holidays have contributed greatly to reducing its occurrence.
Cognitive Level: Analysis
Nursing Process: Assessment
NCLEX: Safe Physiological Integrity: Pharmacological and Parenteral Therapies
Text Page: 591

10. Answer: 2
Rationale: Although agranulocytosis occurs in only about 1% to 2% of patients, this is a risk 10 to 20 times greater than the risk with standard antipsychotic agents. In addition, even though the risk for this adverse effect decreases substantially after 5 months of taking these drugs, the risk always remains and requires vigilant monitoring. After the first 6 months, blood counts are drawn biweekly, so the nurse in the above situation would want to obtain one today to determine whether the patient is experiencing agranulocytosis or flu. Although this is a serious adverse effect, the nurse will provide specific instructions but endeavor not to alarm the patient. In addition, the fact that this patient is female and of an older age places her at increased risk for agranulocytosis.
Cognitive Level: Application
Nursing Process: Implementation
NCLEX: Psychosocial Integrity
Text Page: 591

11. Answer: 2
Rationale: Increased sensitivity to sunlight is one of most common side effects of antipsychotic agents. The patient will need to be instructed of the importance of using a sunscreen at all times when in the sun. This statement is the only one that refers to the patient's current circumstances, and weight gain actually is among the other common antipsychotic side effects.
Cognitive Level: Analysis
Nursing Process: Assessment
NCLEX: Physiological Integrity: Pharmacological and Parenteral Therapies
Text Page: 591

12. Answer: 2
Rationale: Nonadherence or noncompliance with medication is usually lessened with the decanoate preparation of the antipsychotic medication. The most therapeutic communication is usually the one that helps the patient to share thoughts and feelings. By restating and seeking clarification, the nurse can assist the patient in looking at what he or she is saying. If the nurse focuses, the patient will be able to help with the thinking-through process, which is to communicate that the Prolixin injections are received only 12 to 14 times annually and that they will keep the patient's thoughts clear.
Cognitive Level: Analysis
Nursing Process: Implementation
NCLEX: Psychosocial Integrity
Text Page: 567, 592

13. Answer: 1
Rationale: The most common side effects of antipsychotic medications include the following: dry mouth, blurred vision, nasal stuffiness, weight gain, difficulty urinating, infection, decreased sweating, increased sensitivity to sunlight, yellowing of the eyes (especially the whites of the eyes), breast enlargement/lactation, skin rash, anhedonia, itchy skin, and constipation.
Cognitive Level: Analysis
Nursing Process: Evaluation
NCLEX: Physiological Integrity: Pharmacological and Parenteral Therapies
Text Page: 591

14. Answer: 1
Rationale: Fluphenazine (Prolixin) may cause the side effect of infection, because this medication can reduce the normal bacteria in the patient's mouth and increase sensitivity to infection. A thick white coating on the tongue is indicative of infection and must be treated. Brushing the tongue and teeth is a good preventive measure. The measures the nurse is offering will prevent recurrence if paired with adequate hydration.
Cognitive Level: Analysis
Nursing Process: Implementation
NCLEX: Safe, Effective Care Environment: Management of Care
Text Page: 591

15. Answer: 1
Rationale: Constipation, an anticholinergic side effect, is alleviated by drinking of 6 to 8 glasses of water and eating of bran and green vegetables daily. Prunes and raisins are especially helpful. If the side effect continues, the patient should notify the physician and use a laxative only when medically advised to do so.

Cognitive Level: Analysis
Nursing Process: Planning
NCLEX: Physiological Integrity: Pharmacological and Parenteral Therapies
Text Page: 582

16. Answer: 1
Rationale: Lithium crosses the placental barrier and is excreted in the breast milk, so breast-feeding is not an option. Furthermore, patients who are taking lithium are taught to notify their physician immediately if they are planning to become pregnant or think that they are pregnant.
Cognitive Level: Application
Nursing Process: Implementation
NCLEX: Safe, Effective Care Environment: Management of Care
Text Page: 586

17. Answer: 1
Rationale: The psychiatrist or advanced practice nurse (psychiatric clinical specialist) will wait 2 weeks before changing from a selective serotonin reuptake inhibitor (SSRI) to a monoamine oxidase inhibitor (MAOI). The SSRI should not be administered concomitantly with a MAOI. Foods that contain tyramine (e.g., Chianti, nuts, figs, cheese), a pressor amine, are avoided to prevent hypertensive crisis.
Cognitive Level: Application
Nursing Process: Implementation
NCLEX: Safe, Effective Care Environment: Management of Care
Text Page: 579-580

18. Answer: 1
Rationale: Antidepressant medications can cause orthostatic or postural hypotension, and the nurse will teach the patient the following: Lie down, rest as able, and change positions slowly. Dangle at the side of the bed for 30 seconds or so. Operate heavy equipment and drive a car only with caution. Check and record your blood pressure, both sitting and standing, twice a day.
Cognitive Level: Application
Nursing Process: Implementation
NCLEX: Safe, Effective Care Environment: Management of Care
Text Page: 581

19. Answer: 3
Rationale: Benzodiazepine side effects include drowsiness, confusion, lethargy, dizziness, blurred vision, rash or "itchy skin," unusual nervousness or irritability, headache, and nausea. So, Answers 1 and 4 indicate that the patient is actually obtaining relief from the benzodiazepine, and physiological dependency (Answer 2) is unlikely, whereas psychological dependency can occur if the patient is not taught effective ways to manage anxiety aside from taking a pill.
Cognitive Level: Analysis
Nursing Process: Assessment
NCLEX: Safe, Effective Care Environment: Management of Care
Text Page: 575, 581

20. Answer: 2
Rationale: Although the risk of physiological addiction with benzodiazepines is low, the patient seems to be using the medication first rather than trying more holistic ways of controlling the anxiety. It is the nurse's responsibility to teach complementary and alternative ways to cope with anxiety and stress as a lifetime measure rather than simply using a pill every time the patient identifies anxiety. Mild anxiety may help the individual adapt.
Cognitive Level: Application
Nursing Process: Implementation
NCLEX: Safe, Effective Care Environment: Management of Care
Text Page: 575

21. Answer: 2
Rationale: Pharmacokinetics is the study of how the body affects a drug. It answers the question: how does the body get drugs to and from their intended target? Body functions such as absorption, distribution, metabolism, and elimination all are pharmacokinetics.
Cognitive Level: Comprehension
Nursing Process: Evaluation
NCLEX: Physiological Integrity: Pharmacological and Parenteral Therapies
Text Page: 567

22. Answer: 4
Rationale: Some patients become less responsive to the same dose of a particular drug over time, which is called tolerance, requiring that higher doses of the drug be given over time to obtain the same therapeutic effect.
Cognitive Level: Analysis
Nursing Process: Evaluation
NCLEX: Psychosocial Integrity
Text Page: 568

23. Answer: 1
Rationale: Women are at higher risk for tardive dyskinesia from conventional antipsychotics and for activating side effects caused by antidepressants. All other answers are incorrect.
Cognitive Level: Analysis
Nursing Process: Assessment
NCLEX: Physiological Integrity: Physiological Adaptation
Text Page: 571

24. Answer: 3
Rationale: Many psychiatric disorders are thought to be caused by a dysregulation (imbalance) in the complex process of brain structures communicating with each other through neurotransmission. For instance, psychosis is thought to involve excessive dopamine and serotonin dysregulation.
Cognitive Level: Analysis
Nursing Process: NA
NCLEX: Physiological Integrity: Pharmacological and Parenteral Therapies
Text Page: 572-573

25. Answer: 1
Rationale: In 2003, the National Organization of Nurse Practitioner Faculties (NONPF) published a comprehensive set of competencies defining the scope and practice of psychiatric mental health nurse practitioners (PMHNP). An example of a competency specific to medication prescribing for PMHNP states that the PMHNP "prescribes psychotropic and related medications based on clinical indicators of a patient's status, including results of diagnostic and lab tests as appropriate, to treat symptoms of psychiatric disorders and improve functional health status." Answers 2 and 3 are incorrect, while Answer 4 is specific to only atypical classes of psychotropic medications, but nurses need to know information about all psychotropic medications.
Cognitive Level: Analysis
Nursing Process: NA
NCLEX: Safe, Effective Care Environment: Management of Care
Text Page: 595

CHAPTER 28

1. Answer: 3
Rationale: Patients who receive ECT treatment on an outpatient basis are asked to stay NPO for 6 to 8 hours before treatment to prevent aspiration from general anesthesia. If the patient is taking cardiac, antihypertensive, or H_2 blocker medications, he or she may do so with a small sip of water several hours before the procedure.
Cognitive Level: Application
Nursing Process: Implementation
NCLEX: Physiological Integrity: Reduction of Risk Potential
Text Page: 606

2. Answer: 3
Rationale: The nurse applies equipment necessary for patient monitoring, including blood pressure cuff and oxygen saturation probe. Mild soap is used to cleanse the areas designated for electrode placement, but shampooing of the hair is unnecessary. Results of a 12-lead ECG, which should be performed well before the patient gets to the treatment area, should have been reviewed to determine risks associated with anesthesia. The consent form should be signed earlier, and there is no need to sign another consent form at this time.
Cognitive Level: Analysis
Nursing Process: Implementation
NCLEX: Physiological Integrity: Reduction of Risk Potential
Text Page: 607

3. Answer: 1
Rationale: Although most muscles become completely relaxed during ECT, the nurse uses a bite block between the upper and lower teeth in the patient's mouth to prevent the patient's jaw muscles, which are stimulated directly by ECT, from causing the teeth to clench. This prevents tooth damage and tongue or gum laceration during the stimulus. The nurse removes the bite block after the stimulus has been delivered.
Cognitive Level: Comprehension
Nursing Process: Implementation
NCLEX: Physiological Integrity: Reduction of Risk Potential
Text Page: 606-607

4. Answer: 1
Rationale: Educating the patient and family about ECT is a crucial nursing intervention. During the initial meeting, the nurse performs an assessment to determine the understanding of ECT by the patient and family. The nurse best accomplishes this by asking a direct assessment question that focuses on ECT knowledge. Beginning patient education with a needs-assessment question assists the nurse in organizing an effective teaching-learning plan.
Cognitive Level: Application
Nursing Process: Implementation
NCLEX: Psychosocial Integrity
Text Page: 605

5. Answer: 1
Rationale: Immediately before the patient receives ECT treatment, the nurse instructs the patient to void. This prevents incontinence during the treatment, minimizes the potential for bladder distention, and prevents damage during the procedure.
Cognitive Level: Application
Nursing Process: Implementation
NCLEX: Physiological Integrity: Reduction of Risk Potential
Text Page: 606-607

6. Answer: 1
Rationale: The electrical stimulus causes an observable, brief generalized seizure for 30 to 60 seconds in

the cuffed foot and characteristic EEG changes. If the seizure lasts longer than 120 seconds (2 minutes), it is terminated with diazepam (Valium) or thiopental sodium (Pentothal).
Cognitive Level: Analysis
Nursing Process: Assessment
NCLEX: Physiological Integrity: Reduction of Risk Potential
Text Page: 607

7. Answer: 3
Rationale: Phototherapy has been demonstrated to help patients affected by SAD. However, the question provides no information about whether the patient has been diagnosed as depressed and little data about the clinical manifestations except that the patient speaks of having a depressed mood during the winter. While much of this data fits SAD, it can fit other entities as well. The most therapeutic nursing intervention is the one that attempts to gather more baseline data from the patient rather than one that involves premature intervention.
Cognitive Level: Analysis
Nursing Process: Assessment
NCLEX: Psychosocial Integrity
Text Page: 610

8. Answer: 1
Rationale: Two hours of light therapy at 2500 lux per day appears to be an effective antidepressant treatment that will bring relief of symptoms in 3 to 5 days. It exposes patients to lighting that is 5 to 20 times brighter than indoor lighting. Patients can engage in their activities—reading, writing, or eating—while undergoing light therapy, and a light box may be purchased for about $350 to $500.
Cognitive Level: Analysis
Nursing Process: Implementation
NCLEX: Psychosocial Integrity
Text Page: 610

9. Answer: 2
Rationale: ECT is effective for target behaviors such as catatonia (stupor), hyperemotionality, severe psychosis with acute onset, neuroleptic malignant syndrome, and hypermotility. ECT is used as treatment for major depression in some patients.
Cognitive Level: Analysis
Nursing Process: Assessment
NCLEX: Psychosocial Integrity
Text Page: 605

10. Answer: 3
Rationale: It is helpful to have the patient speak with another individual who has undergone ECT therapy to alleviate anxiety. The motor seizure induced as part of the ECT treatment should last about 20 seconds but should not exceed 2 minutes to prevent a postictal state. Family should be encouraged to come with the patient for at least the first few treatments. Memory loss is temporary in most cases, but any residual memory impairment is not due to brain damage.
Cognitive Level: Application
Nursing Process: Implementation
NCLEX: Psychosocial Integrity
Text Page: 607-608

11. Answer: 4
Rationale: Adverse behaviors associated with ECT treatment include prolonged periods of confusion or disorientation, recurrent nausea or headaches, and elevated blood pressure that does not remit after several hours following ECT treatment.
Cognitive Level: Application
Nursing Process: Evaluation
NCLEX: Physiological Integrity: Reduction of Risk Potential
Text Page: 607-608

12. Answer: 2
Rationale: The post-treatment recovery room for ECT should contain oxygen and suctioning equipment, an emergency cart (not an intubation tray alone), a pulse oximeter, and vital-sign monitoring equipment. A chest tube insertion kit or straight catheter kit is unnecessary.
Cognitive Level: Analysis
Nursing Process: Implementation
NCLEX: Physiological Integrity: Reduction of Risk Potential
Text Page: 606

13. Answer: 3
Rationale: The nurse is caring for a patient who has just received her first ECT treatment. The most therapeutic nursing communication is the one in which the nurse does the following: greets the patient by the name he or she prefers; identifies the nurse and his or her purpose; orients the patient to the surroundings; reassures the patient of his or her status; and provides anticipatory guidance by telling the patient that his or her confusion is only of short duration.
Cognitive Level: Application
Nursing Process: Implementation
NCLEX: Psychosocial Integrity
Text Page: 607

14. Answer: 1
Rationale: Patients who undergo ECT treatment often worry about the possibility of electrocution. However, it is best if the patient identifies fears by the facilitative communication technique of the nurse. The most therapeutic technique is that which provides information using a matter-of-fact communication style and a sense of authority that is reassuring but not overbearing.

Trivialization is disrespectful, and using the word "electrocution" prematurely can often create anxiety rather than alleviate it. It is important for the patient to identify concerns rather than for the nurse to identify them; talking to a supportive nurse will alleviate a patient's anxiety.
Cognitive Level: Application
Nursing Process: Implementation
NCLEX: Psychosocial Integrity
Text Page: 605-606

15. Answer: 3
Rationale: Responders to light treatment are characterized by atypical symptoms such as hypersomnia, afternoon and evening slump, reverse diurnal variation (evenings are worse with respect to depression), anxiety, and carbohydrate craving.
Cognitive Level: Analysis
Nursing Process: Assessment
NCLEX: Psychosocial Integrity
Text Page: 610-611

16. Answer: 2
Rationale: The patient has asked a legitimate question that reflects some reluctance about using the same treatment. A sarcastic response is not therapeutic and reflects a lack of respect and mutuality for the patient. Answer 2 shows a respectful consideration of the patient's concern; the most therapeutic communication is the one that investigates the patient's unwillingness to use a treatment that previously worked.
Cognitive Level: Application
Nursing Process: Implementation
NCLEX: Psychosocial Integrity
Text Page: 611

17. Answer: 3
Rationale: TMS, a noninvasive procedure that changes magnetic fields in the brain, has been found to be effective in the treatment of depression. However, patients with pacemakers, screws, plates, shrapnel, and other implants that might create a low-resistance current path are not considered for TMS.
Cognitive Level: Application
Nursing Process: Implementation
NCLEX: Psychosocial Integrity
Text Page: 613

18. Answer: 1
Rationale: The patient's husband is expressing a common concern based on fear about what a loved one may experience. It is important for the nurse to be sensitive to his concerns and encourage their expression. The most therapeutic communication is the one that helps the patient's husband to talk more about his concerns. Use a therapeutic communication such as, "Can you share more about your concerns?" Seeking clarification can be therapeutic. However, Answer 1 is based on research findings. Notice that the nurse uses an analogy to make the point of safety to the patient and asks a question that facilitates communication.
Cognitive Level: Application
Nursing Process: Implementation
NCLEX: Psychosocial Integrity
Text Page: 605-606

19. Answer: 3
Rationale: Memory loss for recent events and confusion are common immediately after ECT treatment. They may persist for several weeks and then remit. The patient requires ongoing orientation for reassurance and safety.
Cognitive Level: Analysis
Nursing Process: Implementation
NCLEX: Physiological Integrity: Reduction of Risk Potential
Text Page: 608

20. Answer: 1
Rationale: Phototherapy is based on biological rhythms and is especially related to light and darkness. Its therapeutic effect seems to be related to the eyes and not to the skin.
Cognitive Level: Analysis
Nursing Process: Implementation
NCLEX: Psychosocial Integrity
Text Page: 611

21. Answer: 2
Rationale: Although up to 60% of depressed patients respond to sleep deprivation therapy immediately, many become depressed again when they resume sleeping even as little as 2 hours a night. Few randomized trials have been conducted in this area, so it is not widely used in clinical practice. Answers 1, 3, and 4 contain false or misleading information.
Cognitive Level: Application
Nursing Process: Implementation
NCLEX: Psychosocial Integrity
Text Page: 611

22. Answer: 3
Rationale: The nurse should check the gag reflex before offering medications and breakfast so that the patient does not aspirate because of the effects of general anesthesia. The nurse should use siderails and assist the patient to walk if unsteadiness is present. Vital signs should be measured every 15 minutes initially, and then less often, but once per shift is insufficient after this procedure. Neurological status should be assessed every 30 minutes while the patient is awake, but the patient should not be awakened. It is thought that sleep helps return the patient to baseline more quickly.

Cognitive Level: Application
Nursing Process: Implementation
NCLEX: Physiological Integrity: Reduction of Risk Potential
Text Page: 608

23. Answer: 1
Rationale: TMS has been studied for a number of indications, but the indication for this therapy most frequently cited in psychiatry has been mood disorders. A few small studies have suggested this treatment also may be helpful for those with obsessive-compulsive disorder and posttraumatic stress disorder.
Cognitive Level: Analysis
Nursing Process: Assessment
NCLEX: Psychosocial Integrity
Text Page: 613

24. Answer: 4
Rationale: The potential for tinnitus or even transient hearing loss caused by the high-frequency noise produced by the treatment apparatus has prompted the routine use of ear plugs for both patient and investigator, thus minimizing the occurrence of this adverse effect.
Cognitive Level: Application
Nursing Process: Planning
NCLEX: Physiological Integrity: Reduction of Risk Potential
Text Page: 613

25. Answer: 2
Rationale: The most compelling use of VNS in psychiatry is in the treatment of affective disorders, particularly depression. Because the vagus nerve has many functions, it should be studied in the future for other conditions such as anxiety disorders, obesity, chronic pain syndromes, addictions, and sleep disorders.
Cognitive Level: Knowledge
Nursing Process: Planning
NCLEX: Psychosocial Integrity
Text Page: 614

CHAPTER 29

1. Answer: 1
Rationale: Nurses must continually learn the research findings related to CAM because nurses play an important role in educating consumers about the evidence supporting these new therapies, as well as about the dangers involved in using some of them. Evidence-based outcomes provide more information about efficacy, tolerability, dosage, safety, and interactions with other treatments.
Cognitive Level: Analysis
Nursing Process: Assessment
NCLEX: Psychosocial Integrity
Text Page: 619

2. Answer: 2
Rationale: Individuals with anxiety and depression use CAM therapies more often than they use conventional mental health treatments.
Cognitive Level: Comprehension
Nursing Process: Assessment
NCLEX: Psychosocial Integrity
Text Page: 619

3. Answer: 3
Rationale: The mechanism of action of hypericum (St. John's wort) is thought to involve monoamine oxidase inhibition and inhibition of reuptake of serotonin, dopamine, and norepinephrine. In addition, regulatory hormones may be reduced by a suspected inhibitory effect on interleukin-6 activity. The nurse needs to investigate all herbs, because many have bioactivity similar to that of medications (kola nut, caffeine; ginkgo biloba and garlic, anticoagulants).
Cognitive Level: Analysis
Nursing Process: Evaluation
NCLEX: Psychosocial Integrity
Text Page: 621

4. Answer: 4
Rationale: Complementary and alternative therapies seem, in some circumstances, to promote well-being. However, research is still a long way from confirming the supportive aspects of these therapies. Because of the adverse effects of these strategies, it is important to teach a patient to discuss any selection of a holistic therapy with the health care provider.
Cognitive Level: Analysis
Nursing Process: Evaluation
NCLEX: Psychosocial Integrity
Text Page: 618-619

5. Answer: 1
Rationale: The nurse, who is often the professional that the patient sees as a health teacher and caregiver, must keep informed about the most contemporary research findings on all kinds of therapies.
Cognitive Level: Knowledge
Nursing Process: Implementation
NCLEX: Psychosocial Integrity
Text Page: 623

6. Answer: 3
Rationale: PMR uses a process of tensing and releasing muscle groups, starting from facial muscles and moving down the body to the muscles in the feet. Patients are taught to perform the technique systematically to gain control over anxiety-provoking thoughts and muscle tension.

Cognitive Level: Knowledge
Nursing Process: Implementation
NCLEX: Psychosocial Integrity
Text Page: 623-624

7. Answer: 1
Rationale: Reflexology is a method based on manipulation and/or movement of the body. The patient is in need of further education about the major domains of complementary and alternative medicines.
Cognitive Level: Comprehension
Nursing Process: Assessment
NCLEX: Psychosocial Integrity
Text Page: 619

8. Answer: 2
Rationale: If a patient is considering CAM therapies, the nurse should teach the patient the importance of checking on the safety and effectiveness of the therapy or treatment with the appropriate persons. The practitioner's credentials also should be checked, and the patient will want to confirm whether the delivery of services meets standards of care that are regulated.
Cognitive Level: Analysis
Nursing Process: Implementation
NCLEX: Psychosocial Integrity
Text Page: 621

9. Answer: 3
Rationale: The mechanism of action of hypericum (St. John's wort) may involve monoamine oxidase inhibition and perhaps serotonin, dopamine, and norepinephrine reuptake inhibition. Other postulated inhibitory effects include inhibition of interleukin-6 activity to reduce regulatory hormones. A 2-week washout period is recommended before starting an antidepressant. Side effects are minimal, but dry mouth, photosensitivity, gastrointestinal symptoms, and dizziness can occur.
Cognitive Level: Knowledge
Nursing Process: Implementation
NCLEX: Psychosocial Integrity
Text Page: 621-622

10. Answer: 3
Rationale: As with most CAM therapies, SAMe has been studied only in small research projects. Tentative findings demonstrate that SAMe is more effective than placebo and as effective as tricyclic antidepressants. The usual oral dose is 200 to 800 mg bid, with most studies examining the use of 1600 mg daily. The high cost of SAMe for a month's supply is a considerable disadvantage of its use.
Cognitive Level: Knowledge
Nursing Process: Implementation
NCLEX: Psychosocial Integrity
Text Page: 622

11. Answer: 1
Rationale: The National Center for Complementary and Alternative Medicine's major domains of complementary and alternative medicine are divided into alternative medical systems, mind-body interventions, biologically based therapies, manipulative and body-based methods, and energy therapies. Meditation, hypnosis, prayer, art, music therapy, and dance therapy are mind-body interventions used to facilitate the mind's capacity to affect bodily function and symptoms.
Cognitive Level: Comprehension
Nursing Process: Planning
NCLEX: Psychosocial Integrity
Text Page: 619

12. Answer: 1
Rationale: Although there are some exceptions, the overall benefits of CAM therapies include less cost, more convenience, fewer side effects, more individualized care, and more practitioner contact.
Cognitive Level: Knowledge
Nursing Process: Implementation
NCLEX: Safe, Effective Care Environment: Management of Care
Text Page: 618-619

13. Answer: 3
Rationale: When a patient inquires about any treatment, it is good practice to first perform a needs assessment. Providing the patient with the most current evidence-based research or directing the patient to an information resource is also good practice. Because of the small research base underlying CAM therapies, conventional medicine has been slow to accept holistic practice as a viable adjunct in the promotion of healing. Patients often have been reluctant to discuss their questions with their medical provider, and the nurse provides a natural communication bridge between the two. Being knowledgeable about the latest holistic practices and their efficacy is an important part of nursing advocacy.
Cognitive Level: Knowledge
Nursing Process: Implementation
NCLEX: Safe, Effective Care Environment: Management of Care
Text Page: 618, 620, 626

14. Answer: 3
Rationale: According to the extant evidence-based research, electroacupuncture has produced significant relief from anxiety, somatization, cognitive processing, and reactive depression.
Cognitive Level: Knowledge
Nursing Process: Implementation
NCLEX: Safe, Effective Care Environment: Management of Care
Text Page: 622-633

15. Answer: 1
Rationale: Evidence-based research has demonstrated that standard auricular acupuncture and biofeedback have reduced drinking days.
Cognitive Level: Knowledge
Nursing Process: Implementation
NCLEX: Safe, Effective Care Environment: Management of Care
Text Page: 625

16. Answer: 1
Rationale: The most therapeutic nursing communication is the one that facilitates the client's expression of feeling and provides an evidence-based practice framework for decision making that is empowering. By presenting the most recent evidence on the topic, the nurse is making a nonjudgmental, nonbiased response that is both professional and therapeutic in its stance. Answer 4 presents the split but does not provide any support (except that the nurse is able to avoid answering the question directly, a strategy that eventually would erode the patient's trust). Answer 3 belittles the patient, and Answer 2 is judgmental and controlling.
Cognitive Level: Analysis
Nursing Process: Implementation
NCLEX: Safe, Effective Care Environment: Management of Care
Text Page: 624

17. Answer: 4
Rationale: Meditation, a relaxation technique, has been beneficial for generalized anxiety and panic disorder. It has been found to be helpful in reducing the severity and frequency of panic attacks and has improved anxiety and depression scores.
Cognitive Level: Knowledge
Nursing Process: Implementation
NCLEX: Psychosocial Integrity
Text Page: 624

18. Answer: 4
Rationale: Guided imagery interventions seem to reduce bingeing and purging and help the patient to self-soothe. Because bulimia nervosa is a disorder of affect and inability to self-soothe, it would seem to hold positive outcomes for patients who use it correctly.
Cognitive Level: Knowledge
Nursing Process: Implementation
NCLEX: Psychosocial Integrity
Text Page: 626

19. Answer: 4
Rationale: Physical exercise that produces cardiovascular benefit has been associated with positive medical benefits, improved mood and self-esteem, a feeling of accomplishment, and renewed energy. Many studies also suggest that depression levels are lower in exercise groups over a longer duration of time. Although other forms of exercise performed on a regular basis may be beneficial, the actual evidence-based research is scarce.
Cognitive Level: Knowledge
Nursing Process: Implementation
NCLEX: Psychosocial Integrity
Text Page: 623

20. Answer: 1
Rationale: EMDR, a recently developed treatment, requires patients to produce a number of rapid lateral eye movements that are paired with the specific traumatic memory or feared stimulus. Positive effects have been reported for patients who experience panic disorder and public speaking anxiety.
Cognitive Level: Knowledge
Nursing Process: Implementation
NCLEX: Psychosocial Integrity
Text Page: 625

21. Answer: 3
Rationale: Ethical concerns about CAM therapies include issues of safety and effectiveness, as well as the expertise and qualifications of the practitioner. Of equal importance is the communication between CAM providers and traditional health care providers.
Cognitive Level: Analysis
Nursing Process: Assessment
NCLEX: Psychosocial Integrity
Text Page: 621

22. Answer: 2
Rationale: The patient would like to take an herbal medicine because she thinks it works well. To encourage the patient to use her self-care skills, you can help her find information and help her present her idea to you, her case manager, and her physician for a discussion. Answer 1 indicates that you expect the psychiatrist to make the decision. Answer 3 sends the message to the patient that she is wrong to ask about this treatment and invokes guilt for asking, and Answer 4 indicates that you are not interested in talking with her about her idea and will not discuss it with her. Encourage the patient to participate in her own care, and especially encourage her to continue to learn and investigate ideas from others and discuss them so that she can utilize the skills she is learning in the psychoeducational group.
Cognitive Level: Analysis
Nursing Process: Planning
NCLEX: Psychosocial Integrity
Text Page: 621

23. Answer: 2
Rationale: Light therapy, or phototherapy, has been shown to be effective for the treatment of seasonal affective disorder (SAD). Phase-delayed sleep brought

on by the reduced sunlight in winter disrupts circadian rhythms.
Cognitive Level: Analysis
Nursing Process: Assessment
NCLEX: Psychosocial Integrity
Text Page: 623

24. Answer: 1
Rationale: The FDA Consumer Advisory and Consumer Reports medical experts have cautioned against the use of kava (Consumer Reports, 2003). Use of kava with other central nervous systems medications can be harmful, and kava may have addictive properties with long-term use.
Cognitive Level: Comprehension
Nursing Process: NA
NCLEX: Psychosocial Integrity
Text Page: 624

25. Answer: 3
Rationale: One of the most widely researched CAM therapies used to treat addiction is acupuncture. Many chemical dependency programs in the United States use auricular acupuncture as an additional therapy. Yoga, therapeutic touch, and Reiki are used mainly for stress and anxiety disorders.
Cognitive Level: Analysis
Nursing Process: Planning
NCLEX: Psychosocial Integrity
Text Page: 625

CHAPTER 30

1. Answer: 4
Rationale: Firm but empathetic limit setting is required in this situation. The patient is splitting, and the nurse needs to set limits and support the consequence that has been administered. By reflecting the patient's psychic distress and providing clear instructions about the behavior that is expected (along with a time limit for that behavior), the nurse is assisting the patient in problem solving more adaptively. In addition, the nurse provides a reward or positive regard when offering a specific time to meet with the patient that occurs after the consequence has been accepted. Answers 1, 2, and 3 also provide similar feedback, but they do not provide specific times that the patient can concretely conceptualize. Mutuality and respect for all patients is required from the therapeutic professional nurse, especially for those patients with impulse-control problems; they may try to enter into a regressive struggle with the nurse, who is trying to set limits on behavior.
Cognitive Level: Analysis
Nursing Process: Implementation
NCLEX: Psychosocial Integrity
Text Page: 642

2. Answer: 2
Rationale: Assertive behavior involves communicating clearly and directly with others. If the assertive individual is conveying negative feelings, thoughts, or issues of concern, the positive aspects are noted in a balance with the negative information, and the individual takes responsibility to state what he or she would like to have done differently or changed. Assertiveness also involves accepting positive and negative input and is used for the purposes of expressing one's feelings, wishes, or desires, but not necessarily as a means of getting one's way or winning. Nursing staff members who are unable to demonstrate appropriate assertive behavior and communications will be unsuccessful role models for their patients.
Cognitive Level: Analysis
Nursing Process: Evaluation
NCLEX: Psychosocial Integrity
Text Page: 639-640

3. Answer: 3
Rationale: In the above communication, the nurse makes a request that describes what she would like the charge nurse to do (i.e., stop calling her "the smart new degree nurse"). This communication is clear and concise, and describes the behavior that the nurse wants to stop. This is assertive. There is not sufficient data provided to predict the charge nurse's subsequent behavior. If the nurse remains calm and simply shares her vulnerability, it is likely that the charge nurse will identify her sarcasm (which may hint at an underlying insecurity and anger) and change the behavior as requested.
Cognitive Level: Analysis
Nursing Process: Evaluation
NCLEX: Psychosocial Integrity
Text Page: 639-640

4. Answer: 1
Rationale: The most therapeutic communication is the one that communicates clearly what the nurse is able to do or, in this case, not to do. Starting by apologizing misses the point, and agreeing to work is passive-aggressive. The charge nurse's job is to provide a nurse for the shift. Assertive people are not afraid to ask for what they want or need. The nurse does not need to apologize, and she does not need to offer an explanation of why she is refusing to work. She would be working overtime, and she has already done quite a bit of overtime.
Cognitive Level: Application
Nursing Process: Implementation
NCLEX: Psychosocial Integrity
Text Page: 639-640

5. Answer: 2
Rationale: The most assertive communication is the one that clarifies any misperceptions and seeks assistance in

a direct manner. Rationalization is not professional. Patients will take their cue from the facilitator of the group. Becoming angry because the psychologist has constructively criticized the nurse's facilitation skills in dynamic supervision is aggressive.
Cognitive Level: Application
Nursing Process: Implementation
NCLEX: Psychosocial Integrity
Text Page: 640

6. Answer: 4
Rationale: There are many dynamic reasons that might be postulated about why alcohol-troubled patients would bring pseudo-alcoholic beverages to the group. The facilitator needs to be assertive and bring the behavior out to the group for its members to examine. It is time to review the purpose of the group and then to assist the group in reflecting on their behavior and its meaning for their sobriety.
Cognitive Level: Application
Nursing Process: Implementation
NCLEX: Psychosocial Integrity
Text Page: 640

7. Answer: 1
Rationale: When dealing with a patient who is escalating, the nurse makes an assessment first of the patient's ability to control himself and to respond to verbal cues. Speaking in a calm, soft voice and calling him by his formal title (unless he has insisted on being called by his first name), the nurse examines whether the patient is able to stop talking loudly and listen to the nurse. If he is able to do so, it is likely that he will be able to take a time-out in his room by himself, and this is always the desired outcome. If a patient has escalated before, this does not mean that he will again, but it does signify a greater risk for violence and acting-out behavior.
Cognitive Level: Analysis
Nursing Process: Implementation
NCLEX: Safe, Effective Care Environment: Management of Care
Text Page: 640

8. Answer: 3
Rationale: The first step in talking with the patient would be to ask the patient if he knows why the nurse has asked to speak with him. If he is unable to assess his behavior accurately (e.g., if he cannot say something like, "I guess I was getting too loud, huh?"), then the nurse would identify what John was doing, assess his mental status, and offer support. In addition, medication might be considered at this point.
Cognitive Level: Analysis
Nursing Process: Implementation
NCLEX: Safe, Effective Care Environment: Management of Care
Text Page: 641

9. Answer: 3
Rationale: Lithium and atypical antipsychotic agents are more effective than stimulants in treating aggression in children and conduct disorders in adolescents.
Cognitive Level: Knowledge
Nursing Process: Assessment
NCLEX: Safe, Effective Care Environment: Management of Care
Text Page: 643

10. Answer: 2
Rationale: The most therapeutic communication is the one in which the nurse assesses the potential for violence by ascertaining the patient's plan, means, and commitment. Depending on the patient's answer to the nurse, the next step would be to determine the meaning of hospitalization to the patient and how that milieu could be achieved in the community.
Cognitive Level: Analysis
Nursing Process: Implementation
NCLEX: Psychosocial Integrity
Text Page: 641

11. Answer: 2
Rationale: It is important that the patient identify his or her own inappropriate behavior. Lecturing to the patient could create defensive behavior. Taking sides with the patient or delivering a threat is not therapeutic. It is a good sign that the patient accepted and completed the consequence, and the nurse will want to comment about this to the patient. It is also important that the nurse deliver the time-out as a consequence in a matter-of-fact manner and not as a punishment. Behavior is altered more adaptively if the consequence (e.g., deduction of tokens, time-out to one's room) is delivered as a support to assist the patient to relearn adaptive ways to behave in problematic situations.
Cognitive Level: Analysis
Nursing Process: Implementation
NCLEX: Psychosocial Integrity
Text Page: 641

12. Answer: 1
Rationale: Working as a crisis team, there is one leader who does all the talking. The crisis team works to provide support to a patient in much the same way that an Ace bandage can support a strained muscle. Having several members of the crisis team talk to the patient is confusing. Furthermore, patients would be more stimulated or confused or would try to "split" the situation. Making judgmental responses to the patient could cause re-escalation. In addition, it is wise to use language that is neutral and not inflammatory.
Cognitive Level: Analysis
Nursing Process: Implementation
NCLEX: Psychosocial Integrity
Text Page: 643-644

13. Answer: 3
Rationale: Contracting is a two-way street. According to the situation presented in this question, the nurse already has received time and understanding from the patient. It takes less than 5 minutes to smoke a cigarette, and the nurse or another member of the staff needs to stop and provide the patient with the cigarette time he has been contracted to receive. The time may be helpful to the nurse, as well, by providing 5 minutes to organize and plan for the unit and two new admissions. It is not the patient's fault if the unit is busy, and the nurse who responds with anger or sarcasm is not being self-aware or mutually respectful of the patient.
Cognitive Level: Application
Nursing Process: Implementation
NCLEX: Psychosocial Integrity
Text Page: 642

14. Answer: 1
Rationale: The most therapeutic communication is the one in which the nurse expresses empathy for the patient and asks the patient to reflect on his or her thinking. In this way, the nurse seeks to determine whether the patient is able to think critically about his or her situation and response and how it appears to others. This eliminates any countertransference in the nurse's behavior. Speaking in clichés is competitive, and lecturing the patient will only stimulate any anger that the patient has. The nurse's goal ought to be to facilitate the patient's expression of feelings so that the patient can begin to reflect and eventually problem solve effectively.
Cognitive Level: Analysis
Nursing Process: Implementation
NCLEX: Psychosocial Integrity
Text Page: 642

15. Answer: 1
Rationale: In assessing the potential for violent behavior, the nurse measures the patient's mental status as well as is possible. A patient who is unable to control talking out loud is not a good participant in a group meeting, whether the behavior is one of manipulation or a sign of potential aggression and disintegration. The most therapeutic nursing intervention is the one that excuses John from the group to protect him from being embarrassed when control is regained. In addition, the time-out may provide a reduction in milieu stimulation and provide needed structure and control. This is a difficult patient behavior even for a seasoned staff member, and the nurse would not delegate the task of dealing with the patient to the patient's peers. The nurse who tries to place responsibility onto the other patients could be considered negligent in her duty.
Cognitive Level: Analysis
Nursing Process: Implementation
NCLEX: Safe, Effective Care Environment: Management of Care
Text Page: 642

16. Answer: 2
Rationale: Despite the fact that everything that could be done in each violent event was done, the staff members are still experiencing high levels of stress more often. If feasible, the nurse will provide ways to manage the staff's higher level of stress during this time. The only selection that offers an avenue for immediate stress management is scheduling frequent breaks.
Cognitive Level: Analysis
Nursing Process: Implementation
NCLEX: Safe, Effective Care Environment: Management of Care
Text Page: 645-646

17. Answer: 1
Rationale: Solitary containment is the use of a fully protective environment with close observation by nursing staff for the purpose of safety or behavior management based on a professional nursing philosophy of concern for human dignity and optimal fulfillment of basic human needs. The scientific rationale for the use of seclusion is based on three principles: containment, isolation, and decrease in sensory input.
Cognitive Level: Analysis
Nursing Process: Assessment
NCLEX: Psychosocial Integrity
Text Page: 642

18. Answer: 1
Rationale: There is no easy way to discuss the use of restraints with a patient who is currently violent. It is important to explain in a nonjudgmental way why restraint is being employed and to open up an avenue of communication so staff members can ensure the patient's optimal well-being during the period of restraint.
Cognitive Level: Application
Nursing Process: Assessment
NCLEX: Psychosocial Integrity
Text Page: 644-645

19. Answer: 3
Rationale: The most therapeutic nursing communication is the one that addresses Mary's concerns more specifically. Often new staff members can offer a new perspective on an issue that will enrich unit operations and provide an expanded approach to effective clinical decision making. Mary may be making an observation that is derived from an idealistic philosophy, but that cannot be determined until Mary has received the opportunity to share her thinking in an open forum. John's response will need to be explored, but it may be explored after letting Mary speak. The nurse facilitator

might then address John as follows: "John, you are out there on the front line with patients, and it sounds as if you are angry that Mary is asking if there might be a better way to approach patients to avoid seclusion." This comment may help process some of John's anger and aggressive drive and proactively avoid any future problematic interactions between John and Mary.
Cognitive Level: Application
Nursing Process: Implementation
NCLEX: Safe, Effective Care Environment: Management of Care
Text Page: 645

20. Answer: 4
Rationale: The most therapeutic communication is the one that does the following:

Addresses the patient by name (assesses the patient's ability to listen and respond to the nurse)

Offers information in a matter-of-fact way (addresses the well part of the patient's communication, that is, the part at which he asks, "When is my doctor coming?"; this is an appropriate communication by the patient and needs to be acknowledged in a respectful manner)

Promotes structure for the patient by offering a plan that suggests he shower (Maslow's hierarchy: The patient will feel better physically while he waits for the doctor.)

Provides breakfast on the unit with the structure of a reduced-stimulus milieu (the patient may be escalating, so it is better to order a tray on the unit if he is usually able to go to breakfast in the cafeteria)
Cognitive Level: Application
Nursing Process: Implementation
NCLEX: Psychosocial Integrity
Text Page: 641

21. Answer: 3
Rationale: Assertive behavior conveys a sense of self-assurance but also communicates respect for the other person. Acknowledging the patient's concern and letting him know that you will meet his needs are considerate and respectful. This response also lets the patient know that you are completing a task and will then meet his needs within a reasonable time. Answers 1, 2, and 4 do not take the patient's feelings into account. They only demean the patient and are not respectful.
Cognitive Level: Application
Nursing Process: Implementation
NCLEX: Psychosocial Integrity
Text Page: 631

22. Answer: 1
Rationale: Clinicians may intentionally or inadvertently precipitate an outbreak of violence because staff attitudes and actions have a powerful effect on patient behavior. Inexperienced staff members, provocation by staff, poor milieu management, understaffing, close physical encounters, inconsistent limit setting, and a norm of violence all may negatively affect the inpatient environment.
Cognitive Level: Analysis
Nursing Process: Planning
NCLEX: Psychosocial Integrity
Text Page: 636

23. Answer: 4
Rationale: The most valuable resource of a nurse is the ability to use one's self to help others. To ensure the most effective use of self, it is important to be aware of personal stress that can interfere with one's ability to communicate therapeutically with patients.
Cognitive Level: Application
Nursing Process: Implementation
NCLEX: Psychosocial Integrity
Text Page: 637

24. Answer: 1
Rationale: Because it is much less dangerous to prevent a crisis than to respond to one, every effort should be made to carefully monitor patients who are at risk for violent behavior and intervene at the first possible sign of increasing agitation.
Cognitive Level: Analysis
Nursing Process: Assessment
NCLEX: Psychosocial Integrity
Text Page: 640

25. Answer: 3
Rationale: One may manage aggressive behavior more effectively by allowing those at risk to spend time in their rooms away from the hectic day room rather than encouraging them to interact with others in a crowded milieu.
Cognitive Level: Application
Nursing Process: Implementation
NCLEX: Psychosocial Integrity
Text Page: 641

CHAPTER 31

1. Answer: 1
Rationale: The patient is demonstrating cognitive distortions by thinking in extremes and magnifying the problem and solution. The most therapeutic communication is the one that seeks clarification. Presenting the patient's statements back to her allows her to "listen with her third ear" and take a view that places the event in perspective. Taking sides is not therapeutic.
Cognitive Level: Application
Nursing Process: Implementation
Client Needs: Psychosocial Integrity
Text Page: 658, 662

2. Answer: 3
Rationale: The patient is demonstrating the cognitive distortion of personalization and arbitrary inference. The therapeutic communication that reflects a cognitive behavioral assessment is the one that first asks, "What is the problem?" Identifying the problem from the patient's perspective in a neutral, nonjudgmental style of communication helps the patient to take this first step. The antecedent and feared consequences also are identified.
Cognitive Level: Analysis
Nursing Process: Implementation
Client Needs: Psychosocial Integrity
Text Page: 658, 662

3. Answer: 3
Rationale: The patient is demonstrating the cognitive distortions of dichotomous thinking (thinking in extremes) and overgeneralization. She is clearly in crisis and may be experiencing suicidal ideation. By identifying the most important problem and giving the patient permission to view one problem at a time with the therapist, the nurse is supporting effective problem solving by the patient. Using a cognitive behavioral approach, the nurse is able to perform a lethality assessment and then help the patient to expand alternatives and become a more flexible thinker.
Cognitive Level: Analysis
Nursing Process: Implementation
Client Needs: Psychosocial Integrity
Text Page: 658-659, 662

4. Answer: 1
Rationale: The patient is demonstrating personalization and engaging in ineffective problem solving. The most therapeutic communication is the one in which the nurse identifies the problem from the patient's perspective and asks how the ineffective problem solving will change things.
Cognitive Level: Analysis
Nursing Process: Implementation
Client Needs: Psychosocial Integrity
Text Page: 658-659, 662

5. Answer: 1
Rationale: The manifestations of relaxation include reduced blood pressure, pulse, peripheral temperature, and respirations; peripheral vasoconstriction; and constricted pupils. Others are listed in Box 31-3 in the textbook.
Cognitive Level: Application
Nursing Process: Evaluation
Client Needs: Psychosocial Integrity
Text Page: 660

6. Answer: 2
Rationale: Interoceptive exposure is used to desensitize patients to specific symptoms that they experience when anxious, such as tachycardia, blurred vision, and shortness of breath. After establishing a hierarchy of the symptoms, the patient does the things that cause him or her to experience extreme anxiety. These are then paired with a movement such as running in place or spinning around. This method has been proved successful with patients whose panic attacks seem spontaneous and unprovoked, which causes increased worry. However, it is not successful for agoraphobic patients.
Cognitive Level: Application
Nursing Process: Planning
Client Needs: Psychosocial Integrity
Text Page: 661

7. Answer: 4
Rationale: In reframing, the nurse changes the meaning of a behavior in order to change the patient's response. In this situation, the nurse helps the father to view his children's behavior as concern for him rather than as an attack against him.
Cognitive Level: Application
Nursing Process: Implementation
Client Needs: Psychosocial Integrity
Text Page: 663

8. Answer: 2
Rationale: Role playing is defined as the process by which patients rehearse problematic issues and obtain feedback about their behavior. In this situation, the patient switches roles with the therapist and is given an opportunity to see issues from another individual's viewpoint.
Cognitive Level: Comprehension
Nursing Process: Implementation
Client Needs: Psychosocial Integrity
Text Page: 663

9. Answer: 4
Rationale: Meditation is used to relax patients and may follow or replace systematic relaxation. Other components that the nurse ensures are a quiet milieu, a passive attitude, and a comfortable position.
Cognitive Level: Analysis
Nursing Process: Implementation
Client Needs: Psychosocial Integrity
Text Page: 660

10. Answer: 2
Rationale: Token economy, a form of positive reinforcement, has been used successfully to reward patients for performing behaviors such as activities of daily living.
Cognitive Level: Knowledge
Nursing Process: Implementation
Client Needs: Psychosocial Integrity
Text Page: 663

11. Answer: 1
Rationale: Social skills training is often helpful for patients who have trouble with assertiveness and with managing their anger.
Cognitive Level: Analysis
Nursing Process: Implementation
Client Needs: Psychosocial Integrity
Text Page: 663

12. Answer: 2
Rationale: Dichotomous thinking is a cognitive distortion that involves thinking in extremes (i.e., things are either all good or all bad).
Cognitive Level: Analysis
Nursing Process: Implementation
Client Needs: Psychosocial Integrity
Text Page: 662-663

13. Answer: 4
Rationale: The patient is projecting perfectionism onto the criteria for college acceptance. Perfectionism is a cognitive distortion, and this is best explored by reflecting the patient's distortion back to have the patient reexamine his or her thinking.
Cognitive Level: Application
Nursing Process: Implementation
Client Needs: Psychosocial Integrity
Text Page: 662-663

14. Answer: 2
Rationale: This is a difficult situation. The patient is cognitively distorting. Catastrophising is thinking the worst about people and events. There may be other distortions, but using cognitive behavioral therapy involves separating issues for the patient to examine.
Cognitive Level: Analysis
Nursing Process: Implementation
Client Needs: Psychosocial Integrity
Text Page: 662-663

15. Answer: 1
Rationale: The patient is cognitively distorting by externalizing her self-worth. The most therapeutic communication is the one that summarizes the patient's viewpoint and reflects it back for the patient to hear in a nonjudgmental way.
Cognitive Level: Analysis
Nursing Process: Implementation
Client Needs: Psychosocial Integrity
Text Page: 662-663

16. Answer: 1
Rationale: Decatastrophising is also called the "what-if" technique. Answer 2 uses an "as-if" technique, but it does not decatastrophise.
Cognitive Level: Application
Nursing Process: Implementation
Client Needs: Psychosocial Integrity
Text Page: 663

17. Answer: 3
Rationale: A positive reinforcement is a rewarding stimulus, such as praise. A negative reinforcement also increases the frequency of the appropriate behavior by reinforcing the power of the behavior to control an aversive, rather than rewarding, stimulus. The behaviors in Answers 1, 2, and 4 are negative reinforcements.
Cognitive Level: Application
Nursing Process: Implementation
Client Needs: Psychosocial Integrity
Text Page: 655

18. Answer: 1
Rationale: Extinction is the process of eliminating a behavior by ignoring it or not rewarding it. Ignoring a temper tantrum is an example of this technique. Answers 2 and 4 are examples of response cost, in which the frequency of a behavior is likely to decrease because of a loss or penalty following the behavior. Answer 3 is an example of punishment, which is an aversive stimulus that occurs after the behavior and reduces its future occurrence.
Cognitive Level: Application
Nursing Process: Implementation
Client Needs: Psychosocial Integrity
Text Page: 656

19. Answer: 2
Rationale: With response cost, the frequency of a behavior is likely to decrease because of a loss or penalty following a behavior. Answer 2 is an example of response cost. Extinction is the process of eliminating a behavior by ignoring it or not rewarding it, which is illustrated in Answer 1. Answers 3 and 4 are examples of punishment, which is an aversive stimulus that occurs after the behavior and reduces its future occurrence.
Cognitive Level: Application
Nursing Process: Implementation
Client Needs: Psychosocial Integrity
Text Page: 656

20. Answer: 1
Rationale: An important characteristic of cognitive behavioral therapy is the mutuality between the therapist and patient (i.e., the collaboration in defining the problem, identifying goals, formulating treatment strategies, and evaluating progress). Other characteristics include an emphasis on an objective assessment process, a supportive rather than curative focus, and a facilitative role of the therapist.
Cognitive Level: Application
Nursing Process: Implementation

Client Needs: Psychosocial Integrity
Text Page: 657

21. Answer: 3
Rationale: The hands are tensed and relaxed first, followed by the biceps and triceps, shoulders, neck, mouth, eyes, breathing, back, midsection, thighs, stomach, calves and feet, and finally toes.
Cognitive Level: Application
Nursing Process: Implementation
Client Needs: Psychosocial Integrity
Text Page: 660

22. Answer: 2
Rationale: With systematic desensitization, the patient must first be able to relax the muscles. Next, the patient constructs a hierarchy of the anxiety-producing situation (insects) by ranking them from 1 to 10. The patient then proceeds to work through the hierarchy, using muscle relaxation to maintain a relaxation response in the face of fearful stimuli.
Cognitive Level: Analysis
Nursing Process: Evaluation
Client Needs: Psychosocial Integrity
Text Page: 660

23. Answer: 4
Rationale: Social skills training is most often used with patients who lack social skills, assertiveness (assertiveness training), or impulse control (anger management), and those with antisocial behavior.
Cognitive Level: Analysis
Nursing Process: Planning
Client Needs: Psychosocial Integrity
Text Page: 664

24. Answer: 1
Rationale: Aversion therapy applies an aversive or noxious stimulus when a maladaptive behavior occurs. Aversion therapy has sometimes been criticized as unethical and detrimental to patients' well-being.
Cognitive Level: Knowledge
Nursing Process: NA
Client Needs: Psychosocial Integrity
Text Page: 664

25. Answer: 3
Rationale: Three basic roles for nurses involved in cognitive behavioral therapy at all levels of practice (novice through generalist and specialist) are: providing patient care, planning treatment programs, and teaching others the use of cognitive behavioral strategies.
Cognitive Level: Application
Nursing Process: Implementation
Client Needs: Psychosocial Integrity
Text Page: 665

CHAPTER 32

1. Answer: 4
Rationale: A screening interview for a therapeutic group is conducted to assess the candidate's appropriateness for the group. This can be accomplished in the following ways:
Cognitive Level: Analysis
Nursing Process: Implementation
Client Needs: Psychosocial Integrity
Text Page: 672

2. Answer: 1
Rationale: In the orientation stage, the group's facilitator clarifies the group's primary tasks and helps the group to agree to the contracted goals.
Cognitive Level: Analysis
Nursing Process: Implementation
Client Needs: Psychosocial Integrity
Text Page: 672

3. Answer: 1
Rationale: Issues that commonly are included in a group's contract include goals, confidentiality, meeting times, honesty, structure, and communication rules.
Cognitive Level: Analysis
Nursing Process: Implementation
Client Needs: Psychosocial Integrity
Text Page: 671

4. Answer: 4
Rationale: The most therapeutic response is Answer 4. The facilitator uses confrontation by indicating that it is true that John has done all the talking in the group today. This is done by a good facilitator in order to spark the other group members into contributing to the statement in a safe environment. Good group facilitators will use active dimensions of empathy, genuineness and confrontation. The above is an example of confrontation without judgment and with genuineness and empathy.
Cognitive Level: Analysis
Nursing Process: Implementation
Client Needs: Psychosocial Integrity
Text Page: 676

5. Answer: 1
Rationale: Patients are screened before admission to a group, so one can assume that it is a therapeutic modality for the patient. Being able to persist in a therapeutic group and work through problems is a successful outcome.
Cognitive Level: Knowledge
Nursing Process: Planning
Client Needs: Psychosocial Integrity
Text Page: 673-674

6. Answer: 3
Rationale: The most therapeutic nursing communication is the one that paraphrases and reflects back the affective domain to the group. When group members express anger or frustration with the group, it is important for the leader to give permission for the group to be angry and for the group to observe that anger does not destroy the leader.
Cognitive Level: Analysis
Nursing Process: Implementation
Client Needs: Psychosocial Integrity
Text Page: 676

7. Answer: 3
Rationale: Group resistance may be observed when members form subgroups, conflict occurs, resistance occurs, or self-disclosure occurs. Other examples include shared silence among members, scapegoating, wishing for magical solutions, and unusual amounts of group dependency.
Cognitive Level: Analysis
Nursing Process: Evaluation
Client Needs: Psychosocial Integrity
Text Page: 674

8. Answer: 2
Rationale: When a member of the group terminates, it is important for the group members to have time to discuss feelings and growth in the group and to reminisce; avoiding this would retard the emotional growth of the group members.
Cognitive Level: Analysis
Nursing Process: Implementation
Client Needs: Psychosocial Integrity
Text Page: 675

9. Answer: 2
Rationale: Individual group member responses are usually placed in the patient's charts, as stated in the stem of this question. Group phenomena belong in the group session notes and include membership (absences, tardiness); pertinent behavior discussed by the group; group themes; important group process issues; and any critical leadership strategies required. The therapist also might predict future strategies and behaviors.
Cognitive Level: Analysis
Nursing Process: Implementation
Client Needs: Safe Effective Care Environment: Management of Care
Text Page: 676

10. Answer: 1
Rationale: The patient is projecting feelings of powerlessness in the group, and this may be a splitting mechanism as well. Fantasies about the co-leaders are only natural, and responding to male and female group members as one has responded with parents or spouses also can occur.
Cognitive Level: Analysis
Nursing Process: Evaluation
Client Needs: Psychosocial Integrity
Text Page: 677

11. Answer: 1
Rationale: Clear group guidelines that have been reviewed during the screening process and with the group will help reduce group resistance. All groups have criteria and accept patients who can work cohesively.
Cognitive Level: Analysis
Nursing Process: Implementation
Client Needs: Psychosocial Integrity
Text Page: 671-672, 674

12. Answer: 1
Rationale: Peer support groups provide an avenue for professional nurses who facilitate stressful groups to share their problems and the stresses related to their work. Appropriate topics include case consultation, sharing of information about educational opportunities, discussion of management skills, general sharing of information, and discussion of strategies to reduce professional isolation. Less appropriate topics for such a group are personal comments that are more social in nature and probing comments that relate to personal rather than professional concerns.
Cognitive Level: Analysis
Nursing Process: Evaluation
Client Needs: Psychosocial Integrity
Text Page: 679

13. Answer: 1
Rationale: The optimum length of time for a group session is 20 to 40 minutes for lower-functioning groups and 60 to 120 minutes for higher-functioning groups, which would include a brief warm-up, work time, and a brief wrap-up.
Cognitive Level: Knowledge
Nursing Process: Planning
Client Needs: Psychosocial Integrity
Text Page: 669

14. Answer: 2
Rationale: Maintenance roles include the roles of "harmonizer" and "rule maker." Answer 2 combines both roles. Answer 1 (individual role) illustrates a latecomer who seeks to invalidate the group's worth. Answer 3 (task role) illustrates a questioner who seeks to clarify the information to be discussed. Answer 4 (individual and task roles) illustrates a moralist and summarizer.
Cognitive Level: Analysis
Nursing Process: Evaluation
Client Needs: Psychosocial Integrity
Text Page: 670

15. Answer: 3
Rationale: The nurse facilitator has a difficult task. It is important that all members of the group agree about the group's confidentiality. John may be displaying aggressive behavior toward Meg, but this feedback might be addressed on a one-to-one basis or later. Not taking sides with one of the group members is an important rule to follow as a group facilitator. By encouraging the group members to share thinking in a matter-of-fact way, the nurse reduces the emotional components and promotes the group's cohesiveness.
Cognitive Level: Analysis
Nursing Process: Implementation
Client Needs: Psychosocial Integrity
Text Page: 671

16. Answer: 2
Rationale: It is important for the nurse leader to provide a safe place for group members to challenge authority. The nurse leader must be clear in the derivation of his or her authority and feel sufficiently comfortable in the leader role to allow it to be humanized. Direct and clear clarification is most helpful here. The nurse can follow the answer with criteria for the leader role and what the group can expect from him or her. Humor can help to diffuse any tension or frustration and allow the group member to feel supported in directly verbalizing feelings within the group. Seeking to control can be manipulative or intimidating, and challenging the group would be aggressive.
Cognitive Level: Analysis
Nursing Process: Implementation
Client Needs: Psychosocial Integrity
Text Page: 673, 676

17. Answer: 1
Rationale: Advantages to Internet group participation include convenience, relating to diverse individuals with similar circumstances, ready access to peer support, and anonymity. Trust may develop differently in this group and so is a major concern for the nurse leader. Other concerns include loss of nonverbal communication assessment, loss of simultaneity in the group, and delay in providing a consequence in a teaching-learning situation.
Cognitive Level: Analysis
Nursing Process: Planning
Client Needs: Psychosocial Integrity
Text Page: 676

18. Answer: 1
Rationale: Activity groups combine psychotherapy and remotivation therapy, which stimulates growth and interaction among members by focusing on simple tasks. It is important for the nurse leader to support the new member's integration into the activity group. It is crucial that the nurse leader respect and encourage all members in performing the task the group has committed to accomplishing. Minimizing the importance of the activity or isolating the new member from sharing in equal member responsibilities diminishes the esteem of each member.
Cognitive Level: Analysis
Nursing Process: Implementation
Client Needs: Psychosocial Integrity
Text Page: 679

19. Answer: 3
Rationale: The goal of brief therapy groups is to identify the ineffective problem-solving approaches and replace them with more adaptive ones. These groups are favored by managed care as a cost-effective method of treatment. The focus is always on the actions that members can take now to improve their situations.
Cognitive Level: Analysis
Nursing Process: Implementation
Client Needs: Psychosocial Integrity
Text Page: 678

20. Answer: 2
Rationale: The primary purpose of support groups is to help members to cope with life stresses. In a support group, members examine dysfunctional thoughts, feelings, and behaviors by sharing and talking things out with other members.
Cognitive Level: Knowledge
Nursing Process: Planning
Client Needs: Psychosocial Integrity
Text Page: 678

21. Answer: 3
Rationale: Nurses often are members of multidisciplinary teams consisting of psychiatrists, psychologists, social workers, rehabilitation counselors, occupational therapists, and so forth. The pooling of all of these resources allows for efficient use of available resources for the benefit of the patient. Having more people on the unit is not a correct answer, nor is to provide more opinions or more effective decisions about nursing care.
Cognitive Level: Comprehension
Nursing Process: Implementation
Client Needs: Psychosocial Integrity
Text Page: 678

22. Answer: 1
Rationale: The goal of psychotherapy group is the treatment of emotional, cognitive, or behavioral dysfunction. Group techniques and processes are used to help members learn about their behavior with other people and how it relates to core personality traits. The intent is for the members to change their behavior, not just understand or seek support for it.
Cognitive Level: Analysis
Nursing Process: Implementation

Client Needs: Psychosocial Integrity
Text Page: 678

23. Answer: 3
Rationale: The only group that would qualify as an educational group is Answer 3. You can use the process of elimination because smoking cessation groups are considered self-help groups. Parents without partners are usually support groups, not educational groups, and living with schizophrenia would not be scheduled for a meeting of 1 hour because members usually are low functioning and could not tolerate a 50-minute group.
Cognitive Level: Analysis
Nursing Process: Planning
Client Needs: Psychosocial Integrity
Text Page: 669, 677

24. Answer: 2
Rationale: The group leader documented observable verbal and nonverbal elements of the group's communication, including spatial and seating arrangements, common themes expressed by the group, how often and to whom members communicate, how members are heard in the group, and what problem-solving processes occur in the group. Answers 1, 3, and 4 do not meet the criteria for documentation of communication patterns during the group process.
Cognitive Level: Analysis
Nursing Process: Evaluation
Client Needs: Psychosocial Integrity
Text Page: 669

25. Answer: 1
Rationale: The work of termination begins during the first phase of the group. However, as the group or individual members approach termination, certain processes are more likely to occur. There are two types of termination: termination of the group as a whole and termination of individual members. A closed group usually terminates as an entire group; in an open group, members (and perhaps the leader) terminate separately. Members and groups may terminate prematurely, unsuccessfully, or successfully. Leadership behaviors include encouraging an evaluation of the group or its terminating members, reminiscing about important events that occurred in the group, and encouraging members to give each other feedback.
Cognitive Level: Application
Nursing Process: Planning
Client Needs: Psychosocial Integrity
Text Page: 675

CHAPTER 33

1. Answer: 2
Rationale: Family advocacy refers to the mutual support, time, energy, and resources needed to advocate for improved services and opportunities for family members with psychiatric illness. It is effective in raising awareness among service providers, legislators, and the public. The other terms in Answers 1 and 4 have no relation to advocacy for family services. Answer 3 is a term used to indicate another advocacy network.
Cognitive Level: Comprehension
Nursing Process: NA
Client Needs: Psychosocial Integrity
Text Page: 683

2. Answer: 3
Rationale: Nurses need to examine their own sociocultural contexts and recognize similarities and differences with those of patients and families. The other choices can be assets, but Answer 3 is a priority for the nurse.
Cognitive Level: Application
Nursing Process: NA
Client Needs: Psychosocial Integrity
Text Page: 683

3. Answer: 3
Rationale: The spouse who maintains peace at any price is said to be in a dysfunctional family system. There is not enough information to make a determination about an adolescent who belongs to a gang, nor is there sufficient information about the pregnant 13-year-old girl. Being a laundry worker has no correlation to family functioning at all.
Cognitive Level: Analysis
Nursing Process: Assessment
Client Needs: Psychosocial Integrity
Text Page: 683

4. Answer: 1
Rationale: A psychiatric diagnosis related to family-related problems is an Axis I diagnosis.
Cognitive Level: Analysis
Nursing Process: NA
Client Needs: Psychosocial Integrity
Text Page: 684

5. Answer: 3
Rationale: According to the risk and protective factors model, this young man has at least one of the risk factors, indicated by his admission of regular drug and alcohol use with an older sibling. Factors indicated in Answers 1, 2, and 4 do not indicate that this adolescent is at risk.
Cognitive Level: Analysis
Nursing Process: Assessment
Client Needs: Psychosocial Integrity
Text Page: 685

6. Answer: 1
Rationale: Answer 1 indicates the use of the risk and protective factors model to assess a youth with a

suspicious bruise. Answers 2, 3, and 4 indicate a diagnosis not based on a sound model of assessment.
Cognitive Level: Analysis
Nursing Process: Assessment
Client Needs: Psychosocial Integrity
Text Page: 685

7. Answer: 1
Rationale: Deciding when family therapy is indicated is not always easy. Resource availability is a factor; many settings do not have family therapists. Some insurance coverage does not include family therapy. In addition, therapist bias may play a role in the use of family therapy as well.
Cognitive Level: Analysis
Nursing Process: Assessment
Client Needs: Psychosocial Integrity
Text Page: 686

8. Answer: 2
Rationale: Answer 2 is correct because when we look at family functioning, one of the reasons to recommend family therapy is the various types of difficulty and conflict that arise between the identified patient (the 17-year-old patient) and other family members (the father). In addition, the family is experiencing transition. The young boy will be graduating from high school and moving on to college.
Cognitive Level: Analysis
Nursing Process: Assessment
Client Needs: Psychosocial Integrity
Text Page: 686

9. Answer: 3
Rationale: Answer 3 is correct because an important component of family therapy, as in all treatments, is to be clear about the targets for therapeutic change.
Cognitive Level: Analysis
Nursing Process: Planning
Client Needs: Psychosocial Integrity
Text Page: 686

10. Answer: 2
Rationale: An essential component of all models of therapy is change.
Cognitive Level: Analysis
Nursing Process: NA
Client Needs: Psychosocial Integrity
Text Page: 686

11. Answer: 4
Rationale: When the therapist is completing a family assessment, it is useful for the therapist to consider meeting with the whole family or just the parents when the presenting problem is with a child.
Cognitive Level: Application
Nursing Process: Implementation
Client Needs: Psychosocial Integrity
Text Page: 687

12. Answer: 3
Rationale: Among the many assessment strategies, it is useful to consider family genogram to capture history, structure, and genetics related to psychiatric disorders and health.
Cognitive Level: Application
Nursing Process: Assessment
Client Needs: Psychosocial Integrity
Text Page: 687

13. Answer: 3
Rationale: Family interventions are aimed at engaging families and encouraging them to be active participants in treatment and rehabilitation, thereby increasing their knowledge and improving coping skills in both patients and their families.
Cognitive Level: Application
Nursing Process: Implementation
Client Needs: Psychosocial Integrity
Text Page: 687

14. Answer: 3
Rationale: Answer 3 would be the most likely program that guidance counselors would find useful for the population that they serve. Answer 1 would probably not be useful because teens would not want to attend a program to learn about family dynamics, nor would their younger siblings probably think that the topic would be useful to them. Answer 2 probably would be better attended in an outpatient, family-planning office, hospital, church, or another family-centered location. Answer 4 does not give information about a program. Competence building is not a skill to be taught, it is the ability to cope; therefore the nurse would not set up a program to teach competence for guidance counselors.
Cognitive Level: Analysis
Nursing Process: NA
Client Needs: Psychosocial Integrity
Text Page: 687

15. Answer: 3
Rationale: The name indicates that the topic of the group is mood disorders and the people in the patient's life that they affect. The term *way of life* tells us that anyone from any culture can learn more about treatment that would be focused on the person's way of life. Answer 1, 2, and 4 indicate a peer group for those with a certain disorder or concern, suicide, alcohol and drugs, or high blood pressure.
Cognitive Level: Analysis
Nursing Process: NA
Client Needs: Psychosocial Integrity
Text Page: 687

16. Answer: 2
Rationale: Direct observation should be used to assess changes in parent/child interactions. Answer 1, 3, and 4 are incorrect answers.
Cognitive Level: Application
Nursing Process: Implementation
Client Needs: Psychosocial Integrity
Text Page: 687

17. Answer: 3
Rationale: Studies of family therapy effectiveness are new; they have been conducted in just the last 20 years.
Cognitive Level: Comprehension
Nursing Process: Implementation
Client Needs: Psychosocial Integrity
Text Page: 687

18. Answer: 4
Rationale: Research on families can include basic family research, family intervention research, and family-related research. In each of these areas of research, the conceptualization, measurement, and analysis aspects view the family as a unit or system and thus contribute to the knowledge of family functioning.
Cognitive Level: Application
Nursing Process: Intervention
Client Needs: Psychosocial Integrity
Text Page: 687

19. Answer: 3
Rationale: The PEPS document is based on the belief that the family is the first line of defense and that there is a need to know which family interventions are effective in preventing substance abuse.
Cognitive Level: Analysis
Nursing Process: NA
Client Needs: Psychosocial Integrity
Text Page: 688

20. Answer: 2
Rationale: The treatment goal of functional family therapy is to modify interaction and communication patterns to foster more adaptive family functioning.
Cognitive Level: Application
Nursing Process: Planning
Client Needs: Psychosocial Integrity
Text Page: 688

21. Answer: 3
Rationale: Marital therapy is the treatment of the distress in a committed relationship, or the education of a couple in regard to what makes healthy relationships, such as good communication skills. This modality has been used in the treatment of depression, substance abuse, sexual dysfunction, divorce, step-family conflict, and trauma. There is strong clinical evidence for the effectiveness of this intervention.
Cognitive Level: Application
Nursing Process: NA
Client Needs: Psychosocial Integrity
Text Page: 689

22. Answer: 4
Rationale: There is much overlap between psychoeducational and family and marital therapy for families with members who have schizophrenia and mood disorders. Psychoeducation is often combined with marital and family therapy. Both psychoeducation and psychotherapy focus on problem solving and communication therapy.
Cognitive Level: Analysis
Nursing Process: Planning
Client Needs: Psychosocial Integrity
Text Page: 689

23. Answer: 2
Rationale: Psychoeducation for families that include persons with severe disorders, such as schizophrenia, major depression, and bipolar disorder, is typically combined with pharmacotherapy.
Cognitive Level: Application
Nursing Process: NA
Client Needs: Psychosocial Integrity
Text Page: 689

24. Answer: 2
Rationale: The goals of a family assessment and subsequent intervention are appraisal, reduction of psychiatric symptoms, increase in family resourcefulness or skills, improvement in individual psychological needs and family interactions, increased family awareness of how family patterns affect the health and satisfaction of their members, and the selection, implementation, and evaluation of treatment. The first step is assessment.
Cognitive Level: Application
Nursing Process: Implementation
Client Needs: Psychosocial Integrity
Text Page: 691

25. Answer: 3
Rationale: Using the family members' sense of humor as a means of bringing family members together and getting them to talk about difficult issues while at the same time reinforcing their affection for one another was a psychiatric nursing skill described as a successful intervention strategy in the Clinical Exemplar of a Psychiatric Nurse.
Cognitive Level: Application
Nursing Process: Implementation
Client Needs: Psychosocial Integrity
Text Page: 691

CHAPTER 34

1. Answer: 1
Rationale: Indications for inpatient hospitalizations include intimations that a person may be dangerous to self or others. Lethality assessment involves the assessment of suicidal plans, ideation, and history of prior attempts. Other indicators include the management of severe clinical manifestations that include confusion, disorganization, and inability to care for self.
Cognitive Level: Analysis
Nursing Process: Assessment
Client Needs: Safe Effective Care Environment: Management of Care
Text Page: 697

2. Answer: 2
Rationale: The stem of the question seeks the outcome that is part of the inpatient process of symptom management. These include teaching the patient and family about the psychotropic medications to be taken, outpatient treatment planning, referral sources, and completion of testing and diagnostic interviewing.
Cognitive Level: Analysis
Nursing Process: Planning
Client Needs: Psychosocial Integrity
Text Page: 697, 706-707

3. Answer: 1
Rationale: Years ago, patients who were admitted were able to remain in inpatient hospitals until symptom remission occurred. Today, stabilization is sought, and then treatment continues in the community. Diagnostic evaluation already would have been performed, and institutionalization (an unwanted passive dependency that develops with long hospital stays) is not an appropriate outcome.
Cognitive Level: Analysis
Nursing Process: Planning
Client Needs: Psychosocial Integrity
Text Page: 699, 705-706

4. Answer: 2
Rationale: When patients are severely confused and unable to care for themselves because of maladaptive coping, the multidisciplinary team will perform a rapid diagnostic evaluation, medicate to calm the patient as needed, and use four-point restraint only if needed to escort a patient to the inpatient unit. There, the goals will include stabilization with safety concerns at the forefront of the discharge planning (which starts with admission).
Cognitive Level: Analysis
Nursing Process: Implementation
Client Needs: Psychosocial Integrity
Text Page: 698-699

5. Answer: 1
Rationale: The priority nursing intervention for such a patient on the inpatient unit would include measures that prevent harm to self or others. Nevertheless, at all times the staff would use the least restrictive care prudently possible. Although laboratory values will assist staff in evaluating nutritional status and should be of concern, if the patient is walking around, these values would be of a lower priority. Remember how frightening invasive procedures can be for confused patients, and keep them to a minimum until the patient's mental status is somewhat cleared and anticipatory guidance can be employed.
Cognitive Level: Analysis
Nursing Process: Implementation
Client Needs: Psychosocial Integrity
Text Page: 700-701, 703

6. Answer: 2
Rationale: Physically destructive behavior is a response that is derived from an unspoken anger or fear. The most therapeutic communication for the situation is the one that validates and supports the underlying feeling but sets limits on the maladaptive action taken. The nurse's task is to help the destructive patient learn more adaptive ways to deal with anger, such as verbalization. Disparagement reflects the nurse's anger, and humiliation is aggressive to patients and nontherapeutic. Enlisting everyone to help clean up is the most therapeutic option, because it promotes cohesion and may encourage patients who did not do the damage to speak up and voice their anger at the offenders for spoiling their activity room. Peer input is always very effective.
Cognitive Level: Analysis
Nursing Process: Implementation
Client Needs: Psychosocial Integrity
Text Page: 702

7. Answer: 2
Rationale: When patients are dysphoric and intrusive on the unit, the nurse will want to protect the patient (who will probably be embarrassed when his or her thinking clears), other inpatients, and self. Probably the best way is to try to distract the patient and enlist cooperation for a time-out before escalation. As the patient's mental status clears, the nurse's sensitivity to the patient will foster trust in the therapeutic relationship.
Cognitive Level: Analysis
Nursing Process: Implementation
Client Needs: Psychosocial Integrity
Text Page: 700

8. Answer: 1
Rationale: It is important to communicate to the patient in a way that helps the patient to view his behavior from others' viewpoints, to observe the catalysts that trigger the behavior, and to view adaptive alternatives. Confrontation can escalate aggression on the unit and is nontherapeutic in that it can promote a regressive struggle between the nurse and the patient.
Cognitive Level: Analysis
Nursing Process: Implementation
Client Needs: Psychosocial Integrity
Text Page: 704

9. Answer: 4
Rationale: Working with dependency strivings is a difficult task and one that requires patience and understanding from the nurse. The most therapeutic nursing intervention is the one that encourages mutual problem solving.
Cognitive Level: Analysis
Nursing Process: Implementation
Client Needs: Psychosocial Integrity
Text Page: 704

10. Answer: 1
Rationale: Open report is a good example of the therapeutic community recommended by Maxwell Jones in 1953. However, it is not effective in today's fast-paced managed-care milieu, where lengths of stay in hospitals have diminished and the focus is on only stabilization.
Cognitive Level: Knowledge
Nursing Process: Implementation
Client Needs: Psychosocial Integrity
Text Page: 700

11. Answer: 1
Rationale: Steps to support patients to be more independent need to be carefully weighed with regard for safety, readiness, and capacity for inner control. By checking the time the next cigarette is due and allowing the patient to clock the time rather than totally removing independence, the nurse is improving the patient's orientation and socialization skills and reducing the amount of dependence and potentially intrusive behavior by the patient.
Cognitive Level: Analysis
Nursing Process: Implementation
Client Needs: Psychosocial Integrity
Text Page: 700

12. Answer: 1
Rationale: The first step is to assess the patient's complaint of sleeplessness. Patients often perceive that they sleep less than they do. Although the other techniques suggested may promote sleep, they would be implemented only if the nurse's assessment confirmed the patient's complaint of sleeplessness. This is one of the advantages of inpatient therapy. Outpatient treatment depends on the nurse's ability to ask the right set of questions to assess the patient's complaints.
Cognitive Level: Analysis
Nursing Process: Assessment
Client Needs: Psychosocial Integrity
Text Page: 705

13. Answer: 1
Rationale: Community resource groups are assigned on the basis of the patient's learning needs. Topics in the group may be provided on a rotating basis to assist patients to use community resources, including the public library, social services, and other agencies. Skills such as reading a newspaper or telephone book are also topics that may be shared. Patients in the group also often share their problem-solving skills about pertinent issues.
Cognitive Level: Analysis
Nursing Process: Planning
Client Needs: Psychosocial Integrity
Text Page: 705

14. Answer: 4
Rationale: An assertive nurse describes the unit situation, asks clearly for what is needed, and describes interim behavior or the consequence. Threatening to quit may constitute abandonment. JCAHO clearly states the staffing patterns that constitute safe standards of care.
Cognitive Level: Application
Nursing Process: Evaluation
Client Needs: Safe Effective Care Environment: Management of Care
Text Page: 707

15. Answer: 2
Rationale: Lethality assessment is the primary reason for using a crisis bed in the hospital. Although the other patients described all would seem to benefit from hospitalization, crisis beds are used for patients who are suicidal and homicidal.
Cognitive Level: Analysis
Nursing Process: Assessment
Client Needs: Psychosocial Integrity
Text Page: 699

16. Answer: 2
Rationale: From the time the patient is admitted, discharge planning begins. Discharge occurs when the client is stabilized. If information that is highly volatile and a likely trigger are uncovered, this might be a consideration for delaying discharge until the patient is informed, the response to the information is assessed, coping skills are evaluated, and additional supports can be provided.
Cognitive Level: Analysis
Nursing Process: Planning

Client Needs: Psychosocial Integrity
Text Page: 705-706

17. Answer: 2
Rationale: Partial hospitalization is not a "rest" for patients. It provides a highly structured and organized treatment plan that is comprehensive and individualized for its patients. Treatment plans include group therapy, education for client and family members, and other treatments to promote continuing stabilization and intermediate-term treatment.
Cognitive Level: Analysis
Nursing Process: Evaluation
Client Needs: Psychosocial Integrity
Text Page: 699

18. Answer: 3
Rationale: Poor hygiene in any patient is a concern. A few of the variables that may be affecting the situation are physical illness associated with age, sociocultural factors, and gender-related issues. The first step in identifying a problem is to explore the underlying factors that contribute to it and then to work with the patient to solve the problem. The other answers, such as teaching or mandating grooming, should be used only after a nonjudgmental assessment has been performed.
Cognitive Level: Analysis
Nursing Process: Implementation
Client Needs: Psychosocial Integrity
Text Page: 705, 708

19. Answer: 1
Rationale: Successful nursing approaches for disorganized patients include reassuring them and working with them to reduce the degree to which their behaviors inhibit therapeutic processes. Analyzing the extent to which fecal smearing from an ileostomy interferes with successful functioning (Maslow's hierarchy) and promoting optimal adaptation constitute primary nursing strategies for such a client. Passivity implies approval or insensitivity. Therapeutic use of self, that is, asking how you would be able to problem solve when so soiled, is a therapeutic approach to deciding nursing action. Answer 1 provides anticipatory guidance, which is an effective teaching approach for all patients. Asking a disorganized patient to make decisions may seem more democratic, but it does not provide support for the patient who is disorganized.
Cognitive Level: Analysis
Nursing Process: Implementation
Client Needs: Health Promotion and Maintenance
Text Page: 705

20. Answer: 1
Rationale: Patients on lithium usually start lithium with blood levels drawn three times a week and then monthly. When the patient is on maintenance medication, the psychiatrist may extend the testing of the blood levels to every 3 to 6 months. Fine hand tremors may be an adverse effect of lithium, but they may indicate the need for medication reduction.
Cognitive Level: Analysis
Nursing Process: Evaluation
Client Needs: Psychosocial Integrity
Text Page: 697, 705-706

21. Answer: 2
Rationale: The scope of contemporary psychiatric nursing practice requires knowledge and expertise in three broad areas: managing the therapeutic milieu; implementing caregiving activities; and integrating and coordinating care delivery. All psychiatric nurses, regardless of education or experience, engage in these activities every day. To do so requires that the nurse be aware of and value the full range of psychiatric nursing activities and know about the changing mental health care delivery system. These three areas of functioning represent both the structure and the process of hospital-based psychiatric nursing care, not just any one of the components; therefore Answer 2 is the only correct answer. Answer 1 relates to only the patient and not to the other areas of care delivered in an inpatient or partial-hospitalization program. Answers 3 and 4 address only certain components of the broad scope of care as well.
Cognitive Level: Analysis
Nursing Process: NA
Client Needs: Safe Effective Care Environment: Management of Care
Text Page: 699

22. Answer: 3
Rationale: Unlike inpatient settings in which the psychiatrist is expected to see patients daily, in most partial hospital programs the patient usually is seen weekly. The psychiatric nurse in most partial hospital programs assumes primary responsibility for assessing and identifying medical issues that may be contributing to the patient's psychiatric condition.
Cognitive Level: Application
Nursing Process: Assessment
Client Needs: Safe Effective Care Environment: Management of Care
Text Page: 699

23. Answer: 3
Rationale: Support includes the staff's conscious efforts to help patients feel better and improve their self-esteem. It is the unconditional acceptance of the patient, whatever his or her circumstances. The function of support is to help patients feel comfortable and secure and reduce their anxiety. It may take many forms, but it falls under the general heading of paying attention to the patient.

Cognitive Level: Application
Nursing Process: Assessment
Client Needs: Psychosocial Integrity
Text Page: 701

24. Answer: 1
Rationale: When barriers have been identified, particular strategies can be incorporated into the teaching plan to help the patient retain and use the information. As with any learner, repeating the information, presenting information in ways that engage multiple sensory avenues, and providing opportunities for practice and feedback promote learning for psychiatric patients.
Cognitive Level: Application
Nursing Process: Planning
Client Needs: Psychosocial Integrity
Text Page: 704

25. Answer: 3
Rationale: With the focus of psychiatric care shifting away from extended inpatient stays, opportunities for activity, group, and program development by psychiatric nurses are great. Nursing programs in social skills development, assertiveness, community-based support, crisis intervention, family preservation, and general health teaching are growing areas of psychiatric nursing responsibility. Patient and family teaching education programs are necessary to prepare family/caregivers for the complex responsibilities that they will face. Common topics for education include symptom recognition and management, desired effects and potential side effects of medication, relapse prevention, and importance of and plans for aftercare.
Cognitive Level: Application
Nursing Process: Implementation
Client Needs: Psychosocial Integrity
Text Page: 704, 705

CHAPTER 35

1. Answer: 2
Rationale: According to the report from the New Freedom Commission on Mental Health, *Achieving the Promise: Transforming Mental Health Care in America*, (NFCMH, 2003), evidence shows that offering a full range of community-based alternatives is more effective than hospitalization and emergency room treatment.
Cognitive Level: Analysis
Nursing Process: NA
Client Needs: Psychosocial Integrity
Text Page: 710

2. Answer: 4
Rationale: The goal of the fifth service of the Community Mental Health Centers Act of 1963 is consultation and education. One focus for education is primary prevention.
Cognitive Level: Analysis
Nursing Process: Planning
Client Needs: Psychosocial Integrity
Text Page: 710-711

3. Answer: 3
Rationale: Major amendments to the Community Mental Health Centers Act in 1975 required that community mental health centers continue to offer all five areas of service with less funding. Because of the funding cuts, the service that most community mental health centers reluctantly reduced is their preventive efforts, and they focused more resources on the care of people with diagnosed mental illness.
Cognitive Level: Application
Nursing Process: Outcome Identification
Client Needs: Psychosocial Integrity
Text Page: 711

4. Answer: 2
Rationale: The only correct answer is 2. Deinstitutionalization refers to the transfer of a patient hospitalized for extended periods of time to a community setting. At the mental health care system level, it refers to a shift in the focus of care from long-term institution to the community, accompanied by discharging long-term patients and avoiding unnecessary admissions.
Cognitive Level: Application
Nursing Process: NA
Client Needs: Safe Effective Care Environment: Management of Care
Text Page: 711

5. Answer: 2
Rationale: Soon after deinstitutionalization began, it became clear that policymakers had seriously miscalculated both the service needs of this population and the ability of communities to accommodate the large numbers of people with mental illness who had been discharged from the state. Often these former patients had to be readmitted to state hospitals.
Cognitive Level: Analysis
Nursing Process: NA
Client Needs: Safe Effective Care Environment: Management of Care
Text Page: 711

6. Answer: 3
Rationale: A special federal initiative was launched to help states and communities develop comprehensive services for the psychiatric population. This initiative was led by the National Institute of Mental Health (NIMH), which began to fund

demonstration programs for community support systems in all states.
Cognitive Level: Analysis
Nursing Process: NA
Client Needs: Psychosocial Integrity
Text Page: 711

7. Answer: 1
Rationale: A systems model of community mental health operates on the philosophy that all aspects of a person's life need care—basic human needs, physical health needs, and needs for psychiatric treatment and rehabilitation—if a person is to live successfully in the community.
Cognitive Level: Application
Nursing Process: Assessment
Client Needs: Safe Effective Care Environment: Management of Care
Text Page: 711

8. Answer: 2
Rationale: The court found that "confinement in an institution severely diminishes the everyday life activities of individuals, including family relations, social contacts, work options, economic independence, educational achievement, and cultural enrichment." Answers 1 and 3 have some validity to them, and Answer 4 is partly correct. But Answer 2 is the globally correct answer for this question.
Cognitive Level: Analysis
Nursing Process: NA
Client Needs: Safe Effective Care Environment: Management of Care
Text Page: 711

9. Answer: 4
Rationale: Case management involves linking the service system to the consumer and coordinating the service components so that he or she can achieve successful community living. All other answers apply in part, but Answer 4 is the global description of the scope of case management.
Cognitive Level: Analysis
Nursing Process: Outcome Identification
Client Needs: Safe Effective Care Environment: Management of Care
Text Page: 712

10. Answer: 1
Rationale: With the advent of managed care, case management has come to reflect two basic but seemingly contradictory goals, increasing access to services and limiting costs.
Cognitive Level: Analysis
Nursing Process: NA
Client Needs: Safe Effective Care Environment: Management of Care
Text Page: 712

11. Answer: 1
Rationale: According to *Parade*, 70% of Americans saw homeless people in their own communities, and 76% said something should be done to reduce homelessness in America.
Cognitive Level: Analysis
Nursing Process: NA
Client Needs: Psychosocial Integrity
Text Page: 713

12. Answer: 2
Rationale: Mental health professionals have begun to explore the use of new approaches to providing treatment, rehabilitation services, and housing to homeless people with mental illness, a population that often avoids contact with traditional mental health programs. Key components of this focused treatment approach include frequent and consistent staff contact through assertive outreach.
Cognitive Level: Application
Nursing Process: Planning
Client Needs: Psychosocial Integrity
Text Page: 714

13. Answer: 4
Rationale: Rural residents face greater social stigma in regard to seeking mental health care, and basic community services such as transportation, electricity, water, and telephones that are important to providing health care may not be available. Rural suicide rates have surpassed urban suicide rates over the past 20 years.
Cognitive Level: Comprehension
Nursing Process: NA
Client Needs: Psychosocial Integrity
Text Page: 715

14. Answer: 1
Rationale: The rate of serious mental illness in the incarcerated population is about three to four times that of the general U.S. population.
Cognitive Level: Analysis
Nursing Process: Assessment
Client Needs: Psychosocial Integrity
Text Page: 716

15. Answer: 2
Rationale: Mentally ill inmates of both sexes reported higher rates of prior physical and sexual abuse than other inmates, were more likely to have a history of substance abuse, and had higher unemployment before incarceration.
Cognitive Level: Application
Nursing Process: Planning
Client Needs: Psychosocial Integrity
Text Page: 716

16. Answer: 4
Rationale: One of the primary concerns of the Assertive Community Treatment team is relapse prevention. All of the other answers are true if needed by the individual patient, but a primary concern is to keep the individual healthy and out of an inpatient setting.
Cognitive Level: Application
Nursing Process: Implementation
Client Needs: Psychosocial Integrity
Text Page: 716-717

17. Answer: 3
Rationale: The Program of Assertive Community Treatment (PACT) is recognized by the National Alliance of the Mentally Ill (NAMI) as the most effective service-delivery model for community treatment of severe mental illness.
Cognitive Level: Comprehension
Nursing Process: NA
Client Needs: Psychosocial Integrity
Text Page: 718

18. Answer: 1
Rationale: The primary goal of multisystemic therapy is the preservation of the family and prevention of out-of-home placement through the provision of home-based, intensive, and time-limited services to families whose children are at immediate risk of such placement.
Cognitive Level: Comprehension
Nursing Process: NA
Client Needs: Psychosocial Integrity
Text Page: 718

19. Answer: 1
Rationale: Psychiatric home care is available to a broad segment of the population. Factors contributing to the development of the treatment setting include: Continued trend of deinstitutionalization; growth of managed care, which focuses on cost, outcomes, and earlier hospital discharges; and advocacy by consumer groups to find less restrictive and more humane ways of delivering care to people with mental illness.
Cognitive Level: Application
Nursing Process: Implementation
Client Needs: Psychosocial Integrity
Text Page: 719

20. Answer: 1
Rationale: Although changes in Medicare home health reimbursement have limited the growth of psychiatric home care, these programs have proven to be effective in meeting the needs of the psychiatric patient in a cost-effective manner.
Cognitive Level: Analysis
Nursing Process: NA
Client Needs: Psychosocial Integrity
Text Page: 719

21. Answer: 3
Rationale: The advantages of home care in comparison with inpatient treatment include its ability to serve as an enhancement of inpatient treatment through integration of home issues in the inpatient treatment plan.
Cognitive Level: Analysis
Nursing Process: Evaluation
Client Needs: Safe Effective Care Environment: Management of Care
Text Page: 719

22. Answer: 3
Rationale: The only correct answer here is Answer 3. Patients with repeated inpatient or crisis-unit admissions are identified among patients who can benefit from in-home psychiatric nursing services.
Cognitive Level: Analysis
Nursing Process: Assessment
Client Needs: Psychosocial Integrity
Text Page: 720

23. Answer: 2
Rationale: Documentation is one of the most challenging requirements of psychiatric home care. If the nurse's documentation does not reflect the skilled service given, the payment for that service can be denied by Medicare or other payers. Few guidelines are available for documentation of psychiatric home care, but standardized coding and classification systems are preferred. The psychiatric home care nurse must be very organized and detail oriented to successfully manage the extensive and precise paperwork.
Cognitive Level: Application
Nursing Process: Implementation
Client Needs: Safe Effective Care Environment: Management of Care
Text Page: 722

24. Answer: 2
Rationale: The only correct answer is Answer 2. Answer 2 indicates only one goal, while Answer 3 is probably not a realistic view of forensic nursing. Answer 4 does not indicate two conflicting goals but probably indicates a nurse who works in a crisis setting where patients can receive crisis care and/or respite care.
Cognitive Level: Analysis
Nursing Process: Implementation
Client Needs: Psychosocial Integrity
Text Page: 722

CHAPTER 36

1. Answer: 2
Rationale: Nursing interventions that help children learn to delay gratification include a point system to reinforce the behaviors, the use of games with commands like "stop" and "wait," and other activities and strategies that teach self-control.
Cognitive Level: Analysis
Nursing Process: Evaluation
Client Needs: Psychosocial Integrity
Text Page: 746

2. Answer: 4
Rationale: Anxiety, depression, and conduct disorders all share school problems, depression, and altered sleeping patterns. Children with conduct disorders usually demonstrate aggression toward people or animals.
Cognitive Level: Analysis
Nursing Process: Assessment
Client Needs: Psychosocial Integrity
Text Page: 740

3. Answer: 1
Rationale: An outcome is something that is measurable and specific to the individual. Since the only information in the stem of this question is the diagnosis, the most specific outcome is the one that is directly related to family factors, such as parental conflict and poor parenting. Although stealing, learning disability, and verbal abuse all are connected with conduct disorders, they are not measurable and do not exhibit appropriate expectations.
Cognitive Level: Analysis
Nursing Process: Planning
Client Needs: Psychosocial Integrity
Text Page: 740

4. Answer: 3
Rationale: The nurse needs to perform a complete assessment to determine the etiology of the child's problem and the parenting skills of the mother. Determining that the mother has tried to encourage her child to tie her shoes first is the first step in the nursing process.
Cognitive Level: Analysis
Nursing Process: Implementation
Client Needs: Psychosocial Integrity
Text Page: 742

5. Answer: 2
Rationale: It is difficult to assess this situation, but the information in the question demonstrates that the child's parents are concerned about her behavior. The first thing the nurse would want to know is the daughter's response to the incident.
Cognitive Level: Analysis
Nursing Process: Implementation
Client Needs: Psychosocial Integrity
Text Page: 733, 741

6. Answer: 2
Rationale: While the reports of childhood sexual abuse by spiritual leaders describe perpetrators as being well liked and as people who want children to like them, this is not facilitative at this time. The most therapeutic nursing intervention is the one that asks the child to discuss the incident more specifically.
Cognitive Level: Analysis
Nursing Process: Implementation
Client Needs: Psychosocial Integrity
Text Page: 734, 741

7. Answer: 3
Rationale: Management for children with ADHD includes contingency management, stimulant drug therapy, family therapy for conflict, assigning tasks in small steps to channel energy, behavior therapy, parenting-skills training, home help, environmental modification to reduce distractions, and educational programs for learning disabilities.
Cognitive Level: Analysis
Nursing Process: Planning
Client Needs: Psychosocial Integrity
Text Page: 740

8. Answer: 1
Rationale: Being able to tolerate frustration includes being able to persevere despite challenges and resistance. Answer 2 describes an ability to be introspective, and Answer 3 describes passivity. Answer 4 describes an ability to celebrate one's strengths realistically.
Cognitive Level: Analysis
Nursing Process: Evaluation
Client Needs: Psychosocial Integrity
Text Page: 738-739

9. Answer: 3
Rationale: Being able to use one's leisure time and to relax is a skill that must be balanced and learned. Balancing work, love, and play are the challenges that reverberate throughout life for all of us. Too much leisure or daydreaming or excessive use of work as leisure cannot be as adaptive as consistent, balanced activities developed throughout life.
Cognitive Level: Analysis
Nursing Process: Evaluation
Client Needs: Psychosocial Integrity
Text Page: 735, 742-743

10. Answer: 1
Rationale: Being able to lose a game with good sportsmanship is a good indication of social adaptation. Poor concentration and limited attention span can cause the child to interrupt the game or add others to increase distraction. Poor ability to delay gratification would engender demanding behavior and the intolerance of loss.
Cognitive Level: Analysis
Nursing Process: Evaluation
Client Needs: Psychosocial Integrity
Text Page: 734

11. Answer: 2
Rationale: Role playing is an excellent way to teach a child how to verbalize negative and positive feelings without being aggressive or passive. Assertiveness training uses role playing and role reversal to help patients learn how to be appropriately assertive.
Cognitive Level: Analysis
Nursing Process: Implementation
Client Needs: Psychosocial Integrity
Text Page: 742-743

12. Answer: 1
Rationale: Antipsychotics are most often used for rage and violent self-directed or other-directed behaviors in adolescents. Antianxiety agents probably would be avoided for this group of patients, and antidepressants and antihistamines are not specific for violent and rageful behaviors.
Cognitive Level: Analysis
Nursing Process: Planning
Client Needs: Psychosocial Integrity
Text Page: 747

13. Answer: 4
Rationale: Less restrictive interventions for aggressive, hostile, and destructive children include time-outs, open-door seclusion, therapeutic holding, and room programs to reduce inappropriate behavior.
Cognitive Level: Analysis
Nursing Process: Implementation
Client Needs: Psychosocial Integrity
Text Page: 742, 749

14. Answer: 1
Rationale: The child with ADHD will learn best when skills are taught in small steps and when new skills are added only after the child demonstrates mastery and comfort in performing the previous tasks. In addition, it is important to reduce the stimuli in the learning milieu, such as television or radio, to allow the child to concentrate.
Cognitive Level: Analysis
Nursing Process: Implementation
Client Needs: Psychosocial Integrity
Text Page: 749

15. Answer: 2
Rationale: Other symptoms of anxiety disorder include headache, pervasive worry and irritability, restlessness and pervasive fearfulness, and restless sleep and nightmares. Medical illness may be an underlying factor and would need to be excluded; current clinical manifestations are not sufficient to connect the two at this time. Conduct disorders have been related to antisocial personality disorders and early truancy.
Cognitive Level: Analysis
Nursing Process: Diagnosis
Client Needs: Psychosocial Integrity
Text Page: 742

16. Answer: 2
Rationale: The first step is to perform a complete lethality assessment. The nurse begins by asking the child to elaborate on his or her statement. The nurse may need to report the homicidal ideation, but not until the lethality level is determined.
Cognitive Level: Analysis
Nursing Process: Implementation
Client Needs: Psychosocial Integrity
Text Page: 741

17. Answer: 4
Rationale: The clinical manifestations identified by the parents certainly indicate depression, but the nurse cannot assess these without performing a thorough examination and mental status on the child. Parents may not be accurate in describing their observations of their child, so the nurse needs to explore this further.
Cognitive Level: Analysis
Nursing Process: Implementation
Client Needs: Psychosocial Integrity
Text Page: 731-734, 738

18. Answer: 1
Rationale: Certainly parental anxiety disorders, depression, or both have been identified as family factors in children's anxiety disorders, but this would be in the history, not in the plan. Residential treatment would not be the first option in a plan, and individual relaxation may or may not be part of treatment.
Cognitive Level: Analysis
Nursing Process: Planning
Client Needs: Psychosocial Integrity
Text Page: 732-735

19. Answer: 1
Rationale: Children with the medical diagnosis of generalized anxiety disorder may have difficulty establishing trusting relationships because they are very

concerned about their perceived competency. The following questions are used to evaluate this skill:
Does the child enjoy making friends?
Does the child often feel picked on by other people?
Does the child not know what to say when getting to know someone?
Answer 1 is the only correct response. No other answers are indicative of a child's ability to establish a healthy relationship.
Cognitive Level: Analysis
Nursing Process: Implementation
Client Needs: Psychosocial Integrity
Text Page: 734

20. Answer: 4
Rationale: Assessing a child through a biopsychosocial approach should focus attention on the child's biological development, the presence of medical illness, cognitive and personality characteristics, cultural context, and the child's family, school, and social environment. When planning immediate care, the nurse would assess ego competency skills first to determine the child's strengths and the extent of mastery of each skill.
Cognitive Level: Application
Nursing Process: Assessment
Client Needs: Psychosocial Integrity
Text Page: 735

21. Answer: 1
Rationale: A psychiatric illness in children that illustrates the interplay of genetics and environment is ADHD. Children with ADHD usually exhibit excessive activity and have difficulty paying attention. These behaviors are often tolerated by the family. However, when these children begin school, they are identified as problematic because these behaviors interfere with the child's academic performance and peer relationships.
Cognitive Level: Analysis
Nursing Process: Assessment
Client Needs: Psychosocial Integrity
Text Page: 730

22. Answer: 2
Rationale: A child's individual characteristics and early life experiences, as well as protective factors in their social and physical environment, contribute to resilience, their ability to withstand stress. What makes some children more resilient than others? Specific protective or resiliency factors of children have been identified. A sense of autonomy is one resiliency factor. Another factor is adaptive distancing, which occurs when a child is able to distance himself or herself from excessively close involvement with a dysfunctional family, transcend a difficult past, avoid identifying with troubled family members, and select healthy alternatives as they become available.
Cognitive Level: Analysis
Nursing Process: Assessment
Client Needs: Psychosocial Integrity
Text Page: 730

23. Answer: 1
Rationale: If the child's verbal communications are vague or unclear, the nurse needs to ask for additional explanation. Often a child will not respond to a problem-centered line of communication. In this case, the nurse should start by discussing more general aspects of the child's life, such as family members, school, or friends. Children with internalizing disorders such as depression or anxiety are often the best informants about their affective states. Children with externalizing disorders of ADHD or conduct disorder are typically poor informants and generally less cooperative in interview. They tend to blame others, thereby requiring reports from parents, teachers, day care staff, or school personnel to obtain information about problems and progress.
Cognitive Level: Analysis
Nursing Process: Assessment
Client Needs: Psychosocial Integrity
Text Page: 731

24. Answer: 2
Rationale: The child/adolescent can expect on-going timely staff responses to stated cultural health needs. The nurse will monitor and evaluate the response to treatment in an on-going fashion. The nurse will also collaboratively alter treatment approaches to achieve the goal of optimal effective coping and health while preserving cultural values of the client. Adolescents with an anxiety disorder may have difficulty establishing trusting relationships because they are very concerned about their perceived competency. The following questions are used to evaluate this skill:
Does the child enjoy making friends?
Does the child often feel picked on by other people?
Does the child not know what to say when getting to know someone?
The child in this question is obviously showing improvement in social skills and is beginning to trust peers. It is time to change the goals as he improves his communication skills.
Cognitive Level: Application
Nursing Process: Evaluation
Client Needs: Psychosocial Integrity
Text Page: 733-734

25. Answer: 1
Rationale: The only correct answer is Answer 1. Children with low self-esteem will not be motivated to participate in a peer self-help group (Answer 4)

because they usually withdraw and are not motivated to work on goals without guidance and help. Making major goals for the child (answer 3) will probably overwhelm the child, and giving frequent positive statements without foundation (answer 2) will not build self-esteem in the child. Children with low self-esteem express their low self-esteem through infrequent eye contact, lack of motivation, withdrawal, self-deprecating statements, or the use of negative behavior to seek attention. Specific therapeutic activities can be planned to improve a child's self-esteem. Accomplishment of a goal, no matter how small, is very rewarding, and incremental goal setting can be an effective way to provide opportunities for success. All other answers are contraindicated for a child with low self-esteem.
Cognitive Level: Application
Nursing Process: Implementation
Client Needs: Psychosocial Integrity
Text Page: 741

CHAPTER 37

1. Answer: 1
Rationale: The most therapeutic nursing intervention is the one that gives the adolescent the information that adolescence is a time when sexual identity and sexual behavior vary. Answers 2 and 4 are social and not based on a theoretical framework, and Answer 3 is insensitive and probing.
Cognitive Level: Analysis
Nursing Process: Implementation
Client Needs: Psychosocial Integrity
Text Page: 759

2. Answer: 2
Rationale: The nurse must report any violent threats immediately, and the best approach is to assist the girl in telling school authorities. Every school has a protocol for handling such a situation, and the nurse will want to be on hand to consult during the crisis. School nurses know that 6% of teens report carrying a weapon to school in the last 30 days, and that gunshot wounds are the second-most-common cause of death in the 15–24-year age group.
Cognitive Level: Analysis
Nursing Process: Implementation
Client Needs: Psychosocial Integrity
Text Page: 764

3. Answer: 3
Rationale: The occurrence of rampage murders has caused experts to look more closely at lethality among adolescents, and providing a forum that will allow all involved to properly grieve and that will educate them on strategies they can take to prevent further outbreaks would help to reduce their feelings of powerlessness.
Cognitive Level: Analysis
Nursing Process: Implementation
Client Needs: Psychosocial Integrity
Text Page: 764-765

4. Answer: 2
Rationale: The third stage of substance abuse is characterized by progression to midweek use to get high; excitement followed by guilt over use; and regular use progressing from tobacco, alcohol, and marijuana to other substances such as hash oil, tranquilizers, sedatives, and amphetamines.
Cognitive Level: Analysis
Nursing Process: Evaluation
Client Needs: Psychosocial Integrity
Text Page: 767

5. Answer: 1
Rationale: Stage 3 of substance abuse indicates that the adolescent has progressed to midweek use to get high and will benefit from participation in drug-free self-help groups and family therapy. Family intervention is also an important part of treatment, because the issues surrounding the problem of adolescent use must be addressed for the whole family affected.
Cognitive Level: Analysis
Nursing Process: Implementation
Client Needs: Psychosocial Integrity
Text Page: 767

6. Answer: 2
Rationale: Answer 2 demonstrates a cognitive question because it reflects the ability to reason beyond concrete operations. Answer 1 presents a cultural question; Answer 3 reflects a psychoanalytical question; and Answer 4 presents a psychosocial question.
Cognitive Level: Analysis
Nursing Process: Assessment
Client Needs: Psychosocial Integrity
Text Page: 756-757

7. Answer: 1
Rationale: Adolescence is a time for exploration before adulthood. Without any other changes, the youth may just be interested in history, so it would be most therapeutic for the nurse to obtain further information from the parent before seeing the adolescent or recommending help. Answer 2 is not therapeutic but is challenging; Answer 3 is a premature response to insufficient data and breaches confidentiality; Answer 4 is again a premature response to insufficient data and makes an issue of confidentiality at an inappropriate time.
Cognitive Level: Analysis
Nursing Process: Implementation
Client Needs: Psychosocial Integrity
Text Page: 757

8. Answer: 2
Rationale: The mother is upset because she equates the tattoo with negative aspects of growth and may not know that a tattoo is not considered any worse than piercing one's ears to many individuals. Although the parent may elect to educate the child at home (and children often excel scholastically when this happens), such an approach may fail if it lacks the proper purpose for its implementation. Persuading the mother to come in and see the nurse and counselor will help her to problem solve more effectively and view the tattoo in a healthier perspective.
Cognitive Level: Analysis
Nursing Process: Implementation
Client Needs: Psychosocial Integrity
Text Page: 756-757

9. Answer: 1
Rationale: The symptoms the teacher is observing may well be adolescent depression, and the nurse would be most therapeutic to offer this possibility to the teacher as an alternative perspective. All other answers offered to this situation are based on insufficient data and misinformation.
Cognitive Level: Analysis
Nursing Process: Implementation
Client Needs: Psychosocial Integrity
Text Page: 761-762

10. Answer: 1
Rationale: The most therapeutic communication is the one that facilitates more adaptive problem solving, and Answer 1 intimates that there are options other than suicide. Answers 2 and 3 are not therapeutic, and Answer 4 lectures to the patient.
Cognitive Level: Analysis
Nursing Process: Implementation
Client Needs: Psychosocial Integrity
Text Page: 761-762

11. Answer: 3
Rationale: The initial step is to determine what the adolescent says about the schoolbook defacement and then respond from there. The behavior is a cry for help, and the teacher needs to view it correctly and not jump to conclusions.
Cognitive Level: Analysis
Nursing Process: Implementation
Client Needs: Psychosocial Integrity
Text Page: 759-760

12. Answer: 1
Rationale: Answers 2 and 4 describe punitive responses that are not therapeutic. Answer 3 does not address the adolescent's problem, although school authorities have done just this. Answer 1 is the correct answer. It safeguards the adolescent while he is inebriated and seeks assistance that uses a family-centered approach to the adolescent's problems.
Cognitive Level: Analysis
Nursing Process: Implementation
Client Needs: Psychosocial Integrity
Text Page: 765-767

13. Answer: 2
Rationale: The adolescent has suffered a deep loss. The nurse is responsible for identifying adolescents who may be at risk for depression and other problems, so the adolescent should be monitored accordingly.
Cognitive Level: Analysis
Nursing Process: Implementation
Client Needs: Psychosocial Integrity
Text Page: 761-762

14. Answer: 2
Rationale: Answers 1, 3, and 4 indicate that parents are inappropriately applying statistics to their children. The nurse will want to follow-up and carefully clarify each parent's thought processes.
Cognitive Level: Analysis
Nursing Process: Assessment
Client Needs: Psychosocial Integrity
Text Page: 764-765

15. Answer: 2
Rationale: Adolescents can exaggerate situations and issues and often need time and perspective to view issues more objectively. By helping the adolescent view the issues more dispassionately, the nurse will assist him or her to problem solve more effectively and to begin to view issues from the parents' perspective as well.
Cognitive Level: Analysis
Nursing Process: Implementation
Client Needs: Psychosocial Integrity
Text Page: 757

16. Answer: 3
Rationale: The most effective action by the nurse would be to arrange for a family meeting to determine what is happening to cause the girl to feel sick on Fridays. Directly asking her may be too threatening, because she doesn't seem to be able to articulate her concerns except somatically. Suspension simply reinforces school absence, and a telephone call is a superficial intervention for a serious adolescent maladaptive behavior.
Cognitive Level: Analysis
Nursing Process: Implementation
Client Needs: Psychosocial Integrity
Text Page: 761-762

17. Answer: 4
Rationale: Answers 1, 2, and 3 are responses to termination that are within normal range and that

demonstrate readiness for the adolescent to end treatment. The therapist will allow the patient to call but will set limits on the reasons for doing so. Many clients will say they thought they had more sessions, and others will admit to feeling sorry to leave when they feel safe. Expressing doubts about readiness is also within the range of answers, but the therapist will want to work with the adolescent before termination to build support and feelings of confidence.
Cognitive Level: Analysis
Nursing Process: Implementation
Client Needs: Psychosocial Integrity
Text Page: 758

18. Answer: 1
Rationale: The nurse has a duty to report any information that is provided that could present danger to the patients themselves or to others.
Cognitive Level: Analysis
Nursing Process: Implementation
Client Needs: Psychosocial Integrity
Text Page: 771-772

19. Answer: 3
Rationale: Answer 3 acknowledges the patient's concern while still focusing on reality. Answer 1 sets up a situation that may create a regressive struggle. Answer 2 is an overreaction at this point. Answer 4 is premature and may overwhelm an already traumatized adolescent who is hypersensitive.
Cognitive Level: Analysis
Nursing Process: Implementation
Client Needs: Psychosocial Integrity
Text Page: 768

20. Answer: 4
Rationale: Running away may be a cry for help, an attempt to escape from an unbearable living situation, or both. It also can be a solution that would be chosen by an unmotivated youth who may have a conduct disorder.
Cognitive Level: Analysis
Nursing Process: Implementation
Client Needs: Psychosocial Integrity
Text Page: 763-764

21. Answer: 3
Rationale: In response to the changes of puberty that affect their identity and the feelings that are associated with this, adolescents use defenses against these feelings that were helpful in childhood and also experiment with new, more adult-like attempts at mastery. As a result of these attempts to cope, adolescents sometimes act like adults and at other times act like children. Answers 1, 2, and 4 represent some concerns of the adolescent but are unrelated to the issue of this question, which focuses on the overlapping themes of identity and independence.
Cognitive Level: Application
Nursing Process: Implementation
Client Needs: Psychosocial Integrity
Text Page: 757-758

22. Answer: 1
Rationale: Authoritarian parents are oriented toward shaping, controlling, and restricting the adolescent to fixed standards. Obedience is seen as a virtue, and power and responsibility are not shared with the adolescent. Traditional parents value a sense of continuity and order. Democratic parents do not believe that their standards are always right. Laissez faire is not a parenting style identified in the textbook.
Cognitive Level: Analysis
Nursing Process: Assessment
Client Needs: Psychosocial Integrity
Text Page: 758

23. Answer: 4
Rationale: All of the problems described are indicators of depression in adolescents. Although the incidence of depression is twice as great in girls as in boys, the male suicide rate for 15-to-19-year-olds is five times that of the female rate.
Cognitive Level: Analysis
Nursing Process: Assessment
Client Needs: Psychosocial Integrity
Text Page: 761

24. Answer: 2
Rationale: Wearing clothing that hides the effects of self-mutilation is a behavior in which adolescents often engage, but it is not a helpful strategy to prevent the behavior itself. The strategies listed in Answers 1, 3, and 4 are useful in reducing or stopping self-mutilation.
Cognitive Level: Application
Nursing Process: Implementation
Client Needs: Psychosocial Integrity
Text Page: 763

25. Answer: 3
Rationale: Adolescents often test nurses early in the therapeutic relationship to see whether they are anxious, defensive adults or whether they will respond as authority figures. This type of behavior is called resistance. Interestingly, arguing is a way for adolescents to learn. Limits testing is a way for adolescents to see how firm and consistent nurses will be. Embarrassment about being in therapy is common in adolescents and can be discussed openly in a therapy session.
Cognitive Level: Analysis
Nursing Process: Assessment
Client Needs: Psychosocial Integrity
Text Page: 772-773

CHAPTER 38

1. Answer: 1
Rationale: Case management is an effective approach to providing care for the biopsychosocial needs of the elderly. Mental health services can be provided to the elder in diverse care settings, including the patient's own home.
Cognitive Level: Knowledge
Nursing Process: Implementation
Client Needs: Psychosocial Integrity
Text Page: 778

2. Answer: 2
Rationale: The biological programming theory speculates that each cell has stored a biological clock and that the process of aging in DNA is not reversible. In Answer 1, the free radical theory postulates that free radicals damage cell membranes and cause aging, so one would want to eliminate free radicals to retard aging. In Answer 3, the cross-linkage theory speculates that collagen forms bonds between molecular structures and increases rigidity over time. In Answer 4, the immunological theory speculates that the immune system becomes less effective over time, reducing effectiveness of surveillance, self-regulation, and response.
Cognitive Level: Application
Nursing Process: Implementation
Client Needs: Psychosocial Integrity
Text Page: 779

3. Answer: 1
Rationale: ADLs (bathing, grooming, toileting, eating, and dressing) are tasks that can be measured to reflect functional independence. One can ascertain other self-care needs, such as psychosocial ones, by directly asking the patient to recount the activities in which he or she engaged during the previous week.
Cognitive Level: Analysis
Nursing Process: Implementation
Client Needs: Psychosocial Integrity
Text Page: 783

4. Answer: 2
Rationale: A comprehensive health assessment would include oral assessment (checking swallowing, breathing, missing teeth, dry mouth, and any ulcerations in the mouth), poor vision, mental status, and other variables that might affect nutritional status.
Cognitive Level: Analysis
Nursing Process: Implementation
Client Needs: Psychosocial Integrity
Text Page: 784

5. Answer: 1
Rationale: Older adult patients experience sunrise syndrome. This may result from hangover effects of sedative-hypnotics and other nighttime medications that interact with drugs for sleep.
Cognitive Level: Analysis
Nursing Process: Evaluation
Client Needs: Psychosocial Integrity
Text Page: 785-786

6. Answer: 3
Rationale: It is postulated that sundown syndrome is caused by deterioration of the suprachiasmatic nucleus of the hypothalamus. This interferes with the major pacemaker of circadian rhythms. One strategy to ameliorate it is by providing at least minimal exposure to direct sunlight each day to reset circadian rhythm.
Cognitive Level: Application
Nursing Process: Planning
Client Needs: Psychosocial Integrity
Text Page: 785-786

7. Answer: 1
Rationale: The answer that invites the patient to share feelings and perceptions (thus facilitating emotions) is the most therapeutic communication. Saying, "Don't worry" is an example of false reassurance, which is a nontherapeutic communication. Questioning evidence of verbal abuse is premature. Caregivers who have sufficient coping built in (such as respite) do not have to experience negative feelings toward their loved ones.
Cognitive Level: Analysis
Nursing Process: Implementation
Client Needs: Psychosocial Integrity
Text Page: 794

8. Answer: 4
Rationale: All of the above answers are part of the clinical manifestations of relocation stress syndrome, except for a decrease in withdrawal.
Cognitive Level: Analysis
Nursing Process: Evaluation
Client Needs: Psychosocial Integrity
Text Page: 788

9. Answer: 3
Rationale: One can assess the functional ability of mobility and independence by observing the patient's ability to dress, comb hair, shave, and feed self without assistance; to move within the milieu; and to maintain contact with others.
Cognitive Level: Application
Nursing Process: Assessment
Client Needs: Psychosocial Integrity
Text Page: 783

10. Answer: 2
Rationale: Answer 2 supports the disputations about disengagement theory. Instead of thinking that older adults will isolate and reduce socialization, it postulates that active individuals will remain active. The same holds true for sedentary adults, unless they deliberately adapt to bring about increased socialization.
Cognitive Level: Application
Nursing Process: Implementation
Client Needs: Psychosocial Integrity
Text Page: 779

11. Answer: 1
Rationale: Having the patient visit the nursing home before actually moving and having familiar staff visit the patient in the nursing home can reduce relocation stress syndrome.
Cognitive Level: Analysis
Nursing Process: Planning
Client Needs: Psychosocial Integrity
Text Page: 788

12. Answer: 1
Rationale: Whenever there is a concern for lethality, it should be assessed immediately. Lethality risk can be assessed higher when there is a history of a suicide attempt and if the patient is a white male over 65 years of age. Cognitive insight will not bring emotional coping.
Cognitive Level: Analysis
Nursing Process: Implementation
Client Needs: Psychosocial Integrity
Text Page: 787

13. Answer: 1
Rationale: Depression, grief, and loss are common in later life. If mourning and grief are prolonged, they should be treated as depression.
Cognitive Level: Analysis
Nursing Process: Implementation
Client Needs: Psychosocial Integrity
Text Page: 786-787

14. Answer: 2
Rationale: Paranoia, a classic organized and complicated delusional system that is rare in older adults, can be caused by sensory deprivation or loss, medications, social isolation, delirium, and dementia. The older adult with a paranoid personality will exhibit withdrawal, aloofness, fearfulness, oversensitivity, or secretiveness.
Cognitive Level: Analysis
Nursing Process: Assessment
Client Needs: Psychosocial Integrity
Text Page: 786

15. Answer: 2
Rationale: Certainly busy people and those with depression can experience short-term memory loss. Depressed individuals are probably more likely to experience a shorter attention span.
Cognitive Level: Analysis
Nursing Process: Implementation
Client Needs: Psychosocial Integrity
Text Page: 785

16. Answer: 4
Rationale: Until a comprehensive assessment of the patient's family and social support systems is performed, it is impossible to consider any of the other options.
Cognitive Level: Analysis
Nursing Process: Implementation
Client Needs: Psychosocial Integrity
Text Page: 784-785

17. Answer: 1
Rationale: In Answer 2, the risk factors are a move to less familiar surroundings and caring for an active 3-year-old grandchild. In Answer 3, the risk factors include using a cane. In Answer 4, the risk factors include new surroundings and a new relationship. Answer 1 has the following risk factors: stoicism that may indicate an unwillingness to ask for help, a move to unfamiliar surroundings, and increased age (as compared with the other possible choices).
Cognitive Level: Analysis
Nursing Process: Assessment
Client Needs: Psychosocial Integrity
Text Page: 782-783

18. Answer: 2
Rationale: Taking medications that cause sedation (drowsiness) and postural hypotension like antidepressant agents would be the primary risk factor obtained.
Cognitive Level: Analysis
Nursing Process: Assessment
Client Needs: Psychosocial Integrity
Text Page: 783

19. Answer: 1
Rationale: Answers 2, 3, and 4 are all interventions that the nurse might employ over time, but the most effective and timely intervention is the one that provides complete information about the patient's medications.
Cognitive Level: Analysis
Nursing Process: Implementation
Client Needs: Psychosocial Integrity
Text Page: 783

20. Answer: 2
Rationale: The psychological theory of aging states that an individual's personality is established by adulthood and remains stable, although adaptable, over time; any major change may indicate physiological disease (such as brain disease).

Cognitive Level: Knowledge
Nursing Process: Implementation
Client Needs: Psychosocial Integrity
Text Page: 779

21. Answer: 3
Rationale: When interviewing an older adult, questions should be short and to the point, especially if the patient has difficulty with abstract thinking and conceptualization. The nurse should initially rephrase a question if the patient does not answer appropriately or hesitates when answering. Answers 1 and 2 are inappropriate because they do not acknowledge the patient's perplexed look. Answer 4 reads into the patient's lack of verbal response by assuming the lack of response is due to an underlying issue with the move, and also ignores the nonverbal communication (perplexed look) by the patient.
Cognitive Level: Application
Nursing Process: Implementation
Client Needs: Psychosocial Integrity
Text Page: 780

22. Answer: 4
Rationale: Many medications taken by geriatric patients can cause drowsiness, confusion, orthostatic hypotension, uncoordination, or reduced sensation, which in turn can increase risk of falls. The patient taking two antihypertensive medications daily is at great risk for falls caused by orthostatic hypotension. The patient in Answer 1 is at lesser risk because the drug is taken only once per week on average. The patients in Answers 2 and 3 are not taking medications that would cause the side effects listed above.
Cognitive Level: Analysis
Nursing Process: Assessment
Client Needs: Psychosocial Integrity
Text Page: 783

23. Answer: 1
Rationale: Older adults benefit from interesting and appropriate activities, a sense of calm and quiet (soft colors, soothing music, and use of personal articles), a consistent physical layout with no environmental barriers, and a structured daily routine. Answers 2, 3, and 4 all are partially incorrect. Incorrect items include bright colors (Answer 2), rearranging furniture (Answer 3), and varying the daily routine (Answer 4).
Cognitive Level: Analysis
Nursing Process: Implementation
Client Needs: Psychosocial Integrity
Text Page: 790

24. Answer: 2
Rationale: Validation therapy involves searching for emotion and/or meaning in the patient's disoriented or confused words and behavior and validating them verbally with the patient. Answer 1 would be appropriate if the nurse was using reminiscence. Answer 3 reflects reality orientation and Answer 4 is nontherapeutic because it does not address the patient's statement in any way.
Cognitive Level: Application
Nursing Process: Implementation
Client Needs: Psychosocial Integrity
Text Page: 793

25. Answer: 3
Rationale: Slowed response time, benign memory loss, altered gait, and interrupted sleep patterns are a few of the normal changes of aging that elders or their families may interpret as pathological. Depression is a health problem that requires accurate diagnosis and treatment.
Cognitive Level: Analysis
Nursing Process: Evaluation
Client Needs: Psychosocial Integrity
Text Page: 781, 794

CHAPTER 39

1. Answer: 3
Rationale: This question asks that behaviors for intervention be prioritized. First, it is necessary to help the patient identify the problem and to set criteria for future communications. Second, the patient should be taught how to identify verbal abuse and enter into dialogue without being verbally abusive. Along the way, the nurse will seek answers about who provided the verbally abusive model and, in some frameworks; the nurse may set consequences for verbal abuse on which both parties have mutually agreed.
Cognitive Level: Analysis
Nursing Process: Implementation
Client Needs: Psychosocial Integrity
Text Page: 799

2. Answer: 1
Rationale: Answer 1 is an illustration of how the nurse might help the patient to look at her husband's attempt to undermine her sexuality to inappropriately justify his infidelity. This is a form of sexual abuse. Answer 2 helps the patient to place fears (as yet unjustified by the patient's example) in perspective. Answer 3 describes a common parental error when first giving a child an allowance; the nurse will seek to clarify boundaries while remaining alert to the parent's attempts to maintain total control over all financial dealings of the child. Answer 4 describes the child's inability to acknowledge a parent's response as supportive.
Cognitive Level: Analysis
Nursing Process: Implementation
Client Needs: Psychosocial Integrity
Text Page: 809

3. Answer: 3
Rationale: All the other answers are illustrations of myths of abuse survivors.
Cognitive Level: Analysis
Nursing Process: Implementation
Client Needs: Psychosocial Integrity
Text Page: 808-809

4. Answer: 2
Rationale: Answer 2 is a therapeutic reflection that helps the patient to sort out the fears that many battered women have that their children will suffer without the father present. Answer 1 is sarcastic and may reflect the nurse's bias toward the battered woman's ambivalence rather than viewing it as a normal part of the process that battered women experience. Answer 3 is again an example of the nurse's bias in that it is somewhat sarcastic rather than understanding of the battered woman's denial and ambivalence. Answer 4 is incorrect and nontherapeutic because it offers agreement.
Cognitive Level: Analysis
Nursing Process: Implementation
Client Needs: Psychosocial Integrity
Text Page: 810

5. Answer: 2
Rationale: Answer 2 is a therapeutic nursing intervention for a patient with rape trauma syndrome. Mutual goal setting is the key; the patient's plans should not be controlled. Although the nurse can help the patient to make an appointment, the patient would not be enrolled in a group without being given an opportunity to self-select. The patient would be encouraged to discuss the issues with trusted and supportive people who may not be health professionals involved with the patient.
Cognitive Level: Knowledge
Nursing Process: Planning
Client Needs: Psychosocial Integrity
Text Page: 813

6. Answer: 1
Rationale: The first step toward effective intervention with survivors of family violence is the exploration of one's own attitude toward and knowledge about violence.
Cognitive Level: Analysis
Nursing Process: Implementation
Client Needs: Psychosocial Integrity
Text Page: 800-801

7. Answer: 2
Rationale: The most therapeutic communication is the one that facilitates the patient's expression of feelings. This question describes psychological abuse occurring within the family and that reflects struggles for power and control. Answers 1, 3, and 4 reflect ignorance and bias regarding the attempts of the husband to isolate the patient.
Cognitive Level: Analysis
Nursing Process: Implementation
Client Needs: Psychosocial Integrity
Text Page: 813

8. Answer: 4
Rationale: Psychic rape involves an assault on the victim's dignity and self-respect. Examples include verbal assault, street harassment, pornography in the media, and portrayals of violent sex. Answer 1 describes an economic partnership. Answer 2 describes a seduction rape. Answer 3 describes a fear rape.
Cognitive Level: Analysis
Nursing Process: Implementation
Client Needs: Psychosocial Integrity
Text Page: 812-813

9. Answer: 2
Rationale: The acute stage of sexual assault also may appear as one in which the patient is subdued or outwardly calm. Answers 1 and 3 may or may not describe the patient's responses. Answer 4 describes the second stage of sexual assault, which involves long-term reorganization.
Cognitive Level: Analysis
Nursing Process: Implementation
Client Needs: Psychosocial Integrity
Text Page: 813

10. Answer: 1
Rationale: Answer 1 is a direct answer to the patient's question; it teaches more than it is facilitative. The nurse has decided to present evidence-based research and will then facilitate the patient's feelings. Answer 2 is a social response not based on evidence; it provides false reassurance and may slander the late physician's competence. Answers 3 and 4 present half-truths that are twisted.
Cognitive Level: Analysis
Nursing Process: Implementation
Client Needs: Psychosocial Integrity
Text Page: 803

11. Answer: 2
Rationale: There are community groups that help families deal with domestic violence. The nurse works with what is possible and does not impose judgments on the patient. Creative and flexible problem solving is key to successful intervention in domestic violence. The pattern of passivity of battered women is best overcome within a trusting relationship in which the nurse has demonstrated mutuality and tolerance.
Cognitive Level: Analysis
Nursing Process: Implementation
Client Needs: Psychosocial Integrity
Text Page: 810

12. Answer: 4
Rationale: Although most nurses do not actually blame survivors for what has happened to them, research reveals that they are less tolerant of certain behaviors. For example, nurses are more apt to blame a rape survivor if the woman had gone out late at night, not locked her car doors, gone shopping for beer rather than milk for the baby, or did not resist the assault "enough." Studies describe how survivors find the health care system to be unhelpful and even traumatic when they go for help. Nurses often use a paternalistic and individualistic model of helping battered women. The paternalistic model may be contrasted with the empowerment model. The empowerment model is not only more helpful to the survivor, but also more professionallly satisfying for the nurse. Answer 4 is indicative of this rationale and is the correct answer because it is the one that most professionally responds to a colleague who shows evidence of a bias.
Cognitive Level: Analysis
Nursing Process: Implementation
Client Needs: Psychosocial Integrity
Text Page: 800-801

13. Answer: 4
Rationale: Women are four times more likely to be raped by men they know. Contrary to some thinking, if a woman says "no," the partner is responsible for respecting and complying with the request.
Cognitive Level: Analysis
Nursing Process: Implementation
Client Needs: Psychosocial Integrity
Text Page: 802

14. Answer: 1
Rationale: Answer 1 is the most therapeutic nursing intervention. Answer 2 places the nurse in danger. Answer 3 is not a therapeutic nursing intervention and Answer 4 is a judgment and a threat, and may place the nurse in danger.
Cognitive Level: Analysis
Nursing Process: Implementation
Client Needs: Psychosocial Integrity
Text Page: 804-806

15. Answer: 3
Rationale: Although it is often difficult to differentiate elder abuse, bilateral bruising on the upper outer arms is a definitive sign. The nurse is responsible for reporting such findings and to continue vigilant observation of further signs of elder abuse and neglect. It is usually best to inform the family of your intention to report elder abuse with the expressed purpose of obtaining help for both; this makes protective services less threatening and preserves the nurse's therapeutic alliance.
Cognitive Level: Analysis
Nursing Process: Implementation
Client Needs: Psychosocial Integrity
Text Page: 810-811

16. Answer: 3
Rationale: Of all the options, only answer 3 provides no findings that are correlated with witnessing violence and reflecting it in behavior. The young man's comments indicate appropriate problem solving, knowledge, and intent not to be violent again.
Cognitive Level: Analysis
Nursing Process: Implementation
Client Needs: Psychosocial Integrity
Text Page: 807-808

17. Answer: 2
Rationale: Answer 1 indicates that the child was physically abused. Answer 3 involves verbal humiliation and criticism. Answer 4 is a classic response of an elder who is being abused. Answer 2 reflects the fact that many men are conditioned to macho stereotypes and feel vulnerable when they view this as being undermined. However, shame is a more passive response at this time. If handled with sensitivity and reprogramming, the husband will accommodate to a new model.
Cognitive Level: Analysis
Nursing Process: Assessment
Client Needs: Psychosocial Integrity
Text Page: 808-809

18. Answer: 4
Rationale: Answer 1 assumes that the nurse is the more knowledgeable and wise and needs to teach the patient; Answer 2 has the nurse impart knowledge in a one-down style of communication; and Answer 3 places the burden on the survivor. All of these illustrate the use of a paternalistic model of intervention for a battered woman. Answer 4 uses an empowerment model by assuming mutuality in sharing and providing respect for what the survivor knows.
Cognitive Level: Analysis
Nursing Process: Implementation
Client Needs: Psychosocial Integrity
Text Page: 810

19. Answer: 3
Rationale: Answer 3 uses a therapeutic nursing communication to facilitate the abused spouse to view her irrationality. Answer 1 is off-focus, and it is not understandable that someone would not report abuse appropriately. Answer 2 is an angry response that reflects the nurse's bias and is not therapeutic. Answer 4 reflects the myth that the perpetrator needs to be provoked to be abusive.
Cognitive Level: Analysis
Nursing Process: Implementation
Client Needs: Psychosocial Integrity
Text Page: 809

20. Answer: 1
Rationale: Answer 2 is true only because the affluent can afford private assistance and support that is not reported. Answer 3 contains incorrect content and focuses attention on the nurse's response. Answer 4 also contains incorrect content. Answer 1 is a therapeutic nursing communication of reflection; by reflecting back to the patient what she has said, the nurse assists the patient to view the statement in perspective.
Cognitive Level: Analysis
Nursing Process: Implementation
Client Needs: Psychosocial Integrity
Text Page: 807

21. Answer: 3
Rationale: The populations that are particularly at risk for abuse are children, intimate partners, and the elderly. The only group of individuals that fits the criteria is in Answer 3.
Cognitive Level: Analysis
Nursing Process: NA
Client Needs: Psychosocial Integrity
Text Page: 798

22. Answer: 2
Rationale: Social norms and learned family values are sometimes used to justify violence to maintain the family system. For example, a husband's use of violence may be considered legitimate if the wife is having an extramarital affair. Historical attitudes toward women, children, and the elderly; economic discrimination; the nonresponsiveness of the criminal justice system; and the belief that women and children are property are social factors that promote violence.
Cognitive Level: Analysis
Nursing Process: Assessment
Client Needs: Psychosocial Integrity
Text Page: 799

23. Answer: 3
Rationale: Another common factor within the various forms of family violence is the use and abuse of power. In almost all forms of family violence, the abuser has some form of power or control over the victim. Answers 1, 2, and 4 are examples of a self-centered individual feeling victimized and the partner who is able to leave or participate in the situation without becoming a victim. Answer 3 indicates that the husband came home and "picked a fight" about the new recipe that his wife tried. There is a clear indication that the husband has power over his wife as she expresses her lack of ability to "be a good wife."
Cognitive Level: Analysis
Nursing Process: Assessment
Client Needs: Psychosocial Integrity
Text Page: 799-800

24. Answer: 1
Rationale: A characteristic pattern of injuries, especially to the head, neck, face, throat, trunk, and sexual organs has been seen in all forms of family violence. In addition, there is increased anxiety in the presence of the abuser and inappropriate or anxious nonverbal behavior by the abused during the physical exam, for which the nurse will look as well.
Cognitive Level: Application
Nursing Process: Assessment
Client Needs: Safe Effective Care Environment: Management of Care
Text Page: 802, 805

25. Answer: 4
Rationale: School in general is a much safer environment for children and adolescents than their neighborhoods and family homes. A variety of risk factors for school violence are drug use, carrying a weapon, antisocial and impulsive behavior, and family and community disorganization and unresponsiveness. The only correct answer is number 4.
Cognitive Level: Analysis
Nursing Process: Assessment
Client Needs: Safe Effective Care Environment: Management of Care
Text Page: 807

CHAPTER 40

1. Answer: 2
Rationale: Between the development of symptoms and a definitive diagnosis, patients and their family members or loved ones have to endure a time of uncertainty. Often the best way to begin the intervention is to tell the person the behavior or emotion that you are observing and give it a name (shock, disbelief, fear, or sadness). It is important to validate and seek the person's agreement with or refinement of this perception, which makes Answer 2 the best response.
Cognitive Level: Application
Nursing Process: Implementation
Client Needs: Psychosocial Integrity
Text Page: 817

2. Answer: 2
Rationale: Positive attitudes toward advance directives alone do not determine who will or will not complete an advance directive. A recent study found that the majority who completed them were white, female, and over age 65; had less than a high school education; and perceived their health as poor. Most people who had advance directives had specific reasons for doing so.
Cognitive Level: Analysis
Nursing Process: Assessment
Client Needs: Psychosocial Integrity
Text Page: 817

3. Answer: 3
Rationale: Patients and families have concerns immediately after receiving a diagnosis that shows pathology. Concerns frequently include how long people live after diagnosis, emotional effect or inconvenience to family or friends, being a burden, financial concerns, suffering pain or disfigurement, feelings of loss of control, feelings of having so much still to do in life, and dying alone.
Cognitive Level: Application
Nursing Process: Assessment
Client Needs: Psychosocial Integrity
Text Page: 818

4. Answer: 1
Rationale: Ways in which the nurse can respond to patient or family concerns include, among others, listening without interrupting or defending, and providing what is requested if possible. For this reason, the nurse should initially take Answer 1, and should then complete Answer 2. Answer 3 puts the patient's issues on hold, and Answer 4 may be asked at a later time if trying to determine how long call bells are actually ringing before they are answered.
Cognitive Level: Application
Nursing Process: Implementation
Client Needs: Psychosocial Integrity
Text Page: 818

5. Answer: 2
Rationale: The NIH is a reputable and accurate website for obtaining health-related information. The CDC is appropriate for information about communicable diseases. OSHA oversees workplace safety, and the FDA oversees food and drug standards.
Cognitive Level: Application
Nursing Process: Implementation
Client Needs: Psychosocial Integrity
Text Page: 818

6. Answer: 4
Rationale: The patient's symptoms of anxiety need not meet the criteria for a formal psychiatric diagnosis in order to be treated. Pharmacological treatment with benzodiazepines is common practice, and nurses should initiate requests for an order if the patient does not already have one.
Cognitive Level: Application
Nursing Process: Planning
Client Needs: Psychosocial Integrity
Text Page: 819

7. Answer: 3
Rationale: A persistent myth proposes that if a person "has a reason" to be depressed, no treatment is needed because this "functional depression" is a normal response. However, this myth denies the patient needed and effective treatment. For this reason, the nurse should first follow up on the response in Answer 3.
Cognitive Level: Analysis
Nursing Process: Planning
Client Needs: Psychosocial Integrity
Text Page: 819

8. Answer: 1
Rationale: The most therapeutic communication is one that attempts to assess medically the patient who appears depressed. Answer 1 is the only option that attempts to elicit more information about the patient's feelings. Answer 2 patronizes the patient. Answer 3 fails to validate the patient's reason for crying, and Answer 4 does not include any assessment at all.
Cognitive Level: Application
Nursing Process: Assessment
Client Needs: Psychosocial Integrity
Text Page: 819

9. Answer: 2
Rationale: The correct response is one that acknowledges the family member's situation and then explores an alternative. The statements in Answers 1 and 4 try to make the daughter feel guilty. Answer 3 does not allow the daughter to ventilate or to evaluate alternatives to staying in the hospital around-the-clock.
Cognitive Level: Application
Nursing Process: Implementation
Client Needs: Psychosocial Integrity
Text Page: 820

10. Answer: 4
Rationale: The Wong FACES Pain Rating Scale can be used for children ages 3 and above. The patient is asked to point to the face that best describes their pain, from a smiley face to a tearful one.
Cognitive Level: Application
Nursing Process: Assessment
Client Needs: Physiological Integrity: Physiological Adaptation
Text Page: 820

11. Answer: 1
Rationale: Constipation occurs in as many as two thirds of patients receiving palliative care. Patients taking narcotic pain-control agents regularly should have prophylactic treatment for constipation, which could include stool softeners and laxatives.
Cognitive Level: Application
Nursing Process: Planning
Client Needs: Physiological Integrity: Pharmacological and Parenteral Therapies
Text Page: 821

12. Answer: 1
Rationale: Because the nausea and vomiting are anxiety-induced, lorazepam (a benzodiazepine) may be used

to reduce both the anxiety and the nausea and vomiting. The other medications listed are useful in treatment of nausea and vomiting.
Cognitive Level: Application
Nursing Process: Planning
Client Needs: Physiological Integrity: Pharmacological and Parenteral Therapies
Text Page: 821

13. Answer: 2
Rationale: Breath-holding, swallowing a spoonful of sugar, breathing into a paper bag, rapidly drinking a glass of water, and nasopharynx stimulation are noninvasive measures that may relieve hiccups.
Cognitive Level: Application
Nursing Process: Implementation
Client Needs: Physiological Integrity: Physiological Adaptation
Text Page: 821

14. Answer: 4
Rationale: Dyspnea occurs in many chronic and end-stage diseases, and the nurse can assist the patient with shortness of breath by raising the head of the bed to a comfortable position. Bronchodilators may be used as an aid, but positioning is noninvasive and is a first-line intervention. Incentive spirometry, coughing, and deep breathing would prevent atelectasis but would not treat the symptom of dyspnea resulting from the end-stage disease process.
Cognitive Level: Analysis
Nursing Process: Implementation
Client Needs: Physiological Integrity: Basic Care and Comfort
Text Page: 822

15. Answer: 3
Rationale: End-of-life is generally accepted as the probable last 6 months of life.
Cognitive Level: Comprehension
Nursing Process: NA
Client Needs: Psychosocial Integrity
Text Page: 822

16. Answer: 1
Rationale: Having "hope against hope" may not mean that the patient is in denial, but rather that he is using denial as an adaptive defense mechanism. The nurse should first consider what purpose confrontation would serve at this time. Answer 4 may be helpful but is not the first consideration. Answers 2 and 3 do not address the issue of the question, which is the coping response of the patient.
Cognitive Level: Analysis
Nursing Process: Planning
Client Needs: Psychosocial Integrity
Text Page: 822

17. Answer: 1
Rationale: Palliative care includes pain medications, stomach ulcer prevention, skin and mouth care, and other comfort measures. Palliative care does not necessarily include IV hydration (Answer 2) or tube feedings (Answer 4). There is no purpose for doing range-of-motion exercises for this patient.
Cognitive Level: Application
Nursing Process: Implementation
Client Needs: Psychosocial Integrity
Text Page: 823

18. Answer: 4
Rationale: The best interests standard is applied when the patient lacks decisional capacity and there is no other designated health care proxy. This standard is based on what would promote the welfare of the "average" patient. Answer 1 is irrelevant to this question, and Answer 2 does not apply because the patient lacks decisional capacity. Answer 3 is inappropriate because a designated health care proxy would ensure that the patient's wishes were carried out.
Cognitive Level: Application
Nursing Process: Planning
Client Needs: Safe Effective Care Environment: Management of Care
Text Page: 823

19. Answer: 3
Rationale: The patient who wants to withhold further aggressive therapy but not withdraw current therapy would wish to maintain nutrition, hydration, and current treatments such as dialysis. The patient is not likely to maintain full code status (Answer 1), and because the patient is not withdrawing treatment, comfort measures only (Answer 4) is inappropriate.
Cognitive Level: Application
Nursing Process: Planning
Client Needs: Safe Effective Care Environment: Management of Care
Text Page: 823

20. Answer: 1
Rationale: Antibiotics are used to treat infection and therefore would be withheld in the care of a patient who has designated that life-sustaining treatment should be withheld. The medications in the other options promote comfort and would continue to be administered.
Cognitive Level: Application
Nursing Process: Implementation
Client Needs: Safe Effective Care Environment: Management of Care
Text Page: 823

21. Answer: 2
Rationale: Hospice care would not include chemotherapy, which is a therapy generally intended to treat or

cure cancer. Hospice care does involve pain and symptom management, nutritional counseling, physical/occupational/speech therapies, home health services for personal care, psychosocial and emotional support, grief counseling, and crisis care during medical emergencies.
Cognitive Level: Analysis
Nursing Process: Evaluation
Client Needs: Safe Effective Care Environment: Management of Care
Text Page: 824

22. Answer: 4
Rationale: Below the age of 6, attitudes toward death are often a matter of fact rather than emotion.
Cognitive Level: Application
Nursing Process: Implementation
Client Needs: Psychosocial Integrity
Text Page: 824

23. Answer: 3
Rationale: If a nurse finds it difficult to accept a decision a parent has made, professional ethics preclude the nurse from discussing these personal concerns with the parents. The other options are incorrect actions in this situation.
Cognitive Level: Application
Nursing Process: Implementation
Client Needs: Psychosocial Integrity
Text Page: 825

24. Answer: 1
Rationale: It may be challenging for the nurse to maintain professional boundaries when the age of the nurse and patient are near the same. It is advisable for the nurse to discuss the conflict with an experienced nurse or supervisor, or to seek reassignment from that patient until the nurse has learned to adapt emotionally. Answer 2 is not therapeutic; Answer 3 represents suboptimal care; and Answer 4 is excessive.
Cognitive Level: Application
Nursing Process: Implementation
Client Needs: Psychosocial Integrity
Text Page: 825

25. Answer: 2
Rationale: Some reasons why patients may wish to hasten death include loss of autonomy, lack of dignity, unrelieved pain, fatigue, anorexia, fear of the future, and untreated depression. Studies have shown that when pain and depression are adequately treated, patient requests to hasten death diminish.
Cognitive Level: Application
Nursing Process: Assessment
Client Needs: Psychosocial Integrity
Text Page: 825